THE
HISTORICAL DEVELOPMENT
OF BRITISH PSYCHIATRY

Volume 1
18th and 19th Century

THE
HISTORICAL DEVELOPMENT
OF BRITISH PSYCHIATRY

Volume 1
18th and 19th Century

by

DENIS LEIGH

M.D., F.R.C.P.

Physician, The Bethlem Royal and Maudsley Hospitals,
London

PERGAMON PRESS

NEW YORK · OXFORD · LONDON · PARIS

1961

PERGAMON PRESS INC.
122 East 55th Street, New York 22, N.Y.
Statler Center 640, 900 Wilshire Boulevard
Los Angeles 17, California

PERGAMON PRESS LTD.
Headington Hill Hall, Oxford
4 & 5 Fitzroy Square, London W.1

PERGAMON PRESS S.A.R.L.
24 Rue des Écoles, Paris V^e

PERGAMON PRESS G.m.b.H.
Kaiserstrasse 75, Frankfurt am Main

M6241

25|8|81

Set in Bembo 11 on 12pt and printed in Great Britain at
T. AND A. CONSTABLE LTD., EDINBURGH

CONTENTS

	PAGE
LIST OF ILLUSTRATIONS	vii
PREFACE	xi
INTRODUCTION	xiii
THE EIGHTEENTH CENTURY	I
Introduction	I
Psychiatric Hospitals in the Eighteenth Century	5
The Physician as Psychiatrist	15
The Rise of Specialism	47
Some Minor Authors	62
The Insanity of King George III	68
Therapy During the Eighteenth Century	75
A List of Books Dealing with Psychiatric Illness Published in English During the Eighteenth Century	84
JOHN HASLAM, M.D. 1764-1844	94
Student Days	97
Apothecary to Bethlem	103
John Tilly Matthews	107
Disgrace	114
Haslam's Library	115
Minor Works	132
Sketches in Bedlam	134
Haslam and the Discovery of General Paralysis	136
Social Activities	139
Haslam's Place in Psychiatry	144
Bibliography	145
JAMES COWLES PRICHARD, M.D., F.R.S. 1786-1848	148
His Career	148
His Practice	152
Psychiatric Writings	160
Prichard's Position in Psychiatry	186
Prichard's Anthropological Studies	189
Conclusion	200
Minor Works	201
Items from the Catalogue of Prichard's Books	204
Bibliography	207

	PAGE
JOHN CONOLLY, M.D., D.C.L. 1794-1866	210
His Life	211
His Career as a Psychiatrist	222
His Character	227
His Writings	230
On The Method of Securing Lunatics	241
Twelfth Night Entertainment at Hanwell Lunatic Asylum	250
Fancy Fair at Hanwell Lunatic Asylum	253
The Non-Restraint System	260
Minor Writings	264
Conolly's Achievement	267
BIBLIOGRAPHY	268
SUBJECT INDEX	271

ILLUSTRATIONS

FIGURE   PAGE

CHAPTER I

1.   Edward Tyson, M.D., F.R.S., 1650-1708   1
2.   "Physicians Friend" Caricature, 18th Century   3
3.   "Three Friends going on a visit." (Water-colour
     in the author's collection)   4
4.   Bethlem Hospital the second, opened 1676   6
5.   St. Luke's Hospital, opened 1751   10
6.   The Infirmary, Dispensary and Lunatic Asylum,
     Manchester. (From an engraving by J. Davies after
     S. Austin. Impression in the Wellcome Historical
     Medical Museum)   13
7.   George Cheyne, M.D., F.R.S., 1671-1743   22
8.   Sir Richard Blackmore, 1650-1729. (From the
     mezzotint by R. Williams after Closterman. From
     the impression in the British Museum)   29
9.   Georg Ernst Stahl, M.D., 1666-1734   32
10. Robert Whytt, 1714-1766. (The portrait in the Royal
     College of Physicians, Edinburgh)   34
11. William Cullen, M.D., 1710-1790   37
12. William Falconer, M.D., F.R.S., 1744-1824   41
13. James Monro, 1680-1752. Physician to Bethlem
     1728-1752   49
14. John Monro, 1715-1792. Physician to Bethlem
     1752-1792   50
15. Thomas Arnold, M.D., 1742-1816   57
16. William Perfect, M.D., 1740-?   63
17. The Rev. Francis Willis, M.D., 1717-1807   69
18. Bleeding-knives, made of the finest steel and mounted
     on tortoiseshell or mother of pearl handles, and
     contained in a silver bound shagreen case. (From
     the author's collection)   79

FIGURE   PAGE

19.   Bleeding-bowl in Pewter used at Bethlem Hospital in
      the Eighteenth Century. Capacity 14 oz. (From
      the author's collection)   80

20.   Drug jars in use about 1800. (From the author's
      collection, probably Genoese)   81

21.   William Tuke, 1732-1822. (From an engraving of the
      medallion by Adams for the Centenary Presentation
      of 1892. Impression in the Wellcome Historical
      Medical Museum)   83

                        CHAPTER II

1.   John Haslam, M.D., 1764-1844. Apothecary to
      Bethlem 1795-1816   95

2.   George Fordyce, M.D., F.R.S., 1736-1802   98

3.   The Edinburgh Lunatic Asylum. Showing elevation.
      (From an engraving in the Wellcome Historical
      Medical Museum)   102

4.   The Third Bethlem, opened 1815   104

5.   Thomas Monro, M.D., F.R.C.P., 1759-1833.
      Physician to Bethlem 1792-1816   105

6.   James Norris, the American seaman, in his restraining
      harness   108

7.   Edward Thomas Monro, 1790-1856   113

8.   Philippe Pinel, 1745-1826   120

9.   Instrument devised by John Haslam for forced
      feeding. (Reduced by one-half)   123

10.   The attempted assassination of George III at Drury
      Lane in 1800 by James Hatfield   126

11.   Sir Alexander Morison, 1779-1866. (From the
      portrait by Milburn)   140

12.   Alexander Robert Sutherland, 1782-1861. Physician
      to St. Luke's   141

FIGURE   PAGE

CHAPTER III

1.   James Cowles Prichard, M.D., F.R.S., 1786-1848   149

2.   Cupping and scarifying set. (From the author's
     collection)   153

3.   Scarifier. (From the author's collection)   154

4.   Advertisement of lectures given on Egyptology by
     J. C. Prichard   156

5.   Jean Etienne Dominique Esquirol, 1772-1850   168

6.   The Rosetta Stone. (By permission of the Trustees,
     the British Museum)   190

7.   The Sale Catalogue of Prichard's Library   203

CHAPTER IV

1.   John Conolly, M.D., 1794-1866   211

2.   Silver Plate inscribed "To John Conolly, M.D., from
     the inhabitants of Stratford-upon-Avon and its
     neighbourhood as a testimony of their Esteem
     and regard. September 18th, 1828."   218

3.   Dr. John Gideon Millingen. Superintendent of
     Hanwell 1838-39   221

4.   William Charles Ellis. Superintendent of Hanwell
     1831-1838   223

5.   "This Testimonial Commemorative of the Strenuous
     Persevering and Successful labours to Improve the
     Treatment and Ameliorate the Condition OF THE
     INSANE is together with a Portrait of Himself
     Presented by his Admiring and Grateful Contem-
     poraries to John Conolly M.D. Physician to the
     Hanwell Lunatic Asylum. A.D. 1852."   226

6.   Physiognomy. The visage of Satan by Fuseli. From
     Lavater's Essai sur la Physiognomie, 1783   234

7.   Dr. Franz Joseph Gall, 1757-1828. The Founder of
     Phrenology   235

FIGURE   PAGE

8.   Phrenological Inkwell. (Staffordshire Ware. From the
     author's collection)   237

9.   Robert Gardiner Hill, 1811–78   240

1-6 Instruments of Restraint. (From Paul Slade Knight's
     *Observations on the Causes, Symptoms and Treatment
     of Derangement of the Mind* (1827))   242

10. Twelfth-Night entertainment at Hanwell Lunatic
     Asylum   251

11. The Hanwell Asylum 1848   255

Plate I.   Leather instruments of restraint used at Hanwell
                                                      facing page 258

Plate II. Leg locks and Handcuffs attached to abdominal
           belt (Hanwell)   *facing page* 260

PREFACE

In 1949, when I began to write this book, very little had been written specifically on the development of psychiatry in the British Isles. Hack Tuke's *Chapters in the History of the Insane in the British Isles* I found frankly boring; it was almost impossible to picture the kind of men who were our forerunners, how they thought and lived, and whence came their ideas. Zilboorg's book dealt with too large a pattern—and again provided little information about the men themselves. It seemed, indeed, as if the British contribution had been somewhat undervalued. Having been a collector since boyhood, I already possessed the nucleus of a library on the subject, and although the lot of the impecunious collector was becoming more and more difficult, in the restricted field of "early psychiatry" it was still possible to collect the necessary sources. I originally intended to write a history of British psychiatry, but as the years passed, and with the demands of clinical work upon one's time and energy, it became apparent that this would prove a life work. The difficulties in this field also do not allow a speedy conclusion—the rarity of many of the publications, the lack of bibliographical information, and the dearth of learned articles in the historical journals all conspire to make progress slow. It is therefore in the light of these excuses that the following pages must be read, sympathetically I hope, in the knowledge that their contents are imperfect, represent a personal view, and will have served their purpose if they stimulate others to work in this field.

The theme of the book is the development of some aspects of British psychiatry in the eighteenth and early nineteenth centuries. The method is as far as possible biographical; history is made by men, and man is the doctor's study. I have tried to obtain as many illustrations as possible so that names can become faces; the search for illustrations has alone been a time-consuming affair. I hope the book will serve a twofold purpose—that it will interest the psychiatrist with no special leanings toward history, and that it will provide time saving information for those who specialize in the field. The majority of the works referred to are in my possession; for permission to use those others I am deeply indebted to Dr. Alexander Walk, the librarian of the Royal Medico–Psychological Society. His enlightened policy of loaning rare volumes is almost unique amongst librarians, and yet how otherwise than by study in his own home can a busy clinician work most efficiently? The hours I have spent in various libraries cannot compare in value to the ability to use a book as it should be used, as if it belonged to the reader. So to him I am most grateful. Many others have helped, and it is particularly to the librarians of various learned bodies that thanks are due. Lastly the antiquarian booksellers, through their informative and often scholarly catalogues, have been an invaluable source of information.

For permission to use previously published material on John Haslam I am indebted to the Editors of the *Journal of History of Medicine and Allied Sciences*, and the *British Journal of Delinquency*. For permission to use the portraits of Edward Tyson and of the Monro family I must thank the President of the Royal College of Physicians, London, and for a previously published illustration the Editor of *Medical History* (Fig. No. IV-6). The Royal Medical Society of Edinburgh has allowed me access to John Haslam's *Dissertations*; the President and Fellows of the Royal Society of Medicine have allowed me to take copies of many prints in their collection, the Director of the Wellcome Medical Library has also provided me with illustrations. To Dr. C. R. Birnie, the Medical Superintendent of Hanwell, I am indebted for permission to use the illustrations of the instruments of restraint. To Mr. Barry Richards' energy and interest is due the photographs of these instruments. He has allowed me to use them. Mrs. Dorothy Purves, great-granddaughter of John Conolly, has talked to me about her family, and the Revs. T. E. and E. C. Prichard have given me information about their great-grandfather. Dr. Gilbert M. Tothill, the Medical Superintendent of the Auckland Mental Hospital, supplied me with photographs of the silver formerly belonging to Dr. Conolly, and now entrusted to his care. Mr. P. Jacobs, photographer at the Maudsley Hospital, has cheerfully taken responsibility for many of the illustrations.

Lastly Mr. K. J. Johnson, House Governor of the Bethlem Royal and Maudsley Hospitals, has encouraged me over the years, and helped me to obtain photostats of documents and books.

INTRODUCTION

THE pattern of British psychiatry in the first millennium followed that in other parts of the civilized world. The lunatic was a person possessed by devils, to be dealt with by the witch-doctor, or at a later date by the priest. The Church laid down prescribed methods of Exorcism, and trained certain of its members in the Order of "Exorcists". The English Church possessed one notable practitioner in St. Guthlac, the founder of Croyland Abbey in Lincolnshire. Psychological healing was the first line of attack, but drugs were also used. For instance, treatment might include the singing of seven Masses over various herbs, which the lunatic then swallowed, or a visit to one of the Holy Wells to drink the water or to be immersed. The essentials of the treatment were Faith and the direct influence of a person in authority on the sick person. And that authority was an ecclesiastical one. Although much help and comfort was derived from this type of treatment, many of the mentally sick stubbornly refused to be exorcised or unbewitched. Faith was not enough. They presented as difficult a problem as they do today.

Some went to other sources—to kings to be touched, or to people like Valentine Greatrakes, the stroker, who discovered his healing powers in the mid-seventeenth century. But others encountered a different form of treatment—the rod, and the whip, the chains, and ultimately the stake. The fact that Faith had not been enough was interpreted, both by the Church and by the lunatic's fellow-men, as evidence of heresy, and the work of the Devil. Punishment was indicated. The fifteenth century, which saw the magnificent flowering of the Renaissance, heralded the dark ages for psychiatry. The growth of heterodoxy and the increasing interest in the natural sciences threatened the established structure of the Church, and with it, that of the State. Deviants, such as the heretic, the alchemist and the insane, became grouped together as the earthly agents of the Devil, thus becoming legitimate objects of persecution. So began the great witch hunt which in this country persisted until 1736.

The psychiatric knowledge, so slight and yet so slowly and painfully gathered together, was now brushed aside as this belief in the link between the Devil and the lunatic intensified.

On the European continent no one was safe from the auto-da-fé, the Inquisitor, and the Law. In England, the greater cultural unity, the break with Rome, and the influence of enlightened minds like Sir Thomas More and Erasmus did much to militate against these continental excesses. Witch-hunting there was: James I himself was the author of a book proving that witches should not be regarded as mad, and that pleas of insanity should be rejected by the courts. His *Daemon-ologie*, published in 1597, was written chiefly to refute the opinions of Reginald Scot, the author of the *Discovery of Witchcraft*. Scot was not a physician but was nevertheless the first Englishman to recognize the witch as a mentally sick person, and to castigate the persecutors.

Heralded by William Gilbert, physician to Queen Elizabeth, whose excessively rare book on the magnet was published in 1600, the seventeenth-century physicians—notably Willis and Sydenham—began to emphasize the importance of observation and the collection of facts. Theological and demonological speculation became outmoded and, although treatment was in general of secondary importance, psychiatry owes these men an enormous debt for breaking the hold of the Inquisitor and the Judge.

So far we see an era of belief replaced by disbelief—kindness and religious tolerance by harshness and intolerance. A kind of emotional neutralism now ensued, until with the rise of the Encyclopaedists in France, and philosophers such as Berkeley and Hume, a new attitude began to make itself felt. The eighteenth century is the century of the development of "Moral Treatment". Man was a reasoning, rational creature—God was largely fashioned in the shape of the best type of English country gentleman. In spite of the continued harsh treatment, there was an increasing tendency for moral suasion, as we might now call it, to be used. The care and treatment of the mentally sick had passed into secular hands. Reason was the keynote—although in practice moral suasion was somewhat of a euphemism for the type of treatment employed. A harsh discipline was exerted by the physician or his keepers, the basic element of treatment still consisting of an authoritarian relationship between the patient and his custodian.

It is with the origins in these Islands, of psychiatry as we know it today, that the following pages are concerned.

CHAPTER I

The Eighteenth Century

INTRODUCTION

THE opening in 1676 of the New Bethlem, the most magnificent hospital building in Europe, and the appointment of the much

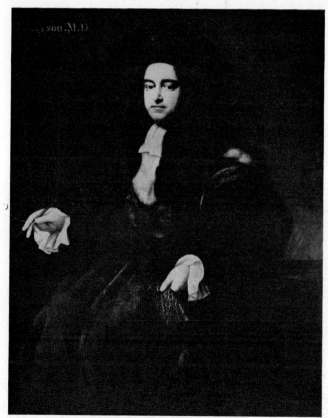

FIG. 1.   Edward Tyson, M.D., F.R.S., 1650–1708

respected Edward Tyson as its Physician (Fig. 1), gave proof of the optimism with which the men of the time planned for the future. Nor

A

did Edward Tyson disappoint them. In an age when the psychiatric literature was chiefly demoniacal, anecdotal or theological in nature, the most eminent position in British psychiatry was held by a man of solid scientific worth, not given to idle speculation. A Fellow of the Royal Society, he was the founder of comparative anatomy in England, the first to describe the anatomy of the chimpanzee, whilst his work on *The Anatomy of a Porpess* "constitutes one of the great landmarks in the history of science". And yet he was a practising physician with a large practice. During his tenure of office (1684–1708) he did more for Bethlem than any of his predecessors, or indeed any of the Monros who took office over the next century. In 1693 a female nurse was hired as an experiment, and in 1700 an out-patient department was organized where former patients could continue their treatment. Tyson realized that physical well-being was just as important as mental well-being, and he found the means wherewith to clothe and otherwise care for his indigent patients on their discharge. He was equally wise and clear-sighted in the medical treatment of his patients, many of whom came to him in dreadful physical condition, emaciated, or too weak to use their limbs; others had developed gangrene of the toes, or dropsy. Tyson's first task was to build up the patient's body, and the sick man was carefully fed, bathed and attended by a trained nurse. Keepers and maids were asked to be as tender as "imaginable". In spite of the blood-letting, purging and emetics with which the mental disorder was tackled, Tyson estimated that two-thirds of his patients recovered. It is a tribute to him that during the golden age of his rule there was a long waiting-list of patients. Unfortunately Tyson has left no written work on mental illness. In fact, it was only on the solicitation of John Strype, at that time collecting material for a new edition of Stow's *Survey of London*, that Tyson drew up a brief account of Bethlem. Strype writes

> the late learned physician Dr. Tyson informed me that for the years 1684 to 1703 (during which time he had been ordinary physician there), there had been in this hospital 1,294 patients, of which number had been cured and discharged 890, which is above two patients in three; that after some years casting up, the number of men and women patients he found them pretty equal and very little difference.

Tyson's death in 1708 was in many ways the end of an era. His work was a presage of the path psychiatry was eventually to take over a

hundred years later. The fine hopes of the time were disappointed—
the scientific fervour of the seventeenth century was replaced by a
period of stagnation. Set against the magnificent vigour of eighteenth-
century literature, art and architecture, psychiatry, and in some
respects medicine, presents a sorry picture. This was the age of the
gentleman, the noble patron, the classicist and the artist. The doctor
was none of these—with a few notable exceptions such as Radcliffe,
Sloane and Mead. A great, fat, coarse, fee-grabbing ignoramus, shelter-
ing behind his few tags of Hippocrates, or Galen—so is he often

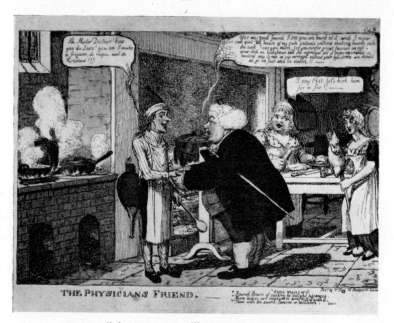

Fig. 2. "Physicians Friend" Caricature, 18th Century.

portrayed in the prints and poems of the period (Figs. 2 and 3). He was
the servant of those who paid him, his position in the social hierarchy
very different from his Victorian successor, who had by then come to
represent an idealization of middle-class longings for respectability,
solid worth, and altruism on a sound financial footing. The great
London hospitals were divided by the rival political factions—
Thomas's and Guy's being Whig, and Bart's and Bethlem, Tory
strongholds. Sir John Hawkins, in his *Life of Johnson*, tells us that

after a physician had chosen his party and his coffee-house, his next business was to be indiscriminately obsequious to all men, to appear much abroad and in public places, to increase his acquaintance and form good connexions; in the doing of which, if he were married, a wife that could visit, play at cards and tattle, was often times very serviceable. A candidate for practice, pursuing these methods, and exercising the patience of a setting dog for half a score of years in the expectation of deaths, resignations and other accidents that occasion vacancies, at the end thereof either found himself a hospital physician, and if of Bethlehem, a monopolist and a very lucrative branch of practice; or doomed to struggle with difficulties for the remainder of his life.

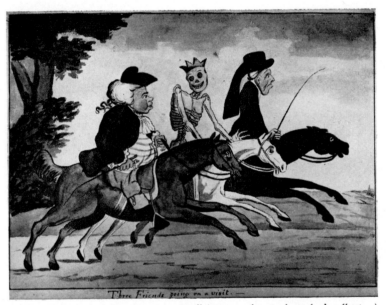

FIG. 3. "Three Friends going on a visit." (*Water-colour in the author's collection.*)

The physician required only a certificate of two years' residence at a regularly constituted University in any country and to have undergone three examinations in Latin before being able to take his degree. The apothecaries, the equivalent of our present-day general practitioner, had undergone an apprenticeship, six months' attendance at hospital, and an examination in the vulgar tongue. Congregating in the coffee-houses, the apothecaries would describe their cases to the physician, who on receipt of a golden guinea would issue the prescription which was thought best suited for the patient. Hospitals, as we know them today, were virtually non-existent at the beginning of the century, the Royal Hospitals of St. Thomas's and St. Bartholomew's alone serving the needs of the metropolis. As the city grew in size and population, so new hospitals were opened, the Westminster in 1720, Guy's in 1724, St. George's in 1733, the London in 1740, and the Middlesex in 1745. In the provinces the bulk of the people were looked after by apothecaries, over whom the London Society had no control, and the first provincial hospital was not founded until the Bristol Infirmary was opened in 1735. The status of medicine depended very greatly on the level of its general practitioners. The comparatively few men of eminence, such as Mead or Radcliffe, or surgeons such as Cheselden, could not greatly affect the general level, and it was only toward the close of the century that the teaching influences of the Hunters and of the Edinburgh School began to raise the standard of medicine. Medical theory was still under the influence of the classical tradition—the vast body of references were to classical authors, and many of the medical works were written in Latin. By the time Johnson died, in 1784, smallpox had been conquered and a new generation of clinicians had come into practice, schooled in observation and experiment. English was now the language of medicine and science, and the increasing spate of books and papers gave testimony to the increasing level of medical education. It is against this background that the development of British psychiatry slowly unfolded over the century.

PSYCHIATRIC HOSPITALS IN THE EIGHTEENTH CENTURY

Psychiatry was indeed comparatively richly endowed. The magnificent second Bethlem had been opened in 1676, more like a palace than a hospital (Fig. 4). Modelled on French architectural principles, it was one of the marvels of the world, although it was feared that such a paradise "might encourage exaltation and make everybody half mad— in order to be a lodger there". Robert Hooke had been its architect, of whom Pepys wrote that he "is the most, though he promises the least, of any man I know", the Governors were eminent and charitable city men, and no expense had been spared. The opening was celebrated by Thomas Jordan in a poem:

This is a structure fair
Royally raised;
The pious founders are
Much to be praised,
    That in such time of need
    When sickness doth exceed
    Do build this house of bread
    Noble New Bedlam

'Tis beautiful and large
In constitution
Deserves a liberal charge
of contribution.
    If I may reach so high
    To sing a prophecy
    Their name shall never die
    That built new Bedlam.

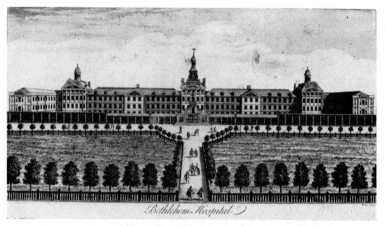

FIG. 4.   Bethlem Hospital the second, opened 1676.

O'Donoghue, historian of Bethlem, must be consulted for the detailed story of the hospital—but it is clear enough that the medical men at Bethlem were in an unrivalled position for the study of mental disorder. Unhappily, from the death of Tyson until John Haslam was appointed Apothecary in 1795, psychiatry in the hospital languished in a sterile conservatism. By good fortune, however, Bethlem presented an enormous attraction to the eighteenth-century artist and man of letters. Defoe was particularly interested in the care of the insane, and had some dealing with Tyson. Dean Swift was elected a Governor of Bethlem in 1714, and in his writings makes frequent use of his experiences at the hospital. In *A Tale of a Tub* there is a section devoted to "A digression concerning the use and improvement of madness in a commonwealth". He considers that persons of genius—great conquerors, politicians and ministers—"have generally been persons whose reason was disturbed". Why not, then, search Bedlam for suitable commanders and politicians—there was a patient swearing and blaspheming, tearing up his bedding and biting his grating—give him a regiment and send him to Flanders? In 1733, inspired by the opening of the incurable wards, he tossed off a satire entitled "A serious and useful scheme to make a hospital for incurables". Jonathan Swift himself was to be eligible as an "incurable scribbler", along with all the other incurable rogues, liars and fools. In a later satire on the Irish House of Commons, which he dubbed the Bedlam of Dublin, there are frequent allusions to the hospital. A letter he wrote to Stella in 1710 tells of a family visit to Bedlam, complete with nursemaids and children. In 1731 he was thinking of endowing a hospital in Dublin, to be called Bedlam, and in 1740 he writes his own epitaph:

> He gave the little wealth he had
> To build a home for fools and mad
> And showed by one satiric touch
> No nation wanted it so much.

Swift's asylum was opened in 1745, and was the first hospital for the charitable care of the insane in Ireland. He bequeathed the whole of his estate for the purchase of the land on which this hospital was built.

Pope, Richardson and Horace Walpole all visited the hospital and wrote about it, whilst on at least two occasions Dr. Johnson visited Bedlam—on one of these visits he was accompanied by Murphy, the dramatist, and Foote, the comedian. Foote afterwards gave an amusing account of Dr. Johnson's interview with a Jacobite patient who imagined he was chastizing the Duke of Cumberland. Johnson himself suffered from various nervous manifestations and said that all his life had been lived on the borderline between sanity and insanity. Walpole knew Dr. Monro personally, and if he disapproved a man's politics would call him an "out-pensioner of Bedlam". Lesser lights such as Tom Brown, and Ned Ward the London Spy, who kept a public-house near the hospital, have left us vivid anecdotes; and lastly there were two writers who were patients—Nathaniel Lee, the dramatist, and Christopher Smart, the poet. Lee had been a successful playwright, who had collaborated with Dryden and Purcell, until drink brought about his ruin. Smart suffered from a "religious mania", but there was little harm in him, and Dr. Johnson considered that Smart ought not to have been shut up. "His infirmities were not noxious to society. He insisted on people praying with him; and I'd as lief pray with Kit Smart as anyone else. Another charge was that he did not love clean linen; and I have no passion for it." Smart wrote the "Song of David" —later a favourite of Browning.

The best description of Bethlem has come down to us from the artists—pre-eminently Hogarth. In the spring of 1733 Hogarth was painting the eighth scene of his *Rake's Progress* in the new incurable wards at Bethlem. This wonderful painting faithfully portrays the incurable ward, with its cells and staircase. Thomas Rakewell has reached his last stage of degradation—his head has been shaved, and a keeper is putting him in irons. Surrounding him are other lunatics— would-be popes, kings and astronomers. In the background two visitors, a lady of fashion and her maid, observe their wretched fellow-creatures with no trace of compassion on their features. Sarah Young, the Rake's mistress whom he had deserted, is the only person in this dreadful scene to feel pity for the madman's plight. Piratical editions as well as parodies of this picture were soon on the market. Hogarth himself was harshly lampooned, particularly in connection with his *Analysis of Beauty*—a rather incoherent book in which he upheld the serpentine line as the sole canon of grace and beauty. In one caricature he is seen as a patient in Bedlam, chained by the leg, fantastically dressed and painting a wall of his cell with religious pictures.

Rowlandson and Gillray used Bedlam as a motif for their merciless caricatures of the politician of the day. Gillray pictured Burke in a cell being shaved by Major Scott, the agent of Warren Hastings, his legs fettered by a chain of letters recording the verdict of the Lords and Commons on his speeches. Rowlandson also pilloried Burke in a similar type of caricature, and Fox was shown in a strait-jacket being examined by Dr. John Monro, following the success of Pitt over Fox in the election of 1784.

Bethlem was the only public institution caring for lunatics in the whole kingdom at the beginning of the eighteenth century, although numerous private asylums existed. The scandals and abuses which occurred in some of these houses were animadverted upon by Defoe in *The True Born Englishman* and by lesser lights in the journals of the day. Little attempt, however, was made to control these houses, although the elder Pitt and Fox were both members of a Committee of the House of Commons which sat in 1763 to enquire into the state of the private madhouses. Their report showed that sane people were often committed to asylums, and that a troublesome wife or daughter was often dealt with in this way. In spite of this report, no legislation resulted, and in 1765 the *Gentleman's Magazine* again drew attention to these evils—

> Patients often cannot be found out, because the master lets them bear some fictitious name in the house; and if fortunately discovered by a friend, the master or his servants will endeavour to elude his search and defeat his humane intentions by saying they have strict orders to permit no person to see the patient.

Girls were sometimes sent to a madhouse in order to break off a love affair. In 1773 a Bill passed the Commons for the "Regulation of Private Madhouses", but was thrown out by the Lords. The eighteenth century was to draw to its close without any real legislative advance, but by then at last the dawn was in sight. In fact, the only Act of Parliament, up to 1808, relating to the care and protection of the lunatic poor had been passed in 1744 (17 Geo. II, c. 5). This authorized any two justices to apprehend and securely lock and chain the lunatic who might be dangerous!

Out of this general dissatisfaction arose the establishment of St. Luke's Hospital at Moorfields. On 13 June 1750, six gentlemen of the City of London sat down at the Kings Arms Tavern in Exchange Alley to discuss a project for the establishment of a hospital as a further provision for poor lunatics. They were:

Dr. Thomas Crowe, M.D. (in the Chair),
Mr. James Sperling, Merchant of Mincing Lane,
Mr. Richard Speed, Druggist of Old Fish Street,
Mr. Thomas Light, Merchant of Mincing Lane,
Mr. William Prowting, Apothecary of Tower Street, and
Mr. Francis Magnus.

Subscriptions from the public poured in, and the hospital was opened within a very short time (Fig. 5). Dr. William Battie was appointed

physician, and in the first ten years of the hospital's existence 749
patients had been received. Of these, 363 had been discharged cured,

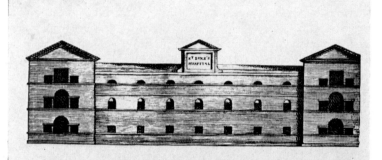

FIG. 5.   St. Luke's Hospital, opened 1751.

198 remained uncured. There were 61 idiots, 33 detained "at the desire
of their friends, 3 for want of necessary clothing and 1 as an improper
object of the Charity; 39 had died". In these early days handcuffs and

leg locks were in use—together with other instruments of restraint, but St. Luke's was never associated with the scandals that beset Bethlem. It was a visit to St. Luke's that directly inspired William Tuke to found "The Retreat"—a decisive event in psychiatric history. In 1782 Mr. Thomas Dunston and his wife were appointed head man and woman Keeper respectively. They came from Bethlem, where they had served for eight years, and remained at St. Luke's for forty-eight years. During that time they established for the hospital and themselves a European reputation, so that in the series of aquatints by Rowlandson and Pugin, St. Luke's was the subject of an interesting picture, whilst Bethlem was not included. William Battie also brought lustre to the hospital, for he was the first London physician to lecture on mental diseases and had opened the practice of the hospital to medical students.

In the provinces, St. Luke's House, Newcastle-upon-Tyne, had been set up as a public hospital in 1764 by Dr. John Hall, with accommodation for nineteen patients. Unfortunately its affairs did not prosper, and the hospital was evidently ill-conducted. An enquiry into its management resulted in a public asylum being built for the pauper patients, but even this new hospital did not improve matters greatly, judging from an account published at Newcastle in 1827; there were "chains, iron bars, dungeon-like cells, many close, dark, cold holes, less comfortable than cow-houses. There was no separation of the sexes, no classification, and for medical treatment, the old exploded system of restraint and coercion."

In Manchester the Trustees of the Public Infirmary had to revise their original decisions with regard to the care of "Poor lunaticks". In 1763 they met to consider a plan to "provide for and cure such patients as are disordered in their senses" and went on to explain their reasons in a pamphlet entitled "An Account of the Rise and Present Establishment of the Lunatic Hospital in Manchester".

> The Trustees of the Publick Infirmary in Manchester, raised in the year 1752, in forming their first and general Plan, found it extremely inconvenient to admit Poor Lunaticks as In-Patients; upon Account First of the great Expence which would necessarily be incurred by Building a Ward or Wards proper for their Reception; and Secondly, in maintaining a Governor and other Servants whose whole Care would be entirely taken up in guarding and securing these unhappy Wretches from those Violences which they frequently commit upon themselves and others.

They had, however, been long solicited

> to take the Care of Poor Lunaticks once more under Consideration, upon
> Account chiefly of their being denied admission into all other Infirmaries.
> As they were Promised generous contribution to any extraordinary
> Expence which might be so incurred, in addition to contributions to the
> General Hospital itself, they were at length prevailed upon to set about
> this desirable Work, to which they were strongly urged by the following
> motives:
>
> In the first Place, they apprehended that no Cases could be more truly
> deplorable than those of Poor Lunaticks, who only wanted a proper place
> for their reception, and a suitable Guard and Attendance upon their
> Persons; Conveniences only to be found in three public Foundations in
> the Kingdom, to wit, the Hospital of Bedlam, and that of St. Luke's, both
> in our great Metropolis, together with one at Newcastle-upon-Tyne.
>
> Secondly, the large Expence which these unhappy Objects necessarily
> bring upon their Parishes to maintain and secure them; and this commonly
> without any Prospect of a Cure, Confinement alone, without a proper
> Regimen, merely serving to keep them alive, to the great Terror and
> Concern of their Neighbours.
>
> Not the least consideration, was the Assistance which they might hope
> to give many Persons of middling Fortune, who may have Relations thus
> terribly afflicted, by preserving them from the Impositions of those who
> keep private Mad-Houses, and thus supplying what is so much wanted
> in this Part of the Kingdom, an Hospital for Lunaticks, upon the most
> moderate Terms.

This statement well exemplifies the attitude of the enlightened
eighteenth-century mind—there was no question of treatment, the
emphasis being on the care and protection of the lunatic. The plan was
adopted, the building opened on 10 May 1766, and within the first
year thirty-two patients had been treated (Fig. 6). Of these, thirteen
were discharged as cured and two as much relieved. The manner in
which the hospital was constructed is shown in the hospital rules:

> Every patient, upon admission, was carefully examined, and if there were
> any wounds, sores, or bruises, the Physician or Surgeon was informed of
> them.
>
> No stripes or beatings, then so freely used by keepers, no coercion
> whatever more than what was necessary, to restrain the Furious from
> hurting themselves or others, were to be inflicted or made use of by the
> Keeper, or any of his Servants; and no medicines were to be forcibly
> administered unless by special Order in Writing from the Physician, upon

pain of expulsion. The feet of those in straw, or chains were carefully examined, gently rubbed, night and morning, and covered with flannel during the winter season, and notice given to the Physician or Surgeon if any injury had taken place.

The male and female patients were kept separate, upon different stories of the Hospital; and commodious apartments were appointed for the convalescents so that they were not disturbed by the noisy or violent patients.

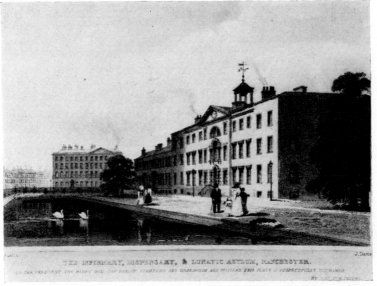

Fig. 6. The Infirmary, Dispensary and Lunatic Asylum, Manchester. (*From an engraving by J. Davies after S. Austin. Impression in the Wellcome Historical Medical Museum.*)

All were aired in the different yards appointed for the purpose, as often as possible.

As the hospital was designed, in great part, to help persons who could afford to pay for their maintenance and treatment, separate accommodation from that for the paupers was provided for them, and after a few years the part of the hospital which the better-class occupied was called the Asylum.

The House Visitors of the Infirmary visited the Hospital and Asylum daily to observe the behaviour of the Keeper, Matron, and servants towards the patients, and in particular to examine the bedding and nightly accommodation of each patient, for which purpose they occasionally visited in the evening.

There was to be no sightseeing by the curious as in London public hospitals. No relation or friend of a Patient was allowed admittance without an order in writing from one of the managers for the time being, or from one of the Physicians or Surgeons or Weekly Board; and no stranger was admitted but upon the same terms, all which orders had to be filed and kept by the Governor for the inspection of the Trustees.

The Physicians were to visit their respective patients at least twice a week and oftener when necessary. The House Apothecary (the resident medical officer) of the Infirmary was to inspect the whole Hospital and Asylum every day.

Consultations were to be held monthly or more Frequently by the Physicians concerning the cases of the patients by which experience and knowledge could reciprocally be communicated in a disease of all others the most perplexing and obscure. Regular journals and records were to be kept. No patient was to be discharged without consultation of the physicians.

These precautions for ensuring the humane treatment of the insane were a great improvement on those in force generally in many public institutions and private houses. They prevented, at Manchester, the occurrence of such abuses as were revealed in 1805 and 1816 before Committees of the House of Commons appointed to enquire into the treatment of the insane and the better regulation of madhouses in England. No criticism of the conduct of the Manchester Asylum was made at either enquiry, although many other institutions were seriously called to task for the conditions in which their patients lived and were treated.

The hospital met a demand, and by 1773 it was enlarged to "forty-two wards, several of them commodious for the higher sort of people". There were also four different yards to air the patients in, two for the men and two for the women, in which they were suffered to walk "according to their class". In 1787, when 120 patients, half of them men and half women, were treated, the hospital was enlarged to accommodate 80 persons, with the necessary administration rooms. This extension sufficed until the end of the century, when, with over 100 beds, it reached its largest size. At this time it was still the only public institution of its kind in the north-west of England, and too small for all those who sought admission to it.

Bethlem, St. Luke's and the Manchester Lunatic Hospital were primarily concerned with lunatics. Luckily, psychiatry has had wider interests than madness alone, and the general physician has always had a considerable influence on psychiatric thought. This was particularly so during the eighteenth century, and not until its closing years did the professional psychiatrist come into prominence. As the history of the period unfolds, so we may follow the influence on psychiatry first of the physicians, then of the psychiatrists, and lastly of the quacks.

THE PHYSICIAN AS PSYCHIATRIST

At the beginning of the century British clinical medicine was still in thrall to the ideas of Hippocrates, Celsus, Galen and other classical writers. Willis and Sydenham, and to a lesser extent Harvey, had set their contemporaries thinking along new paths. Sydenham in particular, by his insistence on clinical observation, and his distrust of theorizing, exerted a considerable influence on the development of psychiatry. His views are worth stating, representing as they do the ideas of the most outstanding clinician of the seventeenth century. A Dr. Cole had asked him, in a letter, to write to him upon the treatment of smallpox, and on the subject of hysteria—

> You have observed some rare facts concerning the so-called hysterical diseases. These have long exercised (and tired) the wits of the physicians. They have also (alas) eluded the recognised methods of treatment; well showing how unsafe it is in our philosophy to trust the simple reason except in those matters of which we may ascertain the certainty by means of our senses. Well will you deserve, most worthy Sir, both of the present age and of posterity, if you will condescend to publish what you have considered upon these points.

The result was an *Epistolary Dissertation to Dr. Cole* published in 1682. Sydenham began in a manner with which anyone who has written on the subject can sympathize.

> I now gird up my loins to comply with your second request, and to explain what I have as yet discovered by observation concerning the hysterical diseases. I admit at once, that of all diseases, these present the obscurest diagnosis, and the most uncertain treatment. Still I will meet your wish, and within the brief limits of a letter state my opinion. Indeed I am forced to be short, since, so shaken is my health, especially at this time of year, that if I were to indulge in any very deep train of thought, I

should bring on an attack of gout. I will, therefore, despatch my subject briefly; keeping to my usual method.

First, will come a short history of the disease according to the phenomena of Nature.

Secondly, my method of practice: as taught by no untrustworthy instructress—Experience.

Of all chronic diseases hysteria—unless I err—is the commonest; since just as fevers—taken with their accompaniments—equal two thirds of the number of all chronic diseases taken together, so do hysterical complaints (or complaints so called) make one half of the remaining third. As to females, if we except those who lead a hard and hardy life, there is rarely one who is wholly free from them—and females, be it remembered, form one half of the adults of the world. Then, again, such male subjects as lead a sedentary or studious life, and grow pale over their books and papers, are similarly afflicted; since, however much antiquity may have laid the blame of hysteria upon the uterus, hypochondriasis (which we impute to some obstruction of the spleen or viscera) is as like it, as one egg is to another. True, indeed, it is that women are more subject than males. This, however, is not on account of the uterus, but for reasons which will be seen in the sequel.

The frequency of hysteria is no less remarkable than the multiformity of the shapes which it puts on. Few of the maladies of miserable mortality are not imitated by it. Whatever part of the body it attacks, it will create the proper symptom of that part. Hence, without skill and sagacity the physician will be deceived; so as to refer the symptoms to some essential disease of the part in question, and not to the effects of hysteria.

However, of all phenomena, the most peculiar and inseparable is this—that the patients, at various times, void a great quantity of limpid urine, clear as the water from the rock. By detailed inquiries I have ascertained that, for hypochrondriasis of males, as well as for the hysteria of females, this sign is pathognomonic. In males, even a few seconds after passing water of the true straw-coloured hue, a sudden and violent mental emotion may produce the discharge of an abundant flow of urine—not straw-coloured, but of crystalline clearness. As long as the urine is of this colourless character, the fit is on the patient, and he suffers accordingly.

The affection which I have characterised in females as hysteria, and in males as hypochondriasis, arises (in my mind) from a disorder (ataxy) of the animal spirits. This precipitates them on the different parts of the system; so that bearing down violently and multitudinously upon particular organs they excite spasm and pain wherever the sensations are exquisitely acute; deranging and perverting the functions both of the parts they leave, and of the parts they fall on. No wonder. The irregularity of the distribution is opposed to nature; and the economy takes therefrom no small damage.

Of this derangement, or ataxia, the origin and antecedent cause is the weakened crasis of the spirits, whether natural or adventitious. Hence, the slightest occasion dissipates them, and the system is pulled down without difficulty. Just as the outer man is built up as a framework of parts visible to the outward sense; so, also, is it the inner man similarly constituted— of parts, however, consisting in the due and proper arrangements of the spirits, an arrangement cognisable only to the eye of reason; an arrangement, too, which is so united and intimately combined with the temper of the body, that it stands or falls according to the firmness of the constituent principles. For this reason we see more females than males, hysterical; the female being endowed by Nature with a more fine and delicate habit of body, as being destined to a life of more refinement and care. Man, on the contrary, is born to labour at the tillage and pasture of the earth, and at the capture of beasts for food. This makes him of a stronger and more muscular body.

That this ataxia is the true cause may be proved by the phenomena already described; of these I will treat upon the chief; beginning with the well-known hysterical affection called the strangulation of the womb. Here the spirits congregated into a mass in the lower belly, rush in a troop, and with all their impetus upon the fauces, exciting spasm along the whole tract that they traverse, and blowing up the belly to the size of a vast globe. This, however, is nothing more than the convolution and conglobation of the part affected with spasm, which can only be restrained and repressed by the exertion of considerable force. Meanwhile, the external parts, and the mass of the flesh are so deprived of their due share of spirits (these being diverted elsewhere), as to become as cold as death— a phenomenon which occurs in all other forms of hysteria as well as this. This, however, has been already stated. The pulse remains natural; and, unless the chill has been preceded by any enormous evacuation, there is no danger to life.

It is clear then, to me, that it is not any corruption of either the semen or the menstrual blood, to which, according to the statements of many writers, this disease is to be referred. It is rather the faulty disposition of the animal spirits. There is no malignant halitus towards the parts affected, no perverse depravation of the juices, no congestion of acrid humours. There is the cause I have assigned, and no other.

However much it may be clear that the origin of hysteria is by no means lodged in the humours, it must, nevertheless, be admitted that the ataxia of the spirits, to which the disease is due, begets an accumulation of putrid humours, whereby the function of the parts whereon they are so violently

B

borne, and the parts from which they are removed is wholly perverted. Such parts are chiefly organs of separation, designed for the recrementitious parts of the blood. Hence, if their functions be impaired, it follows, per-force, that a vast colluvies of impurity must accumulate. Had the organs done their duty, this would have been eliminated, and the blood purified accordingly.

With this view I bleed. I then purge for three or four mornings running. Meanwhile, the patient is so far from improving that she gets worse. Such is the disorder excited by the evacuations. Hence I warn her against being dispirited; to which the nature of the disease leads her. Be this, however, as it may, the vicious humours which we suppose to have become accumulated during the disease must, in some degree, be drawn off, before we can well satisfy our primary intention.

After these evacuations, I comfort the blood and the spirits belonging to it by giving a chalybeate thirty days running. This is sure to do good. To the worn-out and languid blood it gives a spur or fillip, whereby the animal spirits, which before lay prostrate and sunken under their own weight, are raised and excited. Clear proof of this is found in the effects of steel upon chlorosis. The pulse gains strength and frequency, the surface warmth, the face (no longer pale and deathlike) a fresh ruddy colour. Here, however, I must remark that with weak and worn-out patients the bleeding and purging may be omitted, and the steel be begun with at once.

This is best given in substance; in which form I have neither seen nor heard of it doing mischief. Nay, the simple substance effects a cure both more surely and more quickly than any of the current preparations. With steel, as with other more famous medicines, the officious sedulity of the chemists had not only failed in adding to its activity, but has succeeded in diminishing it.

Of all the remedies that I know, nothing so cherishes and strengthens the blood and spirits, as riding horseback, long distances, every day. Here all the exercise falls upon the lower belly, and, in the lower belly lie all the excretories which Nature keeps up for eliminating the feculent lodgements of the blood. Now what weakness, or what perversion of function can withstand the innumerable succussions of a day's riding—and that in the open air? Whose natural heat has so cooled down as not to boil afresh at such excitement? What lurking substance can be so unnatural, what juice so depraved, as not, under such exercise, to either return to the state Nature requires, or else to be eliminated, dissipated, dispersed? Surely, the blood thus continually shaken and tossed about, must needs take strength and vigour. Women, perhaps, who, from their sedentary life are liable (especially at first) to be injured, are the less fit of the two sexes for such regimen. For men it is pre-eminently healthy and restorative.

We shall see Sydenham's ideas persisting, albeit in different shapes, throughout the century. Willis, despite his originality, and perhaps because his mechanistic approach, was so sadly distorted by his own theorizing, exerted far less influence. Not one of the eighteenth-century writers on psychiatry followed him in contributing original work on the brain, nor indeed until Haslam was any original clinical work carried out.

"A TREATISE OF VAPOURS", by JOHN PURCELL, M.D. (1702)

The first book to be published in the new century on a psychiatric subject owed more to Willis than to Sydenham, in spite of its author's assertions to the contrary. *A Treatise of Vapours*, "or, Hysterick Fits. Containing An Analytical Proof of its Causes, Mechanical Explanations of all its Symptoms and Accidents, according to the Newest and most Rational Principles: Together with its Cure at large", was written by John Purcell, M.D., and published in 1702. Purcell (1674?–1730) was Shropshire born, and in 1696 became a student of medicine at Montpelier. Here he studied under Pierre Chirac, the Professor of Medicine, attended autopsies, and graduated M.D. on 29 May 1699. He set up in practice in London, became a Licentiate of the College of Physicians of London in 1721, and died in 1730. He published two successful books. The first has been mentioned above; it went into two editions (1702 and 1707). The second was the better known *A Treatise of the Cholick*, first appearing in 1714 (2nd edition 1715), and noted for one of the first descriptions of the dermatitis which the pathologist may develop whilst carrying out an autopsy as a result of contact with peritoneal exudation.

The *Treatise of Vapours* opens with an account of the dilemma facing the physician at the beginning of the century—

> In all Sciences nothing now pleases the Generality, but what is altogether conformable to Modern Philosophy; and again, there are almost as many who condemn whatever deviates from the patterns and footsteps of the Ancients. To please all Men is absolutely impossible, and I am so far from imagining I have done it, that I expect more Cricks upon this Small Treatise, than upon any Book of its kind which has come out these many Years.

Purcell expected censure from mainly two sorts of men, the "Galenick Old-fashioned Doctors", the second "are our Modern Physicians" who are convinc'd that "the Body of Man is a Machine". He hopes to ground his work on the solid and rational principles of Pierre Chirac, and to submit it particularly to those "Ingenious Gentlemen who are well vers'd in Modern Philosophy, Geometry, and the Structure of Mans Body, 'tis them I'd chuse to be my Judges".

Like Sydenham, Purcell subsumed the neuroses and some depressive illnesses under the term "vapours". They were the result of imperfect digestion—food was changed into "Crudities and Indigestions", and these crudities

> by little and little gather together in the Wrinkles and Folds of the Stomach, and Guts; where they lie for some time without much sensible motion of fermentation within themselves; till at last by the Heat of the circumjacent parts, their grosser salts are divided and put in motion; which Fermentation is augmented by the various Juices that flow into the Guts, from the many Glands which are placed in the Lower Belly; and by this means, they are disolv'd and liquify'd, as to enter by the Milky Veines into the Blood, where they produce all these Accidents, which I shall derive from this Cause, and account for Mechanically in the following Chapter.

He considered that his views were confirmed by therapeutic experience:

> Because only Steel Medicines, which are proper to divide the tough glutinous Sulphurs of the Blood, and to Ferment, Volatilize, and render it more Spirituous, can effect an entire Cure.

Purcell desperately tried to throw off the Galenickal influences, but try as he might he had no alternative theory with which to replace these time honoured notions. The lack of any understanding of psychopathology, of what the patient thought or felt, or of neurophysiology, made Purcell's task an impossible one.

In the differential diagnosis he included Syncope, Apoplexy and Epilepsy, and these were to remain the cardinal alternatives in all the works that were to follow. Epilepsy was only "Vapours arriv'd to a more violent degree"; Syncope was distinguished by its cardiovascular manifestations; and Apoplexy by the lack of convulsive movements. A rather macabre ending graces this chapter. Since "Persons in this Distemper lie in Trances for whole Days Motionless, and Senseless

Like Dead Bodies" it is not amiss to consider the signs of life or death
—the mirror held before the mouth, the full glass of water placed on
the chest may both prove useful tests "but that is most secure in this
Case, and what I advise to be done to everyone who is subject to
Vapours, is, to keep them for three or four Days till they are sensibly
perceiv'd to Corrupt". Even at the leisurely pace of practice in the
eighteenth century, this seems a little too much for relatives to have
accepted, and some lurking doubt creeps in as to the extent of Purcell's
experience. In his brief consideration of prognosis one sees the time-
honoured excuses of the physician—he is called in too late, or the
patients have "deprav'd Appetites, and indulge themselves during the
Interval in eating things of bad digestion", or else have something on
their minds which they do not care to divulge to their physician.
Patients were ever thus. Again the chapter reaches somewhat of an
anti-climax when Purcell writes that "if a Patient sneezes whilst she is
in Hysterick Fits, tis a good sign".

As to treatment—

> The cure of the Vapours lies obviously in the removal of the Crudities
> and Indigestions which lie in the Guts and Stomach; to correct the Vices
> which its Ferments hath contracted, and cleanse the Blood of those
> vicious Salts which pervert its Natural Dispositions.

Both internal and external remedies can be used—external stimulation
by tickling, a douche of cold water, burning the fingers and toes, and

> when there is so great a Coagulation of the Blood, that these Remedies
> can produce No Effect, and the Physician has reason to fear the patient
> will die in the Fit, he may then try a last Remedy, which is, to heat a Fire
> shovel red-hot, and hold it to the Head at a convenient distance: this
> seldom fails of wakening the sick Person, and tho' it cures her not, yet it
> gains her some Moments, which are very pretious in this conjuncture, for
> the settling of her Concerns, both as to this, and the next World.

Blood is to be let, followed by a vomit on the second day, a purge
on the third, and then "aperitive broths", into which is put half a dram
of Rust of Iron for the first four days, then alkalis and electuaries. After
these remedies, "Send her to Tunbridge, or some other Waters of the
same nature", then let her go to Bath for the Sulphur Waters, and to
give herself over to "Mirth and Pastime". After all this the patient
must go on a Milk-Diet, visit Bath again, and finally be careful with

her diet, take plenty of exercise, and pass her time in "Divertisements", and Merry Company.

The second edition was published in 1707 larger by eighty pages. Purcell expanded the section on the mechanical explanations of symptoms, changed the prescriptions from English into Latin, and added a brief section on "insignificant Remedies, which Custom and Ignorance have impos'd upon the World, for beneficial in Vapours".

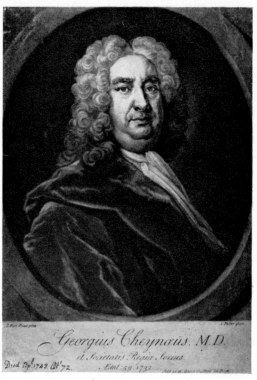

FIG. 7.   George Cheyne, M.D., F.R.S., 1671–1743.

"THE ENGLISH MALADY",
by GEORGE CHEYNE, M.D., F.R.S. (1733)

These same ideas and concepts were taken up at a later date by George Cheyne, who stated and re-stated them in a series of publications (Fig. 7). The book which concerns psychiatry most is *The English*

Malady: "or a Treatise of Nervous Diseases of all Kinds, as Spleen, Vapours, Lowness of Spirits, Hypochondriacal, and Hysterical Distempers, etc.", published in 1733. The title was chosen, Cheyne writes, because it is

> A Reproach universally thrown on this Island by Foreigners, and all our Neighbours on the Continent, by whom Nervous Distempers, Spleen, Vapours, and Lowness of Spirits, are in Derision called the English Malady. And I wish there were not so good Grounds for this Reflection. The Moisture of our Air, the Variableness of our Weather, (from our Situation amidst the Ocean) the Rankness and Fertility of our Soil, the Richness and Heaviness of our Food, the Wealth and Abundance of the Inhabitants (from their Universal Trade) the Inactivity and sedentary Occupations of the better Sort (among whom this Evil mostly rages) and the Humour of living in great populous and consequently unhealthy Towns, have brought forth a Class and Set of Distempers, with atrocious and frightful Symptoms, scarce known to our Ancestors, and never rising to such fatal Heights, nor afflicting such Numbers in any other known Nation. These nervous Disorders being computed to make almost one third of the Complaints of the People of Condition in England.

Cheyne attributed the cause of neurosis to "a siziness or viscidity in the fluids", a sharpness or corrosive quality in the fluids, and a laxity or want of due tone in the fibres or nerves. A milk, seed, and vegetable diet was the rational cure, his own case history being used to illustrate his theories. The 370 pages are far too many for the burden of the book, and Cheyne knew this, for in his preface he acknowledged that his ablest friends had criticized the book as repetitious and unoriginal. In fact, the book is no more than a verbose and rather grandiose piece of padding, although Zilboorg has singled out *The English Malady* as an illustration of the ideas current during this period. Two other writers, in addition to Purcell, are superior to Cheyne in style, material and conception.

"A TREATISE OF THE HYPOCHONDRIACK AND HYSTERIC PASSIONS",
by BERNARD DE MANDEVILLE, M.D. (1711)

First comes Bernard de Mandeville (1670c.–1733), the author of the *Fable of the Bees*. In 1711 he published *A Treatise of the Hypochondriack and Hysterick Passions*, "Vulgarly call'd the Hypo in Men and Vapours in Women; in which the Symptoms, Causes, and Cure of those Diseases are set forth after a Method entirely new" (2nd Edition 1715. 3rd Edition 1730). It is written in the form of three dialogues between the physician Philopirio and his patient Misomedon. The patient recounts his life history—at the age of 37 he developed heart-burn, flushing of the face after meals, wind, belching, and water brash. An eminent physician was called who prescribed bleeding and purging. These measures were worse than the disease and gave him no relief. A course of the Epsom Waters helped him temporarily, but a relapse soon followed. A second physician was called—one of the modern school, in contrast to the first, who had been a Galenist. The modern prescribed emetics—but twelve months of the patient tired him out and he retired from the scene. Two or three other physicians were then consulted—to no satisfaction. The symptoms progressed with the development of headaches, sleeplessness, dreaming, and melancholy. A course of steel was taken, and a visit was made to Bath. By the time de Mandeville was called in the patient had been for twelve years a "hypochondriacus confirmatus". He had begun to study physic himself, which he soon found to be so full of inconsistencies that he became utterly confused. The doctor and patient then begin a general discussion on the different schools of medicine, the training of physicians, their observations, and the gulf existing between theory and practice. The style is witty and amusing, and clearly the work of a more polished writer than the usual medical practitioner.

> MISOMEDON: I have sent for you, Doctor, to consult you about a Distemper, of which I am very well assured, I shall never be Cured.
>
> PHILOPIRIO: Whatever your Case may be, Sir, it is a great misfortune, you entertain so ill an Opinion of it; but I hope, your Disease may prove less desperate than your Fears.
>
> MISOMEDON: It is neither better nor worse than I tell you, and what I say is what I am convinced of by Reason, and not a suggestion of my Fears. But you think perhaps, I'm a Mad-man, to send for a Physician, when I know before-hand, that he can do me no good. Truly, Doctor, I am not far from it; but first of all, Are you in haste, pray?
>
> PHILOPIRIO: Not in great haste, Sir.
>
> MISOMEDON: I am glad of that; for most of your Profession always either are, or at least pretend to be in a great hurry. But tho' you are at leisure, Can you hear a Man talk for half an Hour together, and, perhaps, not always to the purpose, without interrupting him? For I have a great deal

to say to you, several Questions to ask you, and, know I shall be very tedious; but if you can bear with me, I'll consider your Trouble, and pay you for your Time, and Patience both. Can you stay an Hour?

PHILOPIRIO: Yes, Sir, or longer, if there be occasion.

MISOMEDON: Then, pray Sir, sit down—I did not make you come up Stairs because I keep Chamber my self, for I'm abroad every Day, but I thought it best to Discourse you in my Study, because it is the quietest Room in the House, and I hate to be disturbed. That you may be the better acquainted with my Distemper, I'll begin with you ab ove, and give you as short an account as I can, how I have past the greatest part of my Life.

The second dialogue consists of an argument concerning the various hypotheses as to the causes of hypochondria and hysteria. The patient puts forward the views of the authors he has studied, only to have them vigorously demolished by Philopirio. Willis in particular comes in for a severe castigation for his statements regarding the Spleen as the site of the disturbance in hypochondria. After much learned discussion de Mandeville tells the patient about his disputation prior to graduation at Leyden in 1691. Its title was de Chylosi Vitiati and in it he dealt with the correct cause of these conditions, namely a disorder of chylification. As in Purcell's book, this is something of an anticlimax, for de Mandeville's theory is perhaps even more nebulous and less rational than that of Willis. If disorder of the stomach and its ferments is substituted for splenic disturbance, the two theories seem in all other respects almost identical, although Philopirio does take into account life stresses such as excess of venery and excess of study. The primary disorder nevertheless remains an exhaustion of the tone of the spirits as a result of the "robbing of the Stomachick Ferment of what was required for its Volatilization".

Misomedon becomes so impressed by his new physician that he describes both his wife and his daughter's cases to him. The wife is suffering from a neurotic depression, and the daughter with hysteria; the ensuing dialogue is particularly interesting for the account of the treatment of such cases.

MISOMEDON: Pray tell me now, what course of Exercise you would have my Daughter go through.

PHILOPIRIO: Let her every Morning, as soon as she rises, (which I would have her do before Six) be swung for half an Hour, then Eat her Breakfast, and get on Horseback for at least two Hours, either Galloping or

Trotting as much as her Strength will permit her. Immediately after this let her be undrest, and by some Nurse or other chafed or dry rubbed for a considerable time, till her Skin looks red, and her Flesh glows all over: Let her begin to repeat the same Exercises about Three in the Afternoon, and after Supper keep upon her Legs two Hours before she goes to Bed. The Swing I speak of may be made after what manner your Daughter fancies most; that which they call a Flying Horse, makes a very agreeable motion, but if she be apt to be giddy, she may swing in a Chair, or other Seat to which she is fastened, otherwise a Rope tied with both ends to a Beam is sufficient: However strange and absurd this Prescription may appear, I can assure you that I have seen admirable effects of it.

MISOMEDON: What you recommend is no new thing, it is without doubt and consequently the Swing must be either the same with, or else an equivalent for the Petaurus of the Ancients.

PHILOPIRIO: I am not much concerned about either the Name of the Original of Swinging, tho' what you say of it expresses my meaning very well, and that motion which resembles a flying in the Air, is the Exercise I require. A great part of your Daughter's Distemper lies in the Brain and Nerves, and I could never meet with any thing so innocent, that was half so Efficacious in strengthning and reviving the Spirits, as the motion I speak of.

I don't pretend to know any thing of the seat of Quartan Agues, but Experience teaches us, that where they are of long continuance, they generally leave obstructions of the Lower-belly behind them. That this was your Daughter's Case is evident from the Emaciated as well as Cachectick Condition it had reduced her to. Considering every Circumstance, tho' her Ague has left her Four Years, and she gained strength since, and is grown Tall, it is highly probable to think, that all the Miseraick Vessels, the Glandules of the Intestines, and other passages are not yet entirely cleared of those Morbifick remainders, and it is certain, that to remove those obstinate Stoppages in Hypogastrio, there is not a more effectual Remedy than Riding: It is incredible to those that have not observed it, what powerful influence the repeated Succussations of a Horse have upon those Parts, as well to Digest, as to Eliminate whatever Crude, or otherwise Peccant Matter they may contain.

The chafing, or dry rubbing, I speak of does not only Levigate and Beautifie the Skin, open the Pores, and promote Perspiration; but likewise by quickening the Torpid motion of the Blood in the Capillary Vessels, it enlivens the Circulation of its whole Mass, attenuates the Lymphatick Juice, and by squeezing it through the Fibres of the Muscles is a vast help to Nutrition.

MISOMEDON: But might not Marriage be as effectual as all these Exercises?

PHILOPIRIO: Yes, but I never prescribe an uncertain Remedy, that may prove worse than the Disease; for not to speak of the many inconveniences, the advising it often puts People to (praeterquam quod januam aperit nequitae) in the first place it may fail, and then there are two People made unhappy instead of one; Secondly it may but half Cure the Woman, who lingering under the remainder of her Disease, may have half a dozen Children, that shall all inherit it. A Physician has a publick Trust reposed in him: His Prescriptions by assisting some ought never to prejudice others; besides that a Young Lady has no reason with the same Fortune to expect such an agreeable Match, whilst she labours under so deplorable an Infirmity, as if she was in perfect Health; therefore let her either be first Cured, and then Marry without being injurious to her self, her Husband, or her Posterity; or else remain single, with this Comfort at least in her Affliction, that she is not liable of entailing it upon others, that should be no less dear to her than her self.

Although sceptical about the use of medicines, de Mandeville came out strongly in favour of alcohol. "Wine has wrought miraculous Cures in abundance of desperate Cases (of which many Hysterick) and is without doubt, when in perfection, the highest Cordial, and greatest Restorative to the Spirits, that God hitherto has communicated to Mankind."

The book is characterized by an acute and witty style, by the lack of theorizing, and by its peculiar mixture of shrewd empiricism and scepticism. The treatment advocated was in the main psychotherapeutic—the dialogues between physician and patient may even be regarded as very early "recorded interviews". The patients were allowed to ventilate their ideas freely, and to express their hostility to the doctor, a remarkable situation for the early eighteenth century.

Bernard de Mandeville was himself a remarkable man. Of Dutch origin, he had taken his M.D. at Leyden in 1691 before settling in London. Hawkins in his *Life of Johnson* tells us that he lived in lodgings, and never acquired much practice, but some Dutch merchants are said to have provided him with a pension. He moved in literary circles, meeting Benjamin Franklin and Addison, and his own writings were very well thought of by Samuel Johnson. His most famous book, which became a minor classic, was *The Fable of the Bees, or Private Vices Public Benefits*, and first appeared in 1714. By 1755 it had passed into nine editions, and it has often been reprinted since then. Its subject-matter, however, gave great offence and the book was deemed a nuisance by the Grand Jury of Middlesex in 1723. In it de Mandeville put forward the view that man is essentially selfish, his desires evil, and his motives to be regarded with suspicion. Prosperity, he maintained, is increased not by saving, but by spending; virtue was a mere sham, human nature essentially vile. Dr. Johnson was greatly impressed by "the Fable", which, he said, "opened his views into real life very much". Both the Fable and the Treatise provide amusing and interesting reading even today, although their influence on psychiatric thought has been practically negligible.

"A TREATISE OF THE SPLEEN AND VAPOURS", by SIR RICHARD BLACKMORE, M.D. (1725)

In 1725 there appeared *A Treatise of the Spleen and Vapours*: "or, Hypocondriacal and Hysterical Affections", by Sir Richard Blackmore (Fig. 9). Perhaps because of Blackmore's ability as a medical journalist, the book gives a good account of the concepts relating the spleen and mental illness. Blackmore pointed out that for centuries hysteria had been ascribed to noxious fumes rising from the womb, and hypochondria to "dark and windy steams and exhalations elevated from the spleen". The ancients regarded the spleen as a superfluous part of the body, well knowing that life was quite possible without it. Pliny taught that it acted as a strainer separating out the "dark and dreggy" parts of the blood—it was also the seat of intemperate emotion: "hence silly laughter flows; But if cut out, that Passion decent grows". Greek warriors had their chargers' spleens cauterized, to give them greater speed and strength, and even in man, Paulus Aeginatus described a similar procedure, mentioning that the spleen could indeed be excised if necessary. Willis adopted and modified these ideas, believing that in the spleen, after a straining of the blood, the thicker and heavier parts became transformed into a ferment, which was then discharged back into the blood via the splenic veins, or carried to the animal spirits by the nerves. In the blood this ferment "purified and agitated"; by it the animal spirits were refined, stimulated and exalted. Hypochondria was the result of various anomalies in the production of this ferment. Other anatomists conceived splenic function in a purely mechanical light—the organ was so structured as to form a resistance to the blood flow, in order to moderate its velocity.

Blackmore himself considered that the spleen was part of the procreational system, designed not for the preservation of the individual, but of the species.

It performs this office by obstructing the Stream of Blood, and moderating the Rapidity of its Motion, which otherwise might rush into the Parts subservient to Procreation with too great Violence and Abundance; and by that means Communicate to them, by proper Strainers, a greater Measure of prolifick Fluids, than the regular Oeconomy of Nature demands.

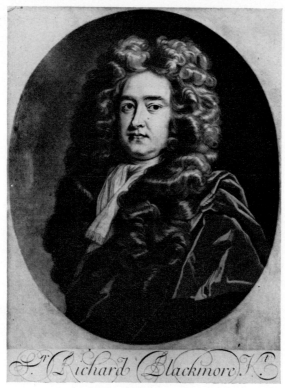

FIG. 8. Sir Richard Blackmore, 1650–1729. (*From the mezzotint by R. Williams after Closterman. From the impresssion in the British Museum.*)

William Cheselden had told him that the blood leaves the spleen eight times slower than it enters, and Purcell had observed that splenectomized dogs were more salacious and prone to venery than before their operation. Suppose, therefore, that individual variations in the size of the spleen and its vessels occur, so the velocity of the blood flow will vary, and consequently the personality may be either sluggish or incontinent and lascivious.

But Blackmore did not consider that the spleen was the cause of psychiatric disorder—rather that "what we call the Spleen, is a distemper belonging to the whole System of the Animal Spirits, and has its Rise immediately from theory". The animal spirits pervade the whole body, but in particular the nervous system; it is the disturbance of these animal spirits which gives rise to the symptoms of hypochondriasis. Hysteria too is not very different, for the "Hysterick as well as Hypochondriacal Passions, act all their tragical parts in the Frame of the Nerves, by the irregular and seditious Motions of the Spirits". Blackmore ends his Essay with some observations on personality. Like a patriotic Englishman he considers that of all the different peoples, French, Italian, Spaniards,

> the temper of the Native of Britain is most various, which proceeds from the Spleen, an Ingredient of their Constitution, which is almost peculiar, at least in the Degree of it, to this Island. Hence arises the Diversity of Genius and Disposition, of which this Sort is so fertile. Our Neighbours have greater Poverty of Humour and Scarcity of Originals than we. The Spaniard sarcastically says of the French, "If you have seen one, you have seen all"; tho' a Frenchman may as justly retort the Raillery on the grave Castilian; and this may be as truly affirm'd of the Italian on each Side of the Appenines, and of the High Dutch and Low. But an Englishman need not go abroad to learn the Humours of these different Neighbours; let him but travel from Temple-Bar to Ludgate, and he will meet . . . in four and twenty hours, the Dispositions and Humours of all the Nations of Europe.

"A NEW SYSTEM OF THE SPLEEN",
by NICHOLAS ROBINSON, M.D. (1729)

Four years after the appearance of Blackmore's book Nicholas Robinson published *A New System of the Spleen, Vapours, and Hypochondriack Melancholy* (1729). Robinson begins by pointing out that there is a "twofold knowledge of natural Beings; the one intuitive, the other experimental; the first relates to the Discovery of new Ideas or Objects, the other their Connections with certain natural phenomena".

As a result of the obscurity which enveloped these disorders, it was of particular importance to consider the natural processes—such as thought and sensation—on which they were superimposed. Moreover, every individual is endowed with a particular constitution, and although as diverse as the different complexions of mankind, in general the four Hippocratic humours, the sanguine, bilious, the phlegmatic and the melancholy, served to distinguish between them. As for the soul, Robinson was a dualist—"the mind can reason, act, and think without any Assistance from the body", the body "digests, assimilates, and nourishes, without any exerted thought of the mind to Commend these operations". Despite this promising beginning, the book rapidly deteriorates, becoming a hotch-potch of Willisian theory, theology, philosophy and imagination. Thus the causes of nervous disorders lie primarily in the dynamics of the "Machinulae" of the Nerves—those "little small Corpuscles of Matter, that Vary their Distance and Motion in every Contraction or Distraction of a Fibre, Muscle or Organ". The state of these Machinulae at any one time may produce different effects in different constitutions—varying from the vapours to "enthusiastic" madness. Therapeutically Robinson was a conservative—he recommends the old-fashioned camphire, hellebore, bleeding, purging, diet and exercise, but tries to integrate their actions into his theory. For instance

> whereas opiate Preparations relax the Brain and Nerves, already too much relax'd, and lets down the Machinulae of their Fibres beneath their Capacity of Sensation; Wine, on the Contrary, if taken in a large Dose, contracts the foregoing Instruments, and prises up their too lax Machinulae, whereby the Fibres are incapable of Conveying those Active Sensations to the Brain and Seat of the common Sensorium: However, both Wine and Opium intercept the Sensations, and infer a Stupor upon all the animal Faculties.

Robinson's book is illustrative of the confusion which may result either from the absence of a sound theory or from faulty clinical observation. Unfortunately this type of work occurs all too frequently throughout the century. There was an over-concern with theory, so much so that the two names on everyone's lips were those of Stahl and Hoffmann. Georg Ernst Stahl (1666–1734) had rebelled against the dualism of Descartes, postulating instead his system of animism (Fig. 9). For Stahl, the anima represented a vital force, the sum of the activities of the organism directing the movements on which life depended. A preoccupation with the difference between the living and dead body, for so long a theological and mystical problem, led Stahl to consider

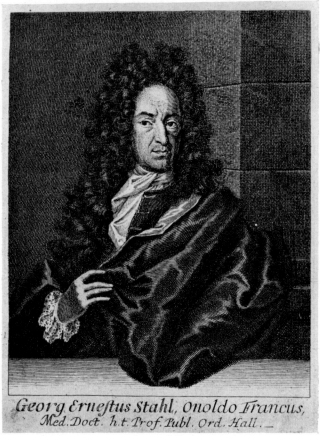

Georg Erneſtus Stahl, Onoldo Francus,
Med. Doct. h. t. Prof. Publ. Ord. Hall. __

FIG. 9.   Georg Ernst Stahl, M.D., 1666–1734.

this central life force or anima as the motive force behind all the manifestations of life. The circulatory system was pre-eminent as the means whereby the anima maintained its activity, and the humoral concept of disease was still adhered to, most diseases arising from the blood, and from a stasis in the blood vessels. His doctrines, which were propounded with a dogmatism which brooked no argument, were as credulously accepted as many another false creed has been accepted in medicine. Zilboorg has given Stahl a prominent place in the development of psychiatric thought, and whilst this is not the place to enter into fuller considerations of the facts, the confused mysticism and logorrhoea of this German Professor in no way appeals. The harm Stahl did to the development of chemistry by his erroneous phlogiston theory is paralleled by the retarding effect of his theories on the advance of neurophysiology, without which, *pace* Zilboorg, psychiatry would have remained within the realms of philosophy and metaphysics.

Frederick Hoffmann's (1660–1742) system was founded on a more mechanistic philosophy. Medicine should be based on reasoning and observation; anatomy, chemistry, physics and the natural sciences were the keystones of knowledge. The influence of the nervous system was pre-eminent, for life depended on movement, and movement was a result of nervous activity. Not however, the nervous activity we recognize today, but one resulting from a "nervous ether", a fluid arising in the brain, and carried to all parts of the body by contraction and dilatation of the meninges. This nervous ether maintained the fibres composing the body in a state of tonus; disease resulted when this tonus became disturbed. Hoffmann's neural concept of disease was to have an important influence on future thought and research, particularly in psychiatry and neurology.

These two systems were very familiar to British psychiatrists, many of whom had received their medical education at Continental Universities. Stahl's way of thinking was alien to the British mind, and two of the greatest eighteenth-century physicians did much to counteract his erroneous ideas. Robert Whytt and William Cullen, both Professors at Edinburgh, exerted an important influence on the course of British psychiatry. From their teaching, their writings and the school they created sprang the first British psychiatrists—men like Arnold, Haslam, Prichard, Conolly and Sir Alexander Morison, to mention but a few.

Robert Whytt (1714–1766) (Fig. 10) was born in Edinburgh, studied under the first Monro, and in 1734 travelled to various clinics, first in London where he was a pupil of Cheselden, then in Paris where he attended Winslow's lectures, and finally in Leyden to study under Boerhaave and Albinus. He took an M.D. at Rheims in 1736, and a year later obtained a similar degree at St. Andrews. After his four years of travelling he set up in practice as a physician at Edinburgh in 1738.

c

His travels had made him familiar with the controversies exercising the minds of Continental physicians, so that he wrote with some authority. He decisively rejected Stahl's doctrine that the rational soul

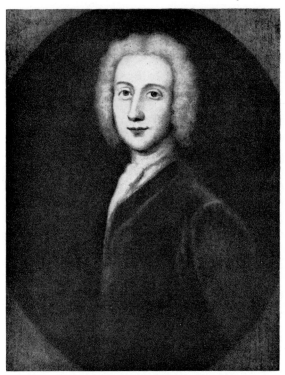

Fig. 10.   Robert Whytt, 1714–1766.   (*The portrait in the Royal College of Physicians, Edinburgh.*)

is the cause of all involuntary motions in his book *On the Vital and other Involuntary Motions of Animals* (1751), and ascribed such movements to "the effect of a stimulus acting on an unconscious sentient principle". Whytt described the pupillary light reflex quite clearly, arguing along those clinico–pathological lines which were later to prove so rewarding to the great neurologists working at the National Hospital, London, toward the close of the nineteenth century.

"OBSERVATIONS ON THE NATURE, CAUSES, AND
CURE OF THOSE DISORDERS WHICH HAVE BEEN
COMMONLY CALLED NERVOUS, HYPOCHONDRIAC
OR HYSTERIC", by ROBERT WHYTT, M.D. (1765)

In 1765 he published his *Observations on the Nature, Causes, and Cure of those Disorders which have been Commonly called Nervous, Hypochondriac or Hysteric*: "To which are prefixed some Remarks on the Sympathy of the Nerves." He begins quite clearly by stating that—

> The disorders which are the subject of the following observations, have been treated of by authors under the name of flatulent, spasmodic, hypochondriac, or hysteric. Of late, they have also got the name of Nervous; which appellation having been commonly given to many symptoms seemingly different, and very obscure in their nature, has often made it to be said, that physicians have bestowed the character of nervous on all those disorders whose nature and causes they were ignorant of. To wipe off this reproach, and, at the same time, to throw some light on nervous, hypochondriac, and hysteric complaints, is the design of the following observations; which are also intended to shew, how far the principles laid down in my Essay on the vital and other involuntary motions of animals may be of use in explaining the nature of several diseases, and consequently in leading to the most proper method of cure.

Then follows an excellent survey of the "Structure, Use and Sympathy" of the Nerves, illustrated by remarkably astute clinical observations. He divided stimuli into those producing voluntary and involuntary motions, proceeding to consider the sympathy between various organs in the body, in most cases giving excellent examples of somatic or of autonomic reflex activity. The emotions of fear, anger, shame, grief, joy and their bodily concomitants are well described before he passes on to discuss nervous disorders in general. Whytt regarded hysteria and hypochondria as identical conditions, the one occurring in woman and the other in man; all else is grouped together under the heading of "nervous disorder".

The causes of nervous disorder Whytt regarded as twofold:

(1) A too great delicacy and sensibility of the whole nervous system.
(2) An uncommon weakness, or a depraved or unnatural feeling, in some of the organs of the body.

Acting on these two are the "particular occasional causes", chiefly

Wind, a tough phlegm (in the stomach and bowels), Worms, "Aliments improper in their quantity or quality, Scirrhosis or other obstructions in the viscera of the lower belly, and Violent affections of the mind". The "general occasional causes", in which he includes "Some morbid matter bred in the blood, the diminution or retention of some accustomed evacuation, and the want of sufficient quantity of blood, or of blood of a proper density", may also produce symptoms.

"Violent affections of the mind" play a comparatively small etiological role, a physical, mechanistic causation being emphasized. As is usual in this period, a long list of symptoms are analysed in the light of the writer's particular theory—and no less than 184 pages are devoted to "cures"—mainly consisting of bitters, quinine, iron and Spa waters. Although starting so well, the book fades out with this somewhat undistinguished pharmaceutics, and adds little to the theories already holding the field.

William Cullen (1710–1790) was 56 when he succeeded Whytt as the Professor of the Institutes of Medicine (Fig. 11). A distinguished career already lay behind him, for he had founded the Glasgow Medical School, occupied the Chair of Medicine there, and at the time of his appointment was Professor of Chemistry at Edinburgh. A man of extraordinary clarity of mind, he was an excellent lecturer and by virtue of his personality exerted a profound influence on the development of British Medicine. His students were devoted to him because

> he was cordially attentive to all their interests, admitted them freely to his house, conversed with them on the most familiar terms, solved their doubts and difficulties, gave them the use of his library, and in every respect treated them with the affection of a friend and the regard of a parent.

Poor students were often admitted free to his lectures, and he introduced the practice of not charging fees for medical attendance on students. He was also on extremely good terms with his co-workers; Joseph Black dedicated his fundamental treatise on fixed air to Cullen, and when the Chair of Chemistry fell vacant at Edinburgh, refused to compete against his friend and master. William Hunter was Cullen's resident pupil from 1737 to 1740 and remained a devoted friend throughout his life, writing of him as "a man to whom I owe most, and love most of all men in the world". Cullen taught his students in

English instead of Latin—his lectures being models of clarity and common sense. No man could be further distant from the dogmatic, somewhat arrogant and aggressive Stahl, nor could his mind be capable of conceiving the kind of theory which Stahl had put forward.

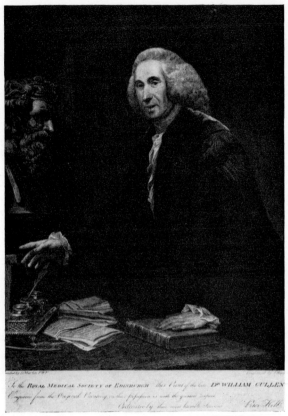

FIG. 11.   William Cullen, M.D., 1710–1790.

"FIRST LINES OF THE PRACTICE OF PHYSIC", by WILLIAM CULLEN, M.D. (1777)

Cullen's two works which concern us here are his *Nosology* and the *First Lines of the Practice of Physic*. He divided diseases into four great categories: (1) Pyrexias, or febrile diseases; (2) Neuroses, or nervous diseases; (3) Cachexiae, or diseases resulting from "bad habit of body"; and (4) Locales, or local diseases. This nosology has the advantage of simplicity and greatly impressed his generation. His most popular work, however, was his *First Lines*, in which he rejected Boerhaave's eclectic system, and came out in favour of Hoffmann. His sponsorship of the neural theory of disease was to influence nearly all of the notable British physicians who were interested in psychiatry.

In the second volume of his *First Lines of the Practice of Physic* he writes that

> almost the whole of the diseases of the human body might be called Nervous but there would be no use for such a general appellation; and on the other hand, it seems improper to limit the term, in the loose inaccurate manner in which it has been hitherto applied to hysteria and hypo-chondriacal disorders, which are themselves hardly to be defined with sufficient precision. In this place I propose to comprehend, under the title of Neuroses, all those preternatural affections of sense or motion, which are without pyrexia as a part of the primary disease; and all those which do not depend upon a topical affection of the organs, but upon a more general affection of the nervous system, and of those powers of the system upon which sense and motion more especially depend. Of such diseases I have established a class, under the title of Neuroses, or Nervous Diseases. These I again distinguish, as they consist, either in the interruption and debility of the powers of sense and motion, or in the irregularity with which these powers are exercised; and have accordingly arranged them under the four orders of Comata, Adynamiae, Spasmi, and Vesaniae.

Hoffmann's influence is clearly to be seen in this passage. As for Cullen's descriptions of psychiatric conditions, he freely admits that his experience had been limited, with the result that his classification is incomplete.

> In my limited views of the different states of insanity, I must go on to consider them under the two heads of Mania and Melancholia; and though I am sensible that these two genera do not comprehend the whole of the species of insanity, I am not clear in assigning the other species, which may not be comprehended under those titles.

He refers to Dr. Arnold's attempts at classification in terms which wounded Dr. Arnold not a little, coming as they did from his old teacher.

> The ingenious Dr. Arnold has been commendably employed in distin-guishing the different species of insanity as they appear with respect to

the mind; and his labours may hereafter prove useful, when we shall come to know something more of the different states of the brain corresponding to these different states of the mind; but at present I can make little application of his numerous distinctions. It appears to me that he has chiefly pointed out and enumerated distinctions, that are merely varieties, which can lead to little or no variety of practice: and I am especially led to form the latter conclusion because these varieties appear to me to be often combined together, and to be often changed into one another, in the same person; in whom we must therefore suppose a general cause of the disease, which, so far as it can be known, must establish the pathology, and especially direct the practice.

But whatever his defects as a psychiatrist, Cullen at least knew brevity, and gave a short, yet full, account of delirium, mania, melancholia, hypochondriasis and hysteria. The development of an adequate psychiatric nosology owes much to Cullen, both directly and indirectly through the efforts of his students and followers.

The day of the physician was almost over when in 1788 two books appeared, one by a medical journalist, the other by a fashionable Spa doctor. The first was a curious compendium by William Rowley, entitled *A Treatise on Female, Nervous, Hysterical, Hypochondriacal, Bilious, Convulsive Diseases; Apoplexy and Palsy*; "with thoughts on Madness, Suicide, etc. In which the principal disorders are explained from anatomical facts, and the treatment formed on several new principles". Rowley had at one time been an army surgeon serving in the West Indies. He travelled widely, and refers to visits he made to Paris, Germany and Vienna, and to meetings with Voltaire and Franklin.

> I remember accidentally meeting and conversing with M. de Voltaire at a famous statuary's in Paris, to whom this philosopher, wit, and satirist had been sitting, his face always represented the sarcastic cynic grin, without disease; but it is easy to conceive that such a face, involuntary convulsed, would naturally assume the muscular actions to which it had been long accustomed.

Rowley was a prolific writer and his publications include *Remarks on Cancerous Diseases, A Treatise on Diseases of Children, Medical Advice to the Army and Navy serving in Hot Climates* and *Schola Medicinae Universalis Nova*. He frequently alludes to his clinical experiences and to his own observations.

> Men acquire professor's chair, sometimes before they have written many prescriptions, before they have had opportunities for great practice and experience; in which case all the knowledge they issue is dependent on the caprices, opinions, or, perhaps, fallacies of their predecessors. Men are not capable of teaching, who are not well taught and experienced themselves; and no man can well comprehend medicine by either hearing lectures, or much reading, but by long practical experience, and observations made by himself, on the force of diseases, and power of medicine. Tuition frequently taints the fancy with numerous prejudices, and a deleterious intoxication; but a multitude of experience in practices sobers the mind again. Trifling medicines would never be prescribed in important cases, nor powerful remedies in trivial diseases, where knowledge is obtained by experiments and observation.

Inasmuch as he recommended clinical observation Rowley was in safe ground, but his theory was a reversion to Purcell, tempered with a sprinkling of the social psychiatry so popular at this period.

> In proportion as the arts, sciences, and luxury increase, so do vices and madness. In countries where the fewest wants and desires are experienced, there are the smallest number of mad persons; in those kingdoms where the greatest luxuries, refinements, wealth, and unrestrained liberty abound, are the most numerous instances of madness. England, according to its size and number of inhabitants, produces and contains more insane than any other country in Europe, and suicide is more common. In other nations mankind are obedient under either military or religious despotism, and are educated from infants in implicit submission and non-resistance; in Britain everyone thinks and acts as he pleases; this produces all that variety and originality in the English character, and causes arts, sciences, and inventions to flourish. The agitations of passions, this liberty of thinking and acting with less restraint than in other nations, force a great quantity of blood to the head, and produce greater varieties of madness in this country, than is observed in others. Religious and civil toleration are productive of political and religious madness; but where no such toleration exists, no such insanity appears.

The second book is of greater interest, for although its author, William Falconer, was again a prolific writer, he was in practice at Bath, where he had unrivalled opportunities to observe the minor psychiatric illnesses. His "Dissertation on the Influence of the Passions upon Disorders of the Body" was the first Fothergillian Medal Prize Essay. The entries had been judged in 1786, and Falconer won—there being no other entry! (Fig. 12). The medal was presented on 6 June

1787 and a long address was given by Dr. J. C. Lettsom. The subject of the Essay was, said Lettsom, "What Diseases may be mitigated or cured, by exciting particular affections or passions of the Mind".

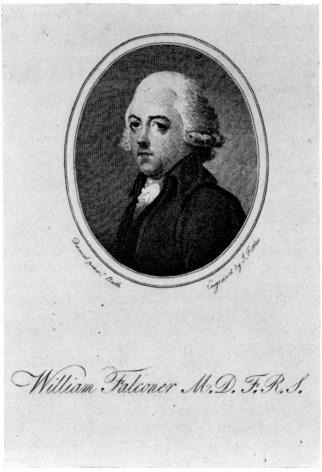

FIG. 12.   William Falconer, M.D., F.R.S., 1744–1824

Every practitioner, therefore, who studies the honour of his profession, and the happiness of his patient, should sedulously endeavour to cultivate an acquaintance with the anatomy of the mind, as well as that of the body. Few subjects can appear of greater importance, in the history of the medical profession, when it is considered that at least, half of the diseases, to which we are prone, originate from the influence of the passions on the human system. It was not designed to introduce the history of diseases, or of the passions which mitigate or cure them—This is the object of the prize dissertation.

Falconer begins his essay by postulating that the mind, when awake, is constantly in a state of action or employment; when its activity is diminished or weakened then sleep occurs. As the mind in action is always active and employed, the only method of banishing one set or train of ideas is by substituting another set in its place. Ideas combine together in such a way that their emotional concomitants are linked together, so that the recollection of one event may be associated with the emotion felt with the original linked "idea". The mind has a tendency to repeat actions and sensations in the same manner, and to "imitation"—the disposition to identify with the thoughts, feelings and behaviour of others. All these aspects of mental functioning are in some respects shared by the bodily organs. Certain periods of life predispose to the manifestations of different aspects of mental functioning.

Falconer divided emotions into two groups, those exciting, and those depressing the "vital system". He described the somatic effects of love, anger, grief, hope, envy, joy and the influence of these emotions on various diseases. These form a curious list ranging from "the intermittent fever" to typhus, by way of scurvy, jaundice, menorrhagia, gout, toothache, headache and several other more clearly psychological disorders such as mania and melancholy.

In general, Falconer was chiefly concerned with the clinical effects of fear or the effects of sudden emotion on a physical state. He quoted Ives, surgeon to Lord Anson, who had noted how the prospect of a battle would empty the sick-bay of its scorbutic occupants, and how a reverse in a ship's fortune might bring death to a certain number of scurvy-ridden sailors as a result of the mental depression ensuing. Falconer also observed that toothache

> is often cured by the application of the artificial magnet; which, whatever the supporters of the imposture of animal magnetism may alledge in its defence, could be only owing to the confidence the patient had in the efficacy of the remedy, which I doubt not was much enhanced by the knowledge of the real powers of that wonderful substance, and its being here applied in a way that gave no information as to the manner in which

it could operate, which added to the impression by increasing the mystery. If the patient's faith be not very strong, the remedy fails of effect. It is more than probable, that several whimsical applications recommended in the rheumatism, as the nine times dyed blue flannel, etc., owe their efficacy, if they have any, to the same cause.

The influence of emotion on mental and physical disease was a popular subject in the eighteenth century, in both medical and non-medical works. The holistic concepts of what is now called psycho-somatic medicine needed no special pleading two centuries ago. Falconer's essay was, in this respect, unremarkable—what is of great interest is his theory of mental functioning. He clearly describes the association of ideas, the binding of affect, and the tendency to repeat old patterns, "the repetition compulsion". Unfortunately this promising beginning did not presage any further studies along similar lines. Falconer, as is so often the case with successful practitioners, was too interested in too many subjects. Born in Chester in 1744, he was the son of the Recorder of Chester. A student of Edinburgh, he took his M.D. there in 1766, and as was then the fashion proceeded to Leyden, where he also took an M.D. In 1767 he returned to Chester, where he settled in practice, was appointed physician to the Chester Infirmary, and soon built up a reputation for himself. Chester proved too small for a man of his talents, and at the suggestion of Dr. John Fothergill, Falconer moved to Bath. Here he again rapidly became successful, and was physician to the Bath General Hospital from 1784 to 1819, when he retired. Bath at the time was the hub of fashion and Falconer was thus in a position to meet many eminent men, mainly in literary and medical circles. At least eleven books on Spa therapy came from his pen; he wrote extensively on theological subjects, on the classics, and contributed many articles to various contemporary journals. He was awarded the Fothergill Medal, and also the Silver Medal of the Medical Society of London for his *Dissertation on the Ischias*; "or the Diseases of the Hip Joint, Commonly called a Hip Case, and on the Use of the Bath Waters as a Remedy in this Complaint", which was published in 1805. He died in 1824.

"AN INQUIRY INTO THE NATURE AND
ORIGIN OF MENTAL DERANGEMENT",
by SIR ALEXANDER CRICHTON (1798)

Sir Alexander Crichton was the last of the general physicians during this century to write on Insanity. *An Inquiry into the Nature and Origin of Mental Derangement*. "Comprehending a Concise System of the Physiology and Pathology of the Human Mind and a History of the Passions and Their Effects", was published in 1798 in two formidable volumes. Although the book attained a wide reputation both in England and abroad, it is largely a compendium of German work, and Crichton shows almost no acquaintance with his English forerunners apart from Dr. Arnold.

> If we except Dr. Arnold, of Leicester, no other author of this country has written fully on the subject of Mental Diseases. Monsieur Dufour is the only author, since the time of Sauvages, who has written systematically on them in France; and although the German press has sent forth a vast number of publications which relate to diseases of the human mind, yet they are only collections of cases, histories of individual diseases, or accounts of new remedies; for no author of that learned nation, at least as far as my knowledge of their literature extends, has written either fully or systematically on Vesaniae.

He related that since 1792 he had been contemplating a work on the relation between mind and body, but

> About the time I am speaking of I received from Germany, among a number of works which had been recommended to me by my esteemed and learned friends, Professor Blumenbach and Professor Arnemann, of the University of Goettingen, one which greatly interested me. It was entitled *Magazine zum Erfahrungsseelenkunde*; which means in English, *Magazine of Psychological Experience*. This work consists of no less than eight volumes, and was first published in numbers under the direction of two learned Psychologists, Charles Philip Moritz and Salamon Maimon. In this work I found what I had not yet met with in any other publication, a number of well-authenticated cases of insane aberration of mind, narrated in a full and satisfactory manner, without a view to any system whatever: for the Magazine is almost entirely made up of cases which are sent to its editors by different hands, and the greatest part of them are without much comment.

He determined therefore to build the framework of his book on this

German magazine. Even Arnold's book, although containing a sufficient number of facts on which to build a system, was unsatisfactory

> inasmuch as it is entirely founded on a gratuitous distinction between ideas
> and notions, and on the apparent variety of these which occur in insanity,
> rather than on the more immediate nature of the diseases themselves.
> Dr. A. makes but one genus of insanity; and of this genus he makes
> several species, which he arranged under two divisions. Mr. Lock had
> observed, that all our ideas are either obtained by means of our external
> senses, or by reflexion; and, accordingly, he says, all our ideas are either
> ideas of sensation, or ideas of reflexion. Dr. A. chooses to confine the term
> idea to the first of these, and to the second class he gives the name of
> notions, and as it appears to him, that in the various species of insanity, the
> disorder exists either in the ideas or in the notions, so he reduces these
> species, as has already been observed, under two general divisions; the
> first he calls Ideal Insanity, the second Notional Insanity. The first is
> characterised by a delirium, arising from an error in the ideas of a person;
> the second, by a delirium arising from an error in his notions.

Crichton considered that this distinction between ideas and notions was in fact irrelevant, for disturbed ideas and disturbed notions can at times be found in the same patient.

The nosology he put forward did in fact represent an advance on Arnold in that Crichton relied on the grouping together of symptoms and signs to form various diagnostic categories. Based largely on a perceptual and association psychology, his classification is as follows:

GENERA AND SPECIES, AND THEIR SYMPTOMS

Class NEUROSES   **Order** VESANIAE

G. 1. **DELIRIUM.** General derangement of the mental faculties, in which diseased perceptions are mistaken for realities; with incoherent language, and unruly conduct.

Species
1. **Mania furibunda.** Delirium, with constant raving, audacity, and fury.
2. **Mania mitis.** Delirium, with raving, and appearance of gaiety and pleasure.
3. **Melancholia.** Delirium, with dejection, despondency, and despair.

G. 2. **HALLUCINATIO, or ILLUSION.** Error of mind, in which ideal objects are mistaken for realities; or, in which real objects are falsely represented, without general derangement of the mental faculties.

Species

1. **Hypochondriasis.** Error, respecting a person's own health or form, with anxiety, apprehension, and dread; flatulency, dyspepsia, palpitation, tremor, and sense of pain.
2. **Daemonomania.** Firm belief in the immediate communication with spirits, or persuasion of the power of working miracles, without other symptoms of general derangement of mind.
3. **Vertigo.** Apparent rotatory motion of external objects, and sense of undulation in the ground, with abolished attention and thought.
4. **Somnambulismus?**

G. 3. **AMENTIA.** Diminished power of the mental faculties.

Species

1. **Fatuitas.** Imbecillity of all the faculties of the human mind, particularly those concerned in associating and comparing ideas; accompanied with want of language, a stupid look, and general bodily weakness.
2. **Memoria imminuta.** Difficulty of recalling thoughts, and incorrectness as to recognizing objects formerly perceived.
3. **Perceptio imminuta.** Difficulty of forming distinct representations.
4. **Vis idearum associandi imminuta.** Deficiency, or total incapability of arranging one's thoughts; giving signs of confusion of intellect.
5. **Vis fingendi imminuta.** Total want of genius, or diminished genius.
6. **Vis judicandi imminuta.** Want of judgment and common sense.

Crichton's etiological theories were still concerned with disturbances of the vessels of the brain and the consequent alteration in the secretion of the nervous fluid. An increased activity of the blood vessels with secretion of fluid occurred in cases of mania, whilst in melancholy the vessels were hypoactive and secretion less. The book owes much to the philosophers, both English and German.

> The most useful of these authors, and their works, I shall now enumerate, in case others, who choose to write on the same subject, may also wish to go to the fountain head. Those of our British Psychologists, such as Loch, Hartley, Reid, Priestley, Stewart and Kaims, need not be mentioned. Of foreign authors, the following are those from whom I have derived most advantage; Unzer, whose work has been already named; Feder, Professor of Moral Philosophy in the University of Gottingen, whose

excellent work on Human Will, it is greatly to be lamented, is not trans-
lated into English. Ewald, on the Human Heart, (*Ueber das Menschleche
Herz*); an interesting work, which does not appear to be much read even
in Germany. Schmidt's *Experimental Seelenlehre,* or *Experimental
Psychology*; Kruger's ditto; Meier *Ueber die Gemüth bewegungen*; Herz
Ueber den Schwindel; Weickhard's *Philosophische Arzt* or *Philosophical
Physician*; Condillic's *Art de Penser*; Tissot's *Works on the Nerves, and on
the Diseases of Men of Letters.*

Crichton himself led a most interesting life. Again a product of
Edinburgh, he was first an apprentice to Alexander Wood the surgeon,
and like many of the Scots, proceeded to Leyden, where he took his
M.D. in 1785. He studied at Paris, Stuttgart, Vienna and Halle, and
then returned to London, where he began to practise surgery. He came
to dislike the operative aspects of surgery, disenfranchized himself
from the Corporation of Surgeons (of which he had become a member
in 1789) and became instead a Licentiate of the College of Physicians.
In 1795 he was elected Physician to the Westminster Hospital, lecturing
there on chemistry, *materia medica* and the practice of physic. In 1804
he was offered the post of Physician-in-ordinary to Alexander I of
Russia, and within a few years of his appointment had become chief
of the civil medical department. The dowager Empress made him her
friend and confidant, and in recognition of his services he received
many honours. He was knighted by George IV in the Pavilion at
Brighton in 1821 and given permission to wear his foreign orders. He
died at the age of 93 in 1856.

THE RISE OF SPECIALISM

At the beginning of the eighteenth century, apart from Bethlem,
the custody of lunatics was largely in private hands. The abuses which
took place in the private madhouses were castigated by Defoe in his
True Born Englishman, and later in the century the *Gentleman's Magazine*
published several accounts of malpractices occurring in such places.
The only Act of Parliament prior to 1808 was that passed in 1744,
which authorized the apprehension and chaining of lunatics on the
authority of two magistrates. Until some degree of specialization
occurred amongst respectable physicians and the monopoly of the
physicians to Bethlem was broken, this was to be the pattern of
psychiatric care. Mid-century, however, saw the rise of the professional

psychiatrist—St. Luke's was opened in 1751, St. Luke's House in Newcastle-on-Tyne in 1764, and the Manchester Lunatic Hospital in 1766.

So far specialist hospital psychiatry has been monopolized by the physicians to Bethlem—all of whom, in the eighteenth century, with the exception of Richard Hale (1670–1728), were members of the remarkable Monro family. Little is known of Hale except that he was a Fellow of the College of Physicians, three times a Censor, and Harveian orator in 1724. His oration was published in 1735, and contains an excellent account of English mediaeval physicians. He was known for his kindness to lunatics, and although his face "wore the look of sternness, characteristic of a mental specialist", Hale considered company, music, jollity and merriment to be very beneficial to the patients of Bethlem—particularly those suffering from melancholia. He was Physician to Bethlem following Tyson's death, from 1708 to 1728, and when he died left £500 to the College of Physicians for the purchase of books.

James Monro was appointed to succeed Hale, and thus started a dynasty which was to provide the Physicians to Bethlem for over a century (Fig. 13). Descended from the chiefs of the Highland Clan of Monro, James was the son of Alexander Monro, D.D., the Principal of the University of Edinburgh. Alexander had been nominated to the Bishopric of Argyle by James II just before the Revolution of 1688, but as his views did not coincide with those of the Government of William III he never took his throne, and was summoned to London in 1691. James, his son, came with him, and was educated in England. He obtained the Oxford M.B. in 1709, but does not appear to have practised in London until middle life, for he did not obtain his M.D. until 1722, when he was 42. In 1728 he was appointed Physician to Bethlem, and held this post until his death in 1752. His only literary work was the Harveian Oration, which he delivered in 1737, and which was solely an eulogy of Harvey, of little grace, and no originality. His policy of refusing students or physicians admission to Bethlem for study came in for bitter criticism from William Battie, and Wesley's mother referred to him as "that wretched fellow, Monro". John Monro answered for his father, and wrote

> He was a man of admirable discernment, and treated this disease (insanity) with an address which will not soon be equalled. He knew very well that the management requisite for it was never to be learned but by observation;

he was honest and sincere, and though no man was more communicative upon points of real use, he never thought of reading lectures upon a subject that can be understood no otherwise than by personal observation: physic he honoured as a profession, but he despised it as a trade. However partial I may be to his memory, his friends acknowledge this to be true, and his enemies will not venture to deny it.

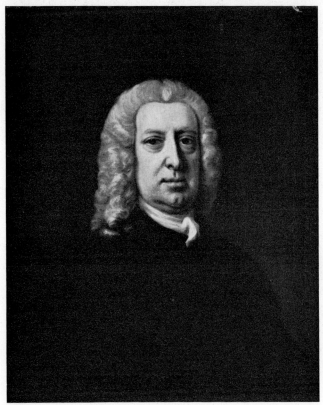

FIG. 13. James Monro, 1680–1752. Physician to Bethlem 1728–1752.

He was succeeded by this son John (1715–1791) (Fig. 14), a man of excellent education—who graduated from Oxford, obtained the Radcliffe Travelling Fellowship, which was then tenable for ten years, and travelled extensively in Europe, permanently returning only in 1751 on his appointment as joint Physician, with his father, to Bethlem. He became full Physician the following year when his father died, in

D

1753 became a Fellow of the College of Physicians—was Censor on seven occasions, and delivered the Harveian Oration in 1757. Battie's remarks stung him into his only other publication, his *Remarks on Dr. Battie's Treatise on Madness*, published in 1758. He took as his motto

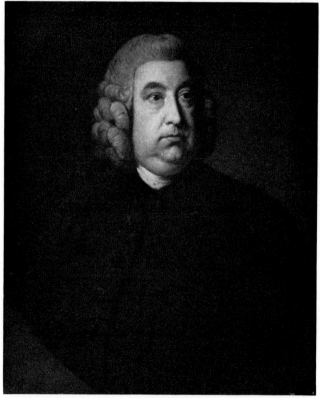

Fig. 14.   John Monro, 1715–1791. Physician to Bethlem 1752–1791.

for the book a quotation from Horace O *major, tandem parcas, insane, minori,* and thenceforth, we are told, Battie was known as Major Battie. Monro wrote,

> Madness is a distemper of such a nature, that very little of real use can be said concerning it; the immediate causes will for ever disappoint our search, and the care of that disorder depends on management as much as medicine. My own inclination would never have led me to appear in

print, but it was thought necessary for me, in my situation, to say something in answer to the undeserved censures which Dr. Battie has thrown
upon my predecessors.

The whole tone of the book follows this pattern—madness is too
difficult to understand, too unpleasant to go deeply into, and after all,
purging, bleeding and vomiting are the most efficacious treatments.
Apart from its minor personal relevance to Battie's career, the book
must surely be one of the poorest pieces of work ever written by a
psychiatrist. It is said that Battie was covered with ridicule as a result
of Monro's replies; reading it today it seems a singularly ineffective
piece of work.

Monro had acquired a taste for the arts on his travels abroad, and
assisted Strutt in the preparation of the latter's *History of Engravers*.
This interest in art was to have an important effect, for it was transmitted to his son Thomas, who became a patron of many of the
English water-colour painters of the late eighteenth and early nineteenth centuries.

Certainly, as an example of a professional psychiatrist, John Monro
was not a shining example to the rest of the medical profession. Not
so was William Battie (1704–1776), a man of great gifts, which were
unfortunately offset by his eccentricity. He was a scholar, became
President of the Royal College of Physicians, was one of the founders
of St. Luke's and its first Physician, and the first to give lectures and
clinical instruction exclusively on mental disorder. He occupies an
important but as yet insufficiently acknowledged position in the history
of British psychiatry.

Born at Modbury, in Devon, his father the Rev. Edward Battie
died when his son was only 10, leaving his widow in straitened circumstances. She managed, however, to send her son to Eton, where he was
a King's Scholar, and from there he entered King's College, Cambridge, in 1722. He obtained his B.A. in 1726 and his M.A. in 1730.
Obtaining a licence to practise medicine, he set up in Cambridge,
where he gave lectures in anatomy. He published an edition of Aris-
totle's *Rhetoric* in 1728 and in 1729 one of Isocrates' 'Orations'—they
cannot have been very popular, for the latter book was ridiculed in
some verses in the *Grub Street Journal* in 1730. About this time he moved
to Uxbridge, where he quickly established himself in practice, so much
so that he decided to move to London. He took his M.D. in 1737,
became an F.R.C.P. in 1738 and occupied successive posts in the

College until in 1764 he was elected President, one of the very few psychiatrists ever to hold that office. He was Harveian Orator in 1746, and Lumleian Lecturer for five years (1749–1754). These lectures were published in 24 separate parts between 1751 and 1757, and a collected edition was issued under the title *De Principiis Animalibus.* A year later his *Treatise on Madness* appeared (1758), and in 1760 his *Aphorismi de Cognoscendis et Curandis Morbis.*

Battie's *A Treatise on Madness* was published in 1758, and was unusual in that it is the first text on insanity which seems to have been written with an eye to the needs of students. He wrote in his "Advertisement"—

> Among the many good reasons offered to the Publick, for establishing another Hospital for the reception of Lunatics, one, and that not the least considerable, was *the introducing more Gentlemen of the Faculty to the Study and Practice of one of the most important branches of Physic.*

Very soon the Governors of St. Luke's, by unanimous votes, "signified their inclination of admitting young Physicians well recommended to visit with me in the Hospital, and freely to observe the treatment of the patients there confined". The experiment succeeded and Battie thus became the first psychiatrist in England, if not elsewhere, to carry out clinical teaching in mental diseases. His book represents a condensation of some of his ideas on the subject presented in a somewhat controversial manner. At the outset he launched an attack on the Monros—though not by name. Madness is as little understood as any disorder that afflicts mankind—

> our defect of knowledge in this matter is, I am afraid, in a great measure owing to a defect of proper communication; and the difficulties attending the care of lunaticks have been at least perpetuated by their being entrusted to Empiricks, or at best to a few select Physicians, most of whom have thought it advisable to keep the Cases as well as the Patients to themselves.

Another difficulty was that madness had not been adequately defined. Philosophy had clouded the issue so that several disorders, really independent of madness, and of one another, were often blended together in "our bewildered imagination". Battie decided that it was best to be content with a "vulgar apprehension of things", and put forward delusion or false perception as the hallmark of insanity. It followed that "natural sensation" must therefore be a primary study—first the nerves which carry sensation, and then the brain. He demolished the theory of a secretion of nervous fluid passing from the brain along the nerves, and exciting either by undulation or retrograde motion all those impulses it receives from external objects. The "molecular" theory of sensation likewise had to go. But as is so often the case with the iconoclast, Battie had really very little to put forward in exchange except that the real cause of natural sensation is a pressure of the medullary substance contained in the nervous filaments.

Battie had some interesting things to say on the relationship between sensation and feeling. Sensation, he maintained, is always accompanied by some degree of pleasure or uneasiness, the latter being of particular value in the preservation of life and health. Motor activity too, as it so often immediately follows sensation, must be regarded as a method whereby the body discharges emotion. There are two types of disordered sensation—anxiety and insensibility, both are related to insanity inasmuch as madness is often preceded by anxiety, and terminates in insensibility.

> New Sensation, which in its most natural and perfect state is sooner or later attended with some degree of uneasiness, may with very little addition be heightened into Anxiety either by the too great or too long continued force of external objects, or by the ill-conditioned state of the nerve itself, whereby it is rendered liable to be too much affected with the usual action of such external objects.

Anxiety is often associated with muscular spasm—presumably what we now call tension—or by its complete opposite—insensibility.

After discussing these different points, Battie comes to the causes of madness—which in his view must have its origin in a disorder of the nervous system. There are two types of madness—original, due to internal causes, and consequential, due to external disorders, such as sun stroke, meningitis, or head injury. The stomach, intestines and uterus, moreover, are frequently the real seats of madness

> occasioned by the contents of these viscera being stopt in such a manner as to compress the many nervous filaments, which here communicate with one another by the mesenteric ganglia, and which enrich the contents of the abdomen with a more exquisite sensation. Thus the glutton who goes to bed upon a full stomach is hagridden in his sleep—thus "Men prove with child as powerful fancy works".

Disturbed haemodynamics will also give rise to insanity—for instance joy, anger, and similar emotions constrict the muscles of the head and

neck, and so force back the blood coming down the jugular veins into
the minutest vessels of the brain. The resulting congestion often produces insanity. Battie gives "spasm" a very important place in the
genesis of madness—on account both of the obstructions to the brain
and nerves and of the secondary effect on the blood vessels.

As for the cure of madness—there is no cure for original madness—
the chief function of the physician being the "management"—the
general care of the patient. Confinement away from friends or familiars
is essential for this purpose, every unruly appetite must be checked, and
a quiet, well-ordered life must be pursued. Other than this, there is
little to be done. But with consequential madness, which we should
today call reactive insanity, relief of pressure is the first desideratum,
and as a result therapy centres around depletion, revulsion, removal
and expulsion, in other words purging, vomiting and bleeding. One
of Battie's etiological hobby-horses seems to have been sun-stroke, and
he seriously considers whether "insolation" might not be possible.
Regretfully he decides against this and recommends the wearing of a
cap of thick paper. The remainder of his book consists of a list of the
various drugs commonly used in the treatment of insanity.

As a simplification of existing theories the book must have served
its purpose; moreover, it has the virtue of a comparative brevity.
Battie was widely read and the lack of classical quotations must have
been deliberate in order to produce a simple text.

Of Battie's other works, the Aphorisms are written in Latin and deal
with a host of conditions, from diabetes to diseases of children. There
are extensive references to the works of other physicians, particularly
those of Hoffmann, Stahl and Boerhaave, and the Aphorisms themselves are clearly written and show a considerable acquaintance with
the practice of medicine. The Lumleian Lectures are of quite another
type—a lengthy physiological and pathological theorizing on the
principles of animal life much according to Hoffmann, although no
references are given.

In these publications, Battie foreshadowed the later cast of eighteenth
and early nineteenth-century psychiatrist—a man of enquiring mind,
concerned with the principles as well as the practice of medicine, and
very literate. In the affairs of life he was equally active. In 1763 he
appeared before the Committee appointed by the House of Commons
to enquire into the state of private madhouses. So did Dr. John Monro.
Battie's evidence is printed in the eleven-page report.

Your Committee being desirous of obtaining every Degree of Assistance and Information which might enable them more perfectly to obey the Orders of the House; they desired the attendance of Doctor Battie, and Doctor Monro, two very eminent Physicians distinguished by their Knowledge and their Practice in Cases of Lunacy.

Dr. Battie gave it as his Opinion to your Committee, that the Private Mad-Houses require some better Regulations; that he hath long been of this Opinion; that the Admission of Persons brought as Lunatics is too loose and too much at large, depending upon Persons not competent Judges; and that frequent Visitation is necessary for the Inspection of the Lodging, Diet, Cleanliness, and Treatment.

Being asked, If he ever met with Persons of sane Mind, in Confinement for Lunacy?

He said, it frequently happened. He related the Case of a Woman perfectly in her Senses brought as a Lunatic by her husband to a House under the Doctor's Direction, whose Husband, upon Doctor Battie insisting he should take home his Wife, and expressing his Surprise at his Conduct, justified himself by frankly saying, He understood the House to be a Sort of Bridewell, or Place of Correction?

Monro agreed with Battie and also instanced cases of wrongful detention, but in spite of the recommendations of the Committee that Legislation should be enacted, nothing was done, for the House of Lords rejected a Bill for the Regulation of Private Madhouses in 1773.

Battie also played a prominent part in the dispute between Dr. Schomberg and the College of Physicians which involved expensive litigation for the College. He was attacked for his part in this affair (a lengthy disciplinary argument between the College and Dr. Schomberg) by Moses Mendez in a poem entitled the "Battiad" (1751):

> First Battas came, deep read in wordly art
> Whose tongue ne'er knew the secrets of his heart
> In mischief mighty, though but mean of size,
> And, like the Tempter, even in disguise.
> See him, with aspect grave, and gentle tread
> By slow degrees approach the sickly bed.
> Then at his club, behold him altered soon
> The solemn doctor turns a low buffoon.
> And he who lately in a learned peak
> Poach'd every lexicon, and publish'd Greek,
> Still madly emulous of vulgar praise
> From Punch's forehead wrings the dirty bays.

The "low buffoon" probably refers to how he is said to have once saved a young man's life.

> He was sent to a gentleman, then only 14 or 15 (who was living in 1782) who was in extreme misery from a swelling of his throat; when the doctor understood what the complaint was, he opened the curtain, turned his wig, and acted Punch with so much humour and success that the lad (thrown into convulsions almost from laughing) was so agitated as to occasion the tumour to break, and a complete cure was the instantaneous consequence (*Nichols Literary Anecdotes*).

His eccentricity was such that

> He affected in the country to be his own daily labourer, and to dress like one. One of Dr. Battie's whims was building. At Marlow he erected a very faulty house of which he forgot the staircase. At high flood the offices below were constantly under water. Another scheme was to have barges drawn up the river by horses, not men. This was unpopular with both rich and poor at the time, and the doctor was very neatly hoisted into the Thames. He always carried pocket pistols about with him after this.

He died worth £100,000, if Walpole is to be believed, having a large town-house and an elegant villa at Twickenham.

After Battie there was an interim period during which the physician still held the field. In 1782, however, Thomas Arnold published the first volume of his *Observations on the Nature, Kinds, Causes, and Prevention of Insanity, Lunacy, or Madness*, a book which heralded a series of publications written by physicians who dealt exclusively with mental disorder. Arnold was born in Leicester in 1742, was educated at Edinburgh, where he was a member of the Royal Medical Society, took an Edinburgh M.D. and became a Fellow of the Royal College of Physicians (Fig. 15). Returning to Leicester, he soon became successful in practice and opened a private house for lunatics. His first book was a considerable advance on anything published to date, and repays a full study.

The growth of natural science toward the close of the seventeenth century had raised hopes that medicine would follow suit and turn from theorizing to observation and experiment. In fact, eighteenth-century medicine was bedevilled by the rankest theorizing—Hoffmann, Stahl, Brown and a host of lesser lights gave full rein to their imagination. The more pragmatic Scottish physicians, so well typified by Cullen, had come to realize the dangers of all this, and to recognize

that one essential basis for a natural science was some mode of classification. Arnold had been educated in Edinburgh under Cullen himself,
so that it was natural for his thoughts to turn largely on this matter of
nosology, for Cullen had admitted that his own experience of mental

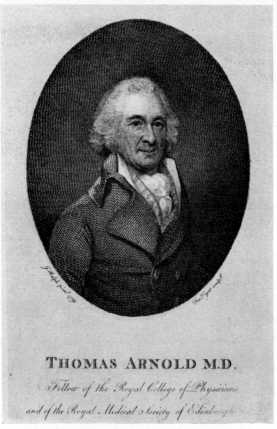

THOMAS ARNOLD M.D.

Fellow of the Royal College of Physicians
and of the Royal Medical Society of Edinburgh

FIG. 15.   Thomas Arnold, M.D., 1742–1816.

disorder was comparatively slight, and that his nosography of the
"vesaniae" left much to be desired. Arnold therefore devoted the whole
of his first volume to the "Definition and Arrangement" of mental
disorder. He writes,

> This part of the work I have endeavoured to execute according to the
> ideas of Sydenham, whose recommendation it was "that every disease

should be reduced to certain, and determinate species, with the same care,
and accuracy, with which we see botanists define, and arrange, the species
of vegetables"—we are indebted for the valuable performances in this way
of Sauvages, Linnaeus, Vogel and Cullen, writers of the first character in
the medical world, who have taken an extensive range through the whole
field of diseases; and whose successful labours in this, and other branches
of medicine, in chemistry, and in natural history, will carry down their
names with honour to the latest posterity.

Arnold divided insanity into Ideal and Notional, but before further
considering them, he could not resist a short chapter on a subject which
recurs time and again in the eighteenth-century literature—the relative
frequency of insanity in England as compared with other countries,
more particularly with France. Sauvages had described a separate
species of insanity, the "Melancholia Anglica", a Gallic taunt which
always provoked the Englishman, and Arnold was no exception. He
hotly replied that the Popish religion, with its confessional and super-
stition, was indeed less likely to give rise to religious melancholy than
Protestantism. In France, too, love is an art, an amusement and not a
tender passion, so that love, which has made more madmen in every
other nation and age than any other emotion, is not so operative a
factor in the French. Nor can many suffer in France from what is a
frequent cause of insanity, the pursuit of riches; the French are, after
all, a nation of slaves, their noblemen petty courtiers. Most important
of all is the national temperament, which shields the French from
attacks of melancholy—

> a lightness of heart, that vivacity and volatility of temper, which will
> seldom suffer them to fix their attention too long, or their affections too
> violently, and seriously, upon any particular object.

After this devastating broadside, Arnold points out, not without
some degree of pride one feels, how common insanity is in Britain,
arising as a result of the wealth and luxury which was almost universal
throughout the land. He shared this view with many laymen; Boswell,
for instance, describes a French novel which began, "In the gloomy
month of November, when the people of England begin to hang and
drown themselves," and continues.

> In Madam Pompadour's letters Britain is called the Gloomy Isles, and
> Groslet, a late traveller, represents our people as under the perpetual
> influence of melancholy. He has no doubt exaggerated considerably; but

his observations at least prove that the Hypochondria is still one of our striking characteristicks. Happy would it be, if there were not so many whose sad experience must bear witness that such is the case in reality, no less than in appearance.

Hypochondria however, is not peculiar to Britain. We may trace it in all countries in one shape or other. Even a French poet though living in a country blessed with the purest air, and whose inhabitants cultivate perpetual gayetym confesses a diseased mind to be universal.

> Tous les hommes sont fous et malgré tous leur soins,
> Ne différent entre Eux que du plus ou du moins.—Boileau.

> All men are mad: disguise it as they please,
> You'll find they differ only in degrees.

After this show of British pride, the mainstream of the work goes forward without further interruption—first the nosology, then the pathology, the etiology, and finally the rules for the prevention of insanity. He starts by reviewing the meanings of the words mania, melancholia and delirium, his sources ranging from Hippocrates, Galen and Areteus the Cappadocian, to Boerhaave and Riverius. No general agreement as to meaning could be discovered, so that after considering these disorders in the light of Locke's philosophy and Hartley's comments, Arnold decided to divide insanity into two types —Ideal and Notional. Under Ideal insanity are grouped what are primarily disorders of perception; Notional insanity consists largely of the delusional disorders. In spite of a wealth of illustrative quotation from Greek, Latin, French, Dutch and German sources (which only tends to cloud the issue), this division has a merit of its own, for under the two different headings Arnold built up various clinical syndromes, largely depending on the form assumed by the hallucinations or delusions and the accompanying affect. His full table is illustrated below. It can be seen that this is chiefly a classification based on symptoms—a derivative of Cullen's teachings. The concept of personality influencing the form of the mental disorder, although age old, had little significance for Arnold, nor indeed, with the methods of clinical study available during the eighteenth century, was much more to be expected of him. He does, however, end the book by briefly considering the interrelations of these different species.

> I have already mentioned that all these species of Insanity may be variously combined, and frequently interchange, one with another. It may be

proper farther to remark, that the same patient sometimes goes through several kinds of insanity—which may be reckoned in such cases, as so many degrees, or stages—during the course of the same illness. Of these combinations, and changes, there is almost an endless variety. One remarkable, and not uncommon transition of Insanity, is from great dejection, and distress, to ease and cheerfulness, and sometimes, to an uncommon flow of spirits. But most frequently it retains its character of liveliness, or anxiety, elevation, or depression. In general, all kinds of Insanity, so far as they arise from mental constitution, and are not the sudden effect of any accidental bodily disease, may be considered as proceeding from two different, and opposite constitutional sources—in one of which the characteristic temperament of mind may properly enough be called Fanciful—and in the other, Thoughtful. The first degree of Insanity in the former case may be called flighty; and the first in the latter melancholy. The following scheme will show the natural progression of these constitutional temperaments of mind from their sound state, if they can ever strictly be said to be in a sound state, to the height of disorder, and Insanity; and from thence again to their ordinary state of sanity.

$$1.\ \text{Fanciful—flighty—} \begin{cases} \text{—maniacal—} \\ \text{—phrenitic—} \\ \text{—maniacal—} \end{cases} \text{flighty—fanciful}$$

$$2.\ \text{Thoughtful—melancholy} \begin{cases} \text{—maniacal—} \\ \text{—phrenitic—} \\ \text{—maniacal—} \end{cases} \text{melancholy—thoughtful}$$

A TABLE OF THE SPECIES OF INSANITY

One Genus—   Insanity.
Two Divisions—   **IDEAL**—and—**NOTIONAL.**

I. **IDEAL INSANITY:**
   Insanity—
                            1. Phrenitic
                            2. Incoherent
                            3. Maniacal
                            4. Sensitive

II. **NOTIONAL INSANITY**
    Insanity—
                            5. Delusive
                            6. Fanciful
                            7. Whimsical
                            8. Impulsive
                            9. Scheming
                            10. Vain or Self-important
                            11. Hypochondriacal
                            12. Pathetic
                            13. Appetitive

The second volume appeared four years later in 1786, its predecessor having been kindly received. Arnold continued with a description of the post-mortem findings in cases of insanity, which unfortunately consists only of a review of the literature, adequately done, but leading to no formulation. The appearances of the various organs in cases of madness were in fact so heterogeneous as to be impossible to codify, and it was not until Haslam published his observations in 1798 that some simplifications could be made.

The causes of insanity are codified under the headings Remote and Proximate; of the remote causes, there are two main subdivisions, the bodily and the mental. There is a remarkably full, and compared with those writings we have previously considered, a remarkably scientific and reasonable list of etiological factors. Brain, body and emotions are all concerned in the production of psychiatric disorder—and Arnold gives an excellent account of the mind–body problem. Although extending over seventy pages of text, his views are summarized in the last two sentences of this section. "In a word, the passions are the principal instruments of the mind's agency on the body. Their effects are various, sudden, and on many occasions, violent." Although diseases of all kinds, both neurological and systemic, are often accompanied by mental illness, none the less Arnold emphasizes the major role played by disturbed emotion. Zilboorg in his history constantly deprecates a "psychiatry without psychology", which he considers that this period was notable for—but certainly Arnold had an excellent conception of the interplay of emotions and the dynamics of mental disorder.

The Prevention of Insanity occupies only 35 of a text of 541 pages, and breaks no new ground. Temperance, exercise, control of the passions and belief in God are held up as the criteria by which we should live and thereby avoid insanity. The book ends with a peroration on the love of God. A somewhat florid and copious style makes the book hard going, but considering the taste of the age, Arnold's work is scholarly and restrained. In addition, by giving a bibliography with precise references, Arnold was again far superior to those authors whose works we have so far considered. His book represents a real advance, and although little more than a nosography, marks the beginning of a new phase in the development of psychiatry, the rise of the professional psychiatrist. Arnold was to write two more books before his death in 1816. *A Case of Hydrophobia successfully Treated* was published in 1793, and *Observations on the Management of the Insane* in 1809. A second edition of the *Observations* appeared in 1806, with a frontispiece portrait of Arnold. In a new preface he recounts how well the first edition had been received, both in England and on the Continent. It had been translated into German by Ackerman, and reviewed with "unreserved approbation" in the *Leipsic Review*. The book itself was substantially unchanged, although in its single binding it now presents a somewhat formidable tome to the reader.

SOME MINOR AUTHORS

There is a miscellaneous group of writers about whom—apart from William Pargeter—I have been able to collect very little information. William Perfect of West Malling enjoyed a contemporary popularity which today is difficult to understand, for his writings are no more than simple case reports (Fig. 16). He was a prolific author, and to the best of my knowledge wrote the following books: *Methods of Cure in Some Particular Cases of Insanity*, 1778; *Cases of Insanity, the Epilepsy, Hypochondriacal Affection, Hysteric Passion, and Nervous Disorders Successfully Treated*, 1781; *An Address to the Public on Insanity*, 1784; *Select Cases in the Different Species of Insanity, Lunacy, or Madness, with the Modes of Practice as Adopted in the Treatment of Each*, 1787; and *A Remarkable Case of Madness, with the Diet and Medicines used in the Cure*, 1791. A German edition of his *Select Cases* was published in Leipzig in 1789, and later in Hanover in 1804. *A Remarkable Case* was also printed in Leipzig in 1794. The case reports are of some little therapeutic interest, illustrating the different methods of treatment employed in what seems to have been a reasonably well-run private house. In addition, Perfect was a poet and wrote "An Elegy on a Storm which happened in West Kent, on the 19th of August 1763", together with a two-volume work *The Laurel Wreath* published in 1766.

William Pargeter (1760–1810) published only one book on psychiatry, but it is of greater interest than Perfect's many books. Pargeter was, like Francis Willis, both clergyman and doctor. He studied at Bart's, took his M.D. at Aberdeen in 1786, and in 1795 joined the Royal Navy as a Chaplain. He served for seven years, took part in the Battle of the Nile aboard H.M.S. *Alexander*, and became Chaplain to the garrison of Malta. He retired from the sea and from medicine in 1802, and passed the remaining years of his life in Oxfordshire. His publications are three in number—*Observations on Maniacal Disorders* was published at Reading in 1792, and in Leipzig a year later; *Formulae Medicamentorum Selectae* was a 58-page pamphlet published in

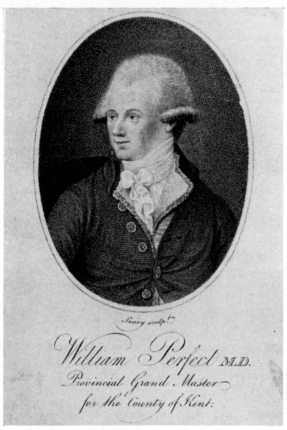

FIG. 16.   William Perfect, M.D., 1740–?

London in 1795; his last publication was "A Sermon, preached in the Protestant Chapel in La Valetta, in the Isle of Malta, on Sunday succeeding the Funeral of Sir Ralph Abercromby, K.B. Commander-in-Chief of his Britannic Majesty's Forces in the Mediterranean, etc. 1801".

Pargeter's rather unusual career, and the fact that he practised little, suggests that he himself had been the subject of a psychiatric illness, for his only work in the field is remarkably astute. He adopted, he tells us, Cullen's nomenclature.

> In doing this, I feel no hesitation; because he not only comes nearer to a right theory of this disorder than any former writer, but I do not think it possible for human understanding to advance any other. Of the authors whose sentiments I have adopted, some I have mentioned, and others I could not call to my recollection. Should the ensuing observations be favourably received, I may probably at some future time, pursue the subject to a greater extent; but if not, I shall never again obtrude myself on the notice of the public.

Pargeter believed that the real cause of madness was a complete mystery—there was, however, some evidence that "the nervous fluid" in cases of insanity has assumed a "certain morbid or irritating principle" and that this is the primary cause of insanity

> with all the unaccountable phenomena which attend it; but what the specific nature of that morbid quality or principle is, it is impossible to conceive, and it will, no doubt, for ever remain a secret.
>
>   —Nec Meus audet
>   Rem tentare pudor, quam vires ferre recusent.
>
> Here our researches must stop, and we must declare, that wonderful are the works of the Lord, and his ways past finding out.

Nevertheless, madness may result from sudden emotion, infections, luxury, the immoderate use of tea, the turning of day into night and night into day, so that "at Length we sink into a fashionable death, the natural consequence of a fashionable life. It is seriously to be remarked, that in this age it is easier to meet with a mad, than a healthy woman of fashion." Fanaticism, too, is a very common cause of madness. Most of the maniacal cases that ever came under his observation proceeded from religious enthusiasm;

> and I have heard it remarked by an eminent physician, that almost all the insane patients, which occurred to him at one of the largest hospitals in the metropolis, had been deprived of their reason, by such strange infatuation. The doctrines of the Methodists have a greater tendency than those of any other sect, to produce the most deplorable effects on the human understanding. The brain is perplexed in the mazes of mystery, and the imagination overpowered by the tremendous description of future torments.

He describes how he visited a woman and found her sitting up in the bed, wrapped about the head, neck and shoulders with cloaks and flannels.

She received me with a smiling countenance, and when I enquired into her complaints, she laughed, and enumerated a great variety of symptoms; but I could not really discover that she had any bodily indisposition, except what was occasioned by lying in bed. In a chair at the bed-side, were, *Wesley's Journal*, *Watt's Hymns*, the *Pilgrim's Progress*, and the *Fiery Furnace of Affliction*. I prescribed according to the usual form, but could do her no good; and I was afterwards informed, that she became so mad as to require confinement. I was told by her husband, that there was not the least predisposition to Insanity before this attack, and it appeared that a Methodist preacher, who had much infested the parish, was frequently in her company, and they were perpetually conversing on religious topics.

I attended a young woman with a peripneumony, occasioned by some tea, or bread and butter passing down the trachea in a fit of laughter; as the symptoms were acute and suspicious, I paid more than ordinary attention, visiting her twice, and often three times a day. I hardly ever went into the room, but I saw a man with a book in his hand, who I afterwards learnt was a Methodist. One day when I called, the girl was exclaiming, "Oh sweet Christ! Dear Christ! I do love Christ!" I asked her what she meant, and she told me "She had seen, and had been talking with, her dear Christ." The patient fortunately lost her complaint, and being enabled to return to her former occupation, her mind was gradually weaned from those delusions, which might probably have terminated in confirmed Mania. The advantage which this fanatic took, of the girl's ignorance and indisposition, may very aptly be compared to the conduct of those inhuman wretches, who avail themselves of the confusion at a fire, to plunder the sufferers. The prevalence of Methodism, with its deplorable effects, in the neighbourhood where this girl resided, might be ascribed to an opulent Tanner, who maintained a preacher in the capacity of a domestic chaplain, a sailor in the last war. He was one day haranging on the subject of Hell flames, and took occasion to observe, that he could not give a description by any means adequate to the horrors of that place, although he had been there eleven months; a wag, whom curiosity had led to hear him, called out, "I wish you had staid there another month, and then you would have gained a settlement." Such dreadful infatuation is the more melancholy, as it tends to augment the number of suicides in a nation, which is supposed to be more generally addicted to this crime, than any other people in Europe: indeed, the French have adopted our word suicide into their language, as an Anglicism. Such consequences, however, from this particular cause, must convince all persons of a sound

E

understanding, of the errors of those tenets, which cause, or very greatly conduce to it; since genuine Christianity must very powerfully deter men from this unnatural violence.

This concern with the effects of Methodism was a general pre-occupation of the educated classes. Wesley exercised an enormous influence over the poor, and over the growing populations in the new industrial areas, rootless and living in squalor. His open-air sermons were attended by multitudes, and it is interesting that on that memorable Sunday, 17 June 1739, when he first preached in the open to a London crowd, it was at Moorfields, in full view of Bethlem Hospital. To the wits and caricaturists Wesley was often linked with Bethlem and even serious writers attributed many cases of lunacy to the influence of his preaching. He was forbidden to enter Bethlem, as an extract in his diary for 22 February 1750 shows, "I went to see a young woman in Bedlam; but I had not talked to her long before one gave me to know that none of the preachers were to come here. So we are forbidden to go to Newgate for fear of making them wicked, and to Bedlam for fear of making them mad!" The extraordinary mental atmosphere of his meetings, with their conversions, and emotional outbursts were no doubt provocative of some psychiatric illness, but not to the degree implied by Pargeter. Wesley was familiar with mental illness and in his *Primitive Physic* devotes some attention to the cure of the different disorders. He advocated both psychological and physical methods of treatment—ranging from the cold douche to religious argument. For one reason or another he was antipathetic to "that wretched fellow, Monro," as Wesley's mother called James Monro—probably because the physician had been largely responsible for barring Wesley from preaching in and visiting the sick in Bethlem.

However, to return to Pargeter—his book continues with a description of the symptoms of melancholy, the text being embellished with quotations from Beaumont and Fletcher, Milton, Cowper and Shakespeare. He very clearly describes how melancholy can pass over into mania. Prognosis he considered a most difficult matter, owing to the ignorance concerning these disorders; the "chief reliance in the cure of insanity must be rather on management than a medicine". He placed great reliance on catching the patients' eye and thus subduing them, and as adjuncts to this so-called moral treatment, used bleeding, arteriotomy in the temples, cupping, carthartics, emetics, setons and blisters, sedatives, camphor, opium, musk, hyoscyamus, medicated snuff, cold bathing, warm bathing, pediluvia and manuluvia, friction, and music! How could his patients fail to get well? The government of maniacs is an art only acquired by long experience and by frequent and attentive observation.

> As maniacs are extremely subdolous, the physician's first visit should be by surprise. He must employ every moment of his time by mildness or menaces, as circumstances direct, to gain an ascendancy over them, and to obtain their favour and prepossession. If this opportunity be lost, it will be difficult, if not impossible, to effect it afterwards; and more especially, if he should betray any signs of timidity. He should be well acquainted with the pathology of the disease—should possess great acumen—a discerning and penetrating eye—much humanity and courtesy—an even disposition, and command of temper. He may be obliged at one moment, according to the exigency of the case, to be placid and accommodating in his manner, and the next, angry and absolute.

Moral management, as it was called, was to be the chief preoccupation of psychiatry over the next thirty years, and in due course led to the rise of the non-restraint school. It is worth quoting Pargeter's methods with patients.

CASE I

> When I was a pupil at St. Bartholomew's Hospital, as my attention was much employed on the subject of Insanity, I was requested by one of the sisters of the house, to visit a poor man, an acquaintance of her's, who was disordered in his mind. I went immediately to the house, and found the neighbourhood in an uproar. The maniac was locked in a room, raving and exceedingly turbulent. I took two men with me, and learning that he had no offensive weapons, I planted them at the door, with directions to be silent, and to keep out of sight, unless I should want their assistance. I then suddenly unlocked the door—rushed into the room and caught his eye in an instant. The business was then done—he became peaceable in a moment—trembled with fear, and was as governable as it was possible for a furious madman to be.

CASE II

> A young lady who resided at a village near the metropolis, had been for some weeks on a visit to a friend, at a distance from home. In a few days after her return, her natural spirits and vivacity gradually forsook her; she became pensive—morose—fond of being in her own room and alone—she would take no nourishment, unless to avoid importunities. After I had informed myself particularly respecting the family—occasional visitors in

her late excursion, etc. I was introduced to her room, and found her in a thoughtful posture, her elbow on the table, and resting her cheek upon her hand. She did not, for some time, seem to know that anybody was in the room; at length she looked up, and the moment I caught her eye, for, till then I had been silent, I told her I was perfectly acquainted with the cause of her complaint, and conversed with her on those topics, I thought most suitable to her case, and at last persuaded her to come down to dinner with the rest of the family, and to drink two or three glasses of wine, and to join in the conversation of the table. I recommended an immediate change of residence—gave directions respecting diet—exercise—amusements—reading—conversation—and had soon the pleasing satisfaction to be informed of the lady's perfect recovery.

Of our next author nothing is known. Andrew Harper wrote *A Treatise on the Real Cause and Cure of Insanity*, published in 1789 and dedicated to Lord Southampton. He set out to show "the extreme absurdity of the common opinion, that Insanity is an hereditary Disease", and to describe what is the real cause of insanity. On the way he makes a large number of mis-statements within the short 69 pages of his book; for instance, epilepsy is never attended with insanity, nor does insanity occur with gout, or from the administration of poisons; the proportion of men afflicted with madness is much greater than the number of women; there is very little connection between mania and melancholy. However, in spite of all this Harper is worth noticing on account of his belief in the "intrinsic" nature of mental disorder, that it is a "positive, immediate discord in the intrinsic motions and operations of the mental faculty, exerted above the healthful equilibrium". His conception of "the intrinsic motions" is that they were a series of modulations of high and low frequency and tone, susceptible to the emotions and particularly to mental causes. In other respects Harper was no more than a pamphleteer compared with the contemporary writers we have reviewed—his book contains no references, and it is difficult to imagine the type of reader for whom it was written.

THE INSANITY OF KING GEORGE III

A psychiatric history of this century would be incomplete without mention of George III's recurrent illnesses. The King had suffered his first attack of madness at the age of 27, five years after his accession to the throne. In this attack, which only lasted a few weeks, he was blooded seven times and three times blistered. A similar mild attack occurred in 1765, but in 1788, when he was 50, a more serious episode began. Thomas Monro was called in, but the care of the patient was

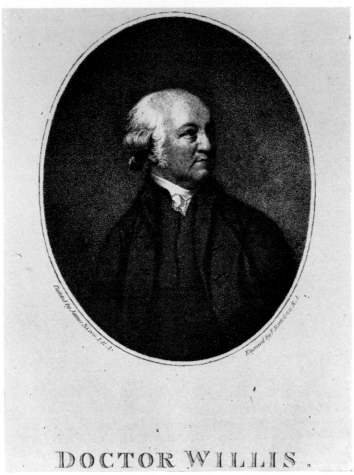

DOCTOR WILLIS.

Fig. 17.   The Rev. Francis Willis, M.D., 1717–1807.

handed over to the Reverend Dr. Willis (Fig. 17). Francis Willis (1717–1807) had for long treated insanity along novel lines in the Lincolnshire village of Gretford, near Stamford, and was a most remarkable character. In obedience to his father he had taken Holy

Orders, but even as an undergraduate had such strong leanings to medicine that he studied and attended the lectures of Nathan Alcock, with whom he had formed a life-long friendship. He married in 1749, settled at Dunston in Lincolnshire, and practised without a licence until 1759, when Oxford conferred on him the M.B. and M.D. In 1769 he was appointed physician to a hospital in Lincoln which he had taken an active part in establishing, and for six years attended here regularly twice weekly, although the hospital was ten miles from his home. His success in the treatment of some cases of mental disorder was particularly striking and soon patients were brought to him from afar. To accommodate them he moved to Gretford. His system relied upon the inculcation of a wholesome sense of fear in a setting of individual attention. Two patients shared a cottage, with a keeper for each. As recovery progressed, long walks and work in the fields were encouraged. A contemporary account described how the village of

> Gretford and its vicinity at that time exhibited one of the most peculiar and singular sights I ever witnessed. As the unprepared traveller approached the town, he was astonished to find almost all the surrounding plowmen, gardeners, threshers, thatchers, and other labourers, attired in black coats, white waistcoats, black silk breeches and stockings, and the head of each *bien poudré, pisé et arrangé.* These were the Doctor's patients: and dress, neatness of person and exercise being the principal features of his admirable system, health and cheerfulness conjoined toward the recovery of every person attached to that most valuable asylum. The Doctor kept an excellent table, and the day I dined with him I found a numerous company. Amongst others of his patients, in a state of convalescence, present on this occasion, there were a Mrs. B., a lady of large fortune, who had lately recovered under the Doctor's care, but declined returning into the world from the dread of a relapse; and a young clergyman, who occasionally read service and preached for the doctor. Nothing occurred out of the Common way till soon after the cloth was removed, when I saw the Doctor frown at a patient, who immediately hastened from the room, taking with him my tail, which he had slyly cut off.

Willis was called in to see the King in December 1788, despite considerable opposition from his regular physicians, for Willis was "considered by some not much better than a mountebank, and not far different from some of those that are confined to his house". George III was not an easy patient, being stubborn and obstinate, incapable of abstract speculation, and unable to tolerate opinions other than his own.

He hated his eldest son, and modelled his whole life on the precept "Fear God and Honour the King". The King was attended at first by Sir George Baker and Dr. Warren, and they were joined by Sir Lucas Pepys, Drs. Reynolds, Gisborne and Addington, of whom the latter alone had some special knowledge of insanity. Warren was the leader of the medical profession in London, and a prominent Whig—the friend of Burke, Fox and Sheridan. The attack did not yield and the Queen and Ministers determined to call in Dr. Willis. He joined the corps of physicians and took up residence on 6 December 1788.

Willis was to have charge of all the domestic arrangements and of the "moral management" of the King. The medical treatment was arranged at the opening consultation and Willis agreed to undertake no decisive measures, either medical or moral, without discussion and general agreement. His son John soon joined him, and two surgeons and two apothecaries were retained. The King asked Willis, when he entered the room, if he, who was a clergyman, was not ashamed of himself for exercising such a profession. "Sir," said Willis, "our Saviour himself went about healing the sick." "Yes," answered the King, "but he had not £700 a year for it." Willis was confident from the first that the King would recover, especially if the "management" were left in his hands. He thought that the attack was produced by weighty business, severe exercise, too great abstemiousness and little rest, and insisted that the moral management of the King required strict seclusion from his family and Ministers, and as far as possible from all other company. Mechanical restraint was frequently used, but it was of a new type "more firm, but not so teasing to the patient". While walking through the palace with an equerry during his convalescence the King saw a strait-jacket lying in a chair. The equerry looked away, but the King said, "You need not be afraid to look at it. Perhaps it is the best friend I ever had in my life." Medical treatment consisted chiefly of "bark and saline" medicines. Blisters were applied to the King's legs but gave rise to considerable irritation and restlessness, and were discontinued.

Willis allowed his patient considerable latitude and gave the King a razor and penknife, for which he was subjected to a hostile cross-examination by a Committee of the House of Commons. Burke and Sheridan were members of this committee and for once they found an adversary who was more than a match for them. Burke asked Willis

what he would have done if the King had suddenly become violent
whilst these instruments were in his hand. Having placed the candles
between them, Willis replied, "There Sir, by the EYE. I should have
looked at him thus Sir—thus!" Whereupon Burke instantly averted
his head and made no reply.

Willis claimed that as a result of taking the medicine he prescribed
"His Majesty had certainly been gradually better from the first six
hours of his taking it". Sheridan stated

> that when he heard Willis assert this and that his physic could in one day
> overcome the effects of seven and twenty years hard exercise, seven and
> twenty years study, and seven and twenty years abstinence, it was im-
> possible for him to keep the gravity fit for the subject. Such assertions put
> him in mind of those nostrums that cure this and that, and also disappoint-
> ments in love and long sea voyages.

Whatever the merits of the system, after five months of the Reverend
Dr. Willis, the King was able to write a sensible letter to Pitt, and soon
to resume the business of State. Willis was rewarded with a pension
of £1,500 per annum for 21 years, surely one of the biggest fees in the
history of medicine. During the King's illness, however, Willis's
character, conduct and practices were subjected to a very searching
scrutiny. His enemies calumnated him, but others found him "the
very image of simplicity, quite a good, plain, old-fashioned country
parson" (Hannah More), or "a man of 10,000, open, honest, dauntless,
lighthearted, innocent and high-minded" (Mde. D'Arblay).

After the King's recovery Willis built a large house at Shillingthorpe, near Gretford, and left the conduct of his practice to two
of his five sons—John and Robert Darling Willis. However, he
was called in to one more Royal Personage, the Queen of Portugal,
and although he pronounced her incurable, he received a fee of
£20,000 for the consultation. He died in 1807 and was buried at
Shillingthorpe.

George III continued in health until 1801, when he broke down
again. On this occasion he was also treated by Willis, but from then
on resolutely refused to see the parson psychiatrist, and Dr. Simmons
of St. Luke's was made responsible for his case. In 1810 the King's
reason became permanently impaired, and for ten years until his death
he was confined to Windsor Castle. His long illness, and the public
knowledge that he was put in a strait-jacket, knocked down and

otherwise severely treated, did much to focus the attention of the public on the care of the mentally sick—and may possibly have stimulated legislation for their protection.

Two of the King's physicians deserve further mention as professional psychiatrists. Thomas Monro (1759–1833) was the third member of the family to be physician to Bethlem. He filled many offices in the College of Physicians, gave the Harveian Oration in 1799, and succeeded his father at Bethlem in 1792. He held the post until 1816, when it passed to his son Edward Thomas Monro. He was chiefly interested in art, being one of the best known connoisseurs of the day, as well as an amateur painter. His house at No. 8 Adelphi Terrace was full of paintings by Gainsborough, Cozens and others, and to it he invited struggling young artists. Here, for their supper and a payment of two shillings or half-a-crown an evening such men as Girtin, Varly and Peter de Wint painted for the doctor, who encouraged them, and cared for them when they fell ill. J. M. W. Turner was a particular friend, and many fine examples of his work were included in Monro's collection. He contributed little to psychiatry and together with Haslam was dismissed from his post at Bethlem in 1816.

Samuel Foart Simmons (1750–1813), although a prolific writer, and physician to St. Luke's, likewise contributed little to psychiatry. He was editor of the *London Medical Journal* from 1781 until 1800.

Lastly comes an unknown, Robert Jones, M.D., who dedicated his book to George III. It was entitled *An Inquiry into the Nature, Causes and Termination of Nervous Fevers*; "together with observations tending to illustrate the Method of Restoring His Majesty to Health, and of Preventing Relapses of His Disease". Jones was a follower of John Brown, the founder of Brunonism, and so opposed to bloodletting and purging, for "all nervous diseases, and fevers in particular, arise more frequently from domestic anxieties, and passions of the mind, such as grief, disappointment, and despair, than from any other cause whatsoever". Jones, of course, considered that all the King's physicians, except Willis, were wrong. If they had proceeded on Brunonian lines, then the King's recovery would have been expedited. Jones tells us of his visit to the "Bissêtre" in 1785 where

> I could not forbear exhibiting my sensibilities, and my feelings, at seeing such a number of unfortunate persons chained down to their solitary abodes, without any other cause, from what I could learn, than the

peculiarity of their conduct, or eccentricity of their behaviour. In the course of my work, and observations, I came to the cell of an Englishman, who had been a captain of a trading vessel from Dover, and who had been captured by a French Privateer in the war before last. I had two English ladies, a French lady and a French gentleman in my company; and as soon as he found that there were English in company, he spoke his mind very freely to us, and told us his story with the most perfect distinctness. His mind was perfectly collected, and he was much disposed to express the fervancy of it during the time we were in conversation with him; but the police of the place rendered it necessary that we should saunter on to another abode of misery, and quit the mansion of this son of misfortune. The pleasure of communicating his sorrowful tale to his country women and myself being thus abruptly interrupted, must unquestionably have affected the feelings of the despairing man: and we could hear him, upon our departure, break out into all the wild language of fury and despair.

This, as well as many other cases which I could place before my reader, during my stay at this place, is a proof that moral causes have as great, if not a greater influence, in creating and perpetuating of nervous diseases of all kinds, than physical causes; and of that disease, called mania, in particular.

The method of restoring the King to his accustomed mental and bodily vigour, is, in my humble opinion, obvious. He ought to be indulged in every rational propensity which is agreeable to his mind. His illustrious consort and family ought to have access to him at all times. He should never be contradicted, nor thwarted in anything that he can request, either in food or drink, unless he calls for vegetable food, and what are called diluting liquors. He should now indulge in animal food, and a proper quantity of wine. Music, provided it is not too loud, will be of great service in the re-establishment of his health. He should refrain from all kind of study and business, unless it is of an agreeable nature. He should avoid going out into the air, until the complaint leaves him entirely, otherwise the smallest chilliness in the air will convey it into the head. His body ought therefore to be kept very warm with flannel cloaths. Soups are very proper. The soups he takes ought to be made very rich of animal food, but much condiment is not necessary in these preparations. His requests ought to be implicitly observed.

Jones' small book of 51 pages is one of the most interesting contemporary accounts of the King's treatment, and shows that he must have had some experience in the treatment of psychiatric illness. Whether he practised as a physician with a particular interest in insanity or in a more specialized role I have been unable to discover.

THERAPY DURING THE EIGHTEENTH CENTURY

A true empiricism is exceedingly rare in the history of medicine: man seems to require a theory on which to base his practice, be it in alchemy, medicine or the physical sciences. The physician has often been the man of science—in the seventeenth century this was especially so—but unfortunately clinical practice has always presented problems which science has been unable to resolve. Sydenham had pointed the way toward clinical excellence, and there is little doubt that the eighteenth-century physician was highly skilled in his clinical practice. But even Sydenham, resist as he might, had been driven to theorise. His successors, living in an age of enlightenment, of rationalism, and of advancing knowledge of the natural sciences, were great theorizers. Unfortunately, medical theory is perhaps more confused during this period than at any other time, for it was an age of transition—there was as yet no solid corpus of observation in medicine on which to build adequate theory, or to replace the knowledge handed down from classical times. The result was a confusion between the old humoral pathology, the iatro-physical and iatro-chemical schools, and philosophical and literary ideas. The natural sciences also were not free from confusion; for instance, until the time of Robert Boyle, chemistry had been largely a servant of medicine, devoted to pharmacy, or an alchemical search for the philosopher's stone. Although chemistry was to become established as a science during this century, the errors of Stahl's phlogiston theory were to distort the path of truth until nearly the end of the period. Therapy was, therefore, under a twofold distraint, the lack of a sound theory of disease, and the absence of a true chemical science which could transform pharmacy into pharmacology.

But an additional problem was inherent in the treatment of psychiatric patients, namely their management. The great resurgence of philanthropy and the waning influence of the Established Church which had its part in producing the Wesleyan revival, led to a more humane treatment of the insane. As the years passed the old nostrums no longer sufficed, and the emphasis shifted entirely to a form of psychological treatment called moral management, which was to preoccupy psychiatry for many years to come. If theory was lacking or unrewarding, then plain common sense must be used, and it is perhaps of some significance that it was the Reverend Francis Willis, both cleric and physician, who first came to use these principles in the treatment of his psychiatric patients.

Owing to the theoretical confusion, treatment was likely to be highly unsystematized. Of the general measures, exercise, particularly horse-riding, was held in high esteem. One of the most popular books of the early eighteenth century was Francis Fuller's *Medicina Gymnastica*, first published in 1705 and which went into nine editions. Here Fuller recounts his own case history, just as Cheyne was to do thirty years later. He had developed a "certain cutaneous infection, more troublesome than dangerous" to which he rashly applied a substance "well charg'd with a dangerous Mineral" for periods of months at a time. Unfortunately his rash remained unhealed and he developed a severe hypochondriasis. In spite of bleeding and a course of the Bath waters, he continued to suffer miseries until he chanced upon the panacea—the somewhat mundane remedy of horse-riding. Arising from this experience with his own illness, he soon began to recommend equitation for most nervous complaints. He found that it was particularly useful in the hypochondriacal and hysterical disorders. It was important, of course, to find a horse that entirely suited the patient's humour,

> and then it will not be easie for him not to delight in a Creature which will perform all he expects from him, that takes Pleasure in what he is put upon, and delights in his Rider; a Creature which (considering the many other Beasts that are Serviceable for Draught or Burden) seems to be made almost only for the Defence, the Pleasure and Health of his Master; and which has so many excellent Qualities above all other Beasts, that there is no Man upon Earth, whose Gravity or Dignity is so great, as not to allow him with Some Pleasure to take Notice of 'em.

But who could fail to get better in the company of such a noble creature, says Fuller, quoting the examples of patients who, at the beginning, had almost to be hoisted into the saddle, and yet after a year were riding forty or fifty miles a day, and were symptom free at that.

Fuller also recommended cold bathing, which had been popularized by Sir John Floyer in his *History of Cold Bathing*, a most curious publication which appeared in 1702. The revival of interest in Spa treatment owed a great deal to this work, and the eighteenth century was to become the great age of the English Spa. In fact water, in one form or another, was the chief therapeutic agent until the close of the century. The Spas held a very special place in the social life of the century, and it would be a fascinating study to trace the effects of hydrotherapy on the manners, customs, architecture and arts, and even on the politics of the period. Until the rise of the professional psychiatrist—heralded by Battie and coming to maturity with Haslam, psychiatric therapy revolved around the Spas. Purcell had recommended Tunbridge Wells, as the waters there were impregnated with particles of iron, and Sydenham had laid great stress on "steel" in psychological illness. Thence the patient was to proceed to Bath, where the acid sulphur waters liquefied and dissolved the blood, and promoted the flow of the Animal Spirits. Bath, too, was a gay place where the patient could set aside brooding care and give herself over to mirth and pastime. This kind of régime was popular and Cheyne devotes most of his books to a discussion of the relative virtues of the different Waters. The regular life, the exercise, and the dieting (or lack of dieting) together with the balls, concerts and other social activities of the spa were perhaps as efficacious as many of our more modern "shocking" therapies. At least the Hippocratic principle of *Primum non nocere* was adhered to.

Diet in a period of excessive eating, at least amongst the educated and monied classes, was a natural gift to the doctors. Normally, light breakfast of tea and rolls was followed by a heavy dinner and supper. Dr. Johnson's appetite was not considered excessive; as an example, Mrs. Thrale tells how he enjoyed a leg of pork, or a veal pie with sugar and plums, chocolate liberally laced with cream, or melted butter. He was so fond of fruit as to usually consume seven or eight peaches before breakfast began, and the like again after dinner. Foreigners observed with astonishment the large quantities of meat eaten at a sitting, and the still larger amounts of port, sack and punch which were drunk. It was little wonder that nervous disorders were attributed to dietary or alcoholic excess, and George Cheyne's milk, seed and vegetable diet acquired a considerable reputation in the cure of these conditions.

These three measures, exercise, diet and hydrotherapy, formed the backbone of the general aspects of treatment. A less popular but interesting remedy was music therapy. Nicholas Robinson devoted a chapter to the "Powers of Musick in Soothing the Passions, and allaying the Tempests of the Soul, under the Spleen, Vapours, and Hypochondriack Melancholy". Robinson considered that the modulations and oscillations of the notes either raised or depressed the motions of the fibres of the brain. Unfortunately, however, grosser and inferior organs such as the spleen and stomach demand a coarser treatment in order to restore the fibres to a regular standard—and thus the physician was driven to the use of medicines. The fullest work on the subject is Richard Brown's *Medicina Musica* published in 1729.

Coupled with these non-specific measures were the medical treatments. Bleeding, vomiting, purging, clysters, cupping and the application of setons or other counter-irritants were the methods chiefly in vogue. The theory that changes in the consistency of the blood were associated with nervous disorders in practice clearly indicated phlebotomy—small quantities of up to six ounces being removed at weekly, monthly or quarterly intervals (Figs. 18 and 19). Then as now, opinions varied as to the details—when should the patient be bled, how much blood removed, and so on. Camphor, mercury, hellebore and iron were the drugs most used. In ancient times, white hellebore (*Helleborus albus*) had been the specific in madness, but owing to its very powerful purgative property it had fallen out of favour and been replaced by black hellebore (*Helleborus niger*) (Fig. 20). This again owed its reputation to the purgative properties of the bark. The prescriptions were works of art, often including a dozen or so items bearing the most fascinating names, and reading like a poem. No doubt the care given to the preparation of the various electuaries, syrups, conserves or mixtures added greatly to their curative functions—how could a patient fail to be impressed by the learning and skill of such physicians? Alas, in our own era of chemo-therapy and antibiotics, medicines have become universal, as good for the colonel's wife as for Mrs. O'Grady, the criterion now being whether the drug is the very latest discovery.

Finally, electricity was introduced into the treatment of nervous disorders. Benjamin Franklin was one of the pioneers in this field—his experiments with the Kite in 1750 was followed, in 1757, by his application of electricity to treatment. Static electrical machines were installed in several hospitals, at the Middlesex Hospital in 1767, St. Bartholomew's in 1777, and at St. Thomas's in 1799. In the provinces an extract from the records of the General Hospital, Nottingham, reads:

July 8, 1783: The Electrical Machine to be paid for, and that any person who may come to the hospital to be Electrified, (that can afford to pay for the same) shall give sixpence each time to the Charity, but the poor to be Electrified gratis.

The machine cost £42.

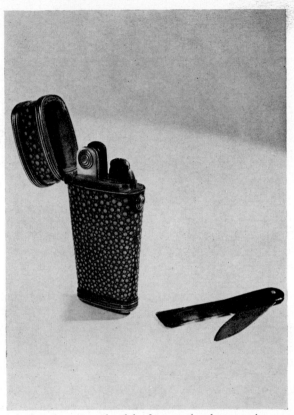

Fig. 18.   Bleeding-knives, made of the finest steel and mounted on tortoiseshell or mother of pearl handles, and contained in a silver bound shagreen case. *(From the author's collection.)*

John Wesley recommended electricity in his *Popular Physic*, and Erasmus Darwin, always up to date, in his book *Zoonomia* (1796) mentioned several patients whom he had so treated. Electricity was either used as current electricity, or by drawing sparks. The latter method was particularly used in eye diseases, but repeated small shocks were passed through the eye in cases of cataract. In nervous afflictions

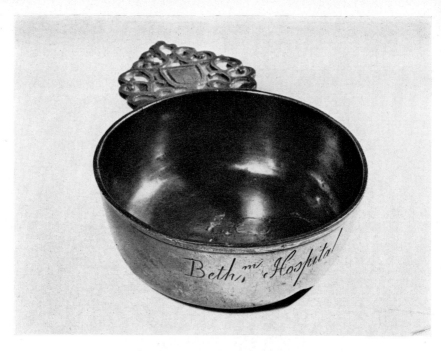

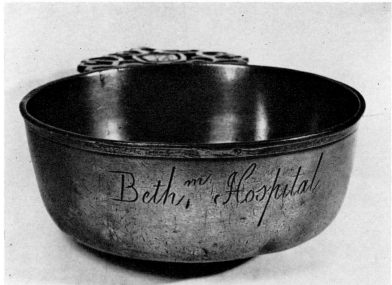

FIG. 19. Bleeding-bowl in Pewter used at Bethlem Hospital in the Eighteenth Century. Capacity 14 oz. (*From the author's collection.*)

resulting in loss of function, electrical shocks were found to be useful, and Darwin mentions the treatment of hysterical aphonia by this method, as well as of suppression of urine, and of cancer of breast. The therapeutic application of electricity was to increase rapidly in

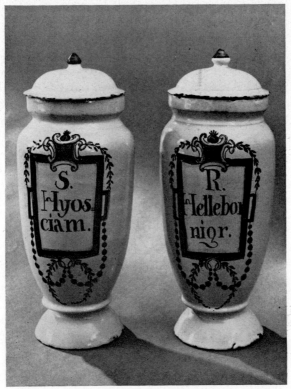

FIG. 20. Drug jars in use about 1800. (*From the author's collection, probably Genoese.*)

the nineteenth century, reaching a triumphant peak with its use in electro-convulsant therapy during the thirties of the present century.

ENVOI

The eighteenth century drew to its close with little change in the care of the lunatic and little advance in psychiatric knowledge. True,

F

the dreadful excesses of the witch hunt were over, and a new spirit was abroad. The pre-occupation of the age with man's relation to man led to the Revolution in France, and to the Reform Movement in England. The lunatic, that most miserable and wretched of mankind, was to benefit directly from a movement springing so largely from the intellectuals of England and France. 1792, the year in which Pinel finally obtained a grudging permission to unchain the maniacs of the Bicêtre, marks the beginning of modern psychiatry.

The first set free was an Englishman. He had been in chains for forty years, no one knew his history except that he had killed one of his keepers with a blow from his manacles. So greatly feared was he, that he was chained more vigorously than any of the other wretches in the Bicêtre. Pinel entered his cell and said, "Captain, I will order your chains to be taken off and give you liberty to walk in the court, if you will promise me to behave well and injure no-one." The chains were removed, and the captain staggered to the door of his cell, his first look was at the sky and he cried, "how beautiful". For the next two years he was in the Bicêtre and had no return of his paroxysms, but indeed helped to rule over the other patients. In a few days Pinel unshackled 53 maniacs, and the success of his experiment was assured.

In England, the same year saw the foundation of The Retreat at York, the first institution in the world devoted to the humane care of the mentally deranged. In 1791 a female of the Society of Friends was placed in the York Lunatic Asylum. Requests were made to the superintendent by acquaintances in the Society to visit this lady, but they were refused on the ground that the patient was not in a suitable state to be seen by strangers. A few weeks later she died. These circumstances "naturally excited reflections on the situation of insane persons" amongst the Friends, and particularly affected one of their number, William Tuke, a citizen of York (Fig. 21). His feeling that something should be done had been strengthened by a visit he had paid to St. Luke's Hospital in London, where he had seen patients lying on straw and in chains. He resolved that an attempt should be made to improve the wretched lot of the Lunatics, and in 1792 he proposed the foundation of an Institution under the government of Friends, "for the care and accommodation of their own members labouring under that most grievous dispensation—the loss of reason". In 1796 the house was opened for the care of patients and Dr. Thomas Fowler was appointed its first physician. In France and England the stage was set for a revolution in the care of the psychiatric patient. It was half a century in coming—some of the story will be told in the following essays on John Haslam and John Conolly.

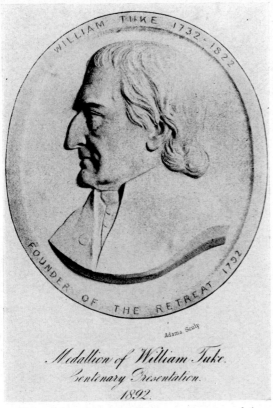

Fig. 21. William Tuke, 1732–1822. (*From an engraving of the medallion by Adams for the Centenary Presentation of 1892. Impression in the Wellcome Historical Medical Museum.*)

A LIST OF BOOKS DEALING WITH PSYCHIATRIC ILLNESS PUBLISHED IN ENGLISH DURING THE EIGHTEENTH CENTURY

[The following bibliography is most probably incomplete. It is drawn from the following sources—my own library, booksellers' catalogues collected over the last twelve years, and Heinrich Laehr's *Die Literatur der Psychiatrie in XVIII Jahrhundert*. The difficulties I have had in compiling this list prompt me to publish it for the use of any future workers, in the hope that it will save them many hours of searching through library catalogues with, as often as not, little to reward them. Such has been my experience.]

ARNOLD, T. *Observations on the Nature, Kinds, Causes, and Prevention of Insanity, Lunacy, or Madness.* G. Ireland, Leicester, Vol. I, 1782; Vol. II, 1786. 2nd edition, 8vo, 298, 314. London, 1806.

ARNOLD, T. *Observations on the Management of the Insane and particularly on the Agency and Importance of Human and Kind Treatment in effecting their Cure.* London, 1809.

BAKER, G. (1755). *De affectibus animi et morbis inde oriundis.* 4to, pp. 34. Cambridge.

BATTIE, W. (1757). *A Treatise on Madness.* 8vo. London.

BATTIE, W. (1757). *De Principiis Animalibus.*

BATTIE, W. (1758). *A Treatise on Madness.* London: Whiston & White.

BATTIE, W. (1760). *Aphorismi de cognoscendis et Curandis Morbis.*

BAYNE, D. (1738). *A new Essay on the Nerves and the Doctrine of the Animal Spirits rationally considered; shewing the great benefit of and true use of bathing, and drinking the Bath waters, in all nervous disorders and instructions; with two dissertations on the gout and on digestion, with the distempers of the stomach and intestines.* Pp. 167. London.

BELCHER, W. (1796). *Belcher's Address to Humanity.* Containing a letter to Dr. Thomas Monro; a receipt to make a lunatic and seize his estate; and a sketch of a smiling hyena. 8vo. London.

BELL, J. (1792). *The general and particular Principles of Animal Electricity and Magnetism. Showing how to magnetise and cure different diseases, to produce crises, as well as somnambulism, or sleep-walking.* 8vo. London.

BILLINGS, P. *Folly Predominant, with a Dissertation on the Possibility of curing lunatics in Bedlam.* 8vo. London.

BLACKMORE, Sir R. (1725) *A Treatise of the Spleen and Vapours: or hypochondriacal and hysterical affections.* London.
    With three discourses on the nature and cure of the cholic, melancholy, and palsies. The 2nd edition to which is added a critical dissertation upon

the spleen, so far as concerns the following question: Whether the spleen is necessary or useful to the animal possessed of it? 2 parts in 1 vol. 8vo, pp. 289. London, 1726.

BLAKEWAY, R. *Essay toward the Cure of Religious Melancholy.* 8vo. London.

BLONDEL, J. A. (1727, 1729). *The Strength of the Imagination in Pregnant Women Examined, and the opinion, that marks the deformities are from them, demonstrated to be a vulgar error.* 8vo. London.

BLONDEL, J. A. (1729). *The Power of the Mother's Imagination over the Foetus Examined, in answer to Dr. Dan Turner's book entitled "A defence of the 12th chapter of the first of a treatise, De morbis cutaneis".* 12mo, pp. 143. London.

BOND, J. (1753). *An Essay on the Incubus or Nightmare.* London, printed for D. Wilson & T. Durham.

BOWEN, T. (1783). *An Historical Account of the Origin, Progress and Present State of Bethlem Hospital, founded by Henry the Eighth, for the cure of lunatics and enlarged by subsequent benefactors, for the reception and maintenance of incurables.* 4to, pp. 16. London.

BRANCH, T. (1737). *Thoughts on Dreaming. Wherein the notion of the sensory, and the opinion that it is shut up from the inspection of the soul in sleep, and that spirits supply us with all our dreams, are examined by revelation and reason.* 8vo, pp. 96. London: for R. Dodsley.

BROWNE, R. (1729). *Medicina Musica, or a mechanical essay on the effects of singing, music and dancing on human bodies, revised and corrected, to which is annexed a new essay on the nature and cure of the spleen and vapours.* 16mo, pp. 125. London.

BRUCKSHAW, S. (1774). *On More Proof of the Iniquitous Abuse of Private Madhouses.* 8vo. London.

BRYDALL, J. (1700). *Non Compos Mentis; or the Law Relating to Natural Fools, Mad Folks, and Lunatick Persons.* 8vo. London.

CHANDLER, G. (1785). *An Inquiry into the various Theories and Methods of Cure in Apoplexie and Palsies.* 8vo. London.

CHEYNE, G. *The English Malady: or a treatise, of nervous diseases of all kinds, as spleen, vapours, lowness of spirits, hypochondriacal, and hysterical, distempers, etc. In three parts: I. Of the nature and cause of nervous distempers. II. Of the cure of nervous distempers. III. Variety of cases that illustrate and confirm the method of cure. With the author's own case at large.* London, 1733.—Dublin, 1733—London, 1735, 1739. 2nd edition, 8vo, pp. 256. London, 1734.

CLARK, W. (1752). *Dissertations Concerning the Effects of the Passions on Human Bodies;* first published in Latin, at Leyden, on the 31st July 1727 . . . and now published in English, with a preface, the aphorismes of Sanctorius to which it refers, and home notes illustrating the object. 8vo. London.

COX, J. M. (1787). *Querdam de mania.* 4to. Lugd. Bat.

CRICHTON, A. (1798). *An Inquiry into the Nature and Origin of Mental Derangement. Comprehending a concise system of the physiology and pathology of the human mind and a history of the passions and their effects.* 2 vols. 8vo.

CULLEN, W. (1777). *First Lines of the Practise of Physic.* London.

ELLIOT, J. (1780). *Philosophical Observations on the Senses of Vision and Hearing.* 8vo. London.

FAITHFUL, A. (1752). *Narrative of the base and inhuman arts that were lately practised upon the Brain of Habbakuk Hilding, justice, dealer, and chapman, who now lies in his house in Covent Garden in a deplorable state of lunacy; a dreadful monument of false friendship and delusion.* By Drawcansir Alexander, fencing master and philomath. 8vo. London.

FALCONER, W. (1781). *Remarks on the influence of climate, situation, nature of country, population, nature of food, and way of life, on the disposition and temper, manner and behavior, intellects, laws and customs, form of government, and religion, of mankind.* 4to, pp. 552. London.

FALCONER, W. *Dissertation on the Influence of the Passions upon the Disorders of the Body.* 8vo, pp. 105. London, 1788, 1796. von. Michaelis, Leipzig, 1789. Paris, 1788.

FALLOWES, T. (1705). *The Best Method for the Cure of Lunatics, with some Accounts of the Incomparable Oleum Cephalicum used in the same, prepared and administered.* 8vo.

FAULKNER, B. (1789). *Observations on the general and improper Treatment of Insanity with a plan for the more speedy and effectual recovery of Insane Persons.* Pp. 26. Printed for the Author. London.

FAWCETT, B. *Observations on the nature, causes and cure of melancholy especially of that, which is commonly called religious melancholy.* 12mo. London, 1779. Leipzig, 1785, 1799.

FERRIAR, J. (1786). *Of Popular Illusions and Particularly of Medical Demonology.* Memoirs of Literary and Philosophical Society. Vol. 3, pp. 23.

FERRIAR, J. *Medical Histories and Reflections.* London, 1792, 1795, pp. 248. London, 1810, 1813, 8vo. Philadelphia, 1816. Leipzig, 1793-97, 1801, pp. 171-86.

FLEMYNG, M. *Neuropathia! Sive de Morbis Hypochondriacis, Hystericis, Libri tres, Poema Medicum, cui praemittitus.* Dissertatio Epistolaris prosaica ejusdem Argumenti. 8vo. York, 1740. Amsterdam, 1741.

FLEMYNG, M. (1755). *Del Mal de Nervi o Sia della Ipocondria, et del Morbo Isterico.* Rome: Stamperia de Rossi.

FLEMYNG, M. (1759). *An Introduction to Physiology, etc.* London, for J. Nourse.

FRINGS, P. (1746). *A Treatise on Phrensy; wherein the cause of that disorder, as assigned by the Galenists, is refuted; and their method of curing the phrensy with their various prescriptions at large are exploded. The true cause set in a clear light, according to Hippocrates, and the most eminent amongst the modern physicians; together with the prescriptions that effectually cure that malady.* Translation from the Latin. 12mo. London.

FULLER, F. (1707). *Medicina Gymnastica.*

HARPER, A. *A treatise on the real cause and cure of insanity, in which the nature and distinctions of the disease are fully explained, and the treatment established on new principles.* London, 1789, 8vo. Marb. 1792, 12mo. 2nd edition, 1798, 8vo, pp. 69.

HARVEY, G. (1703). *Morbus Anglicus, or a theoretick and practical discourse of consumptions and hypochondriack melancholy. Comprising their nature, subject, kinds, causes, signs, prognostics and cures. Likewise, a discourse of spitting of blood, etc.* 12mo, pp. 252. London.

HASLAM, J. *Observations on Insanity, with practical remarks on that disease and an account of the morbid appearance on dissection.* F. & C. Rivington, 8vo. London, 1798, 1809. Stendal. 1800.

HAYGARTH, J. (1800). *Of the Imagination, as a Cause and as a Cure of the Disorders of the Body.* Bath: R. Cruttwell.

HILL, J. (1758). *The Construction of the Nerves and Causes of Nervous Disorders.* 2nd edition, 8vo. London; 1772. *Valerian, on the Virtues of that Root in Nervous Disorders.* 3rd edition, 8vo. London.

HILL, J. (1766). *Hypochondriasis. A practical treatise on the nature and cure of that disorder, commonly the hyp. and hypo.* 8vo, pp. 43. London.

JOHNSTONE, J. (1771). *Essay on the Use of the Ganglions of the Nerves.* 8vo. Shrewsbury.

JOHNSTONE, J. (1795). *Medical Essays and Observations, with Disquisitions relative to the Nervous System.* 8vo. London.

JOHNSTONE, J. (1800). *Medical Jurisprudence. On Madness.* 8vo, pp. 48. Birmingham: J. Belcher.

JONES, R. (1789). *An Inquiry into the Nature, Causes and Termination of Nervous Fevers; together with observations tending to illustrate the method of restoring His Majesty to health, and of preventing relapses of his disease.* Salisbury.

KINNEIR, D. *A New Essay on the Nerves, and the doctrine of the animal spirits rationally considered; shewing the great benefit and true use of bathing, and drinking the Bath waters in all nervous disorders: and obstructions: with two dissertations on the gout, and on digestion, with the distempers of the stomach and intestines.* London, 1738. The second edition with additions. 8vo. London 1739.

KIRKLAND, T. (1774). *A Treatise on Child-bed Fevers, and on the methods of preventing them, being a supplement to the books lately written on the subject. To which are prefixed two dissertations. The one on the brain and nerves; the other on the sympathy of the nerves, and on the different kinds of irritability.* 8vo, pp. 172. London.

LEAKE, J. (1777). *Medical instructions towards the prevention, and care of chronic or slow diseases peculiar to women, especially those proceeding from over delicacy of habit called nervous or hysterical; from female obstructions, weakness, and inward decay; a diseased state of the womb, or critical change of constitution at particular periods of life.* 3rd edition, 8vo, pp. 448. London.

MANDEVILLE, DE B. *A Treatise of the Hypochondriack and Hysterick Passions.* 1st edition, 1711. 2nd edition, London, 1715.

MANNINGHAM, Sir R. (1746). *The Symptoms, Nature, Causes and Cure of the Febricula, or Nervous or Hysteric Fever, Vapours, Hypo, or Spleen.* 12mo, pp. 112. London.

MASON, S. (1747). *Pract. Obs. in Physic, wherein is exhibited the aetiology, or the rise and nature, of the most prevalent distempers, with a plain, rational and concise method of treating them. With a new hypothesis concerning the cure of apoplexies, palsies and many nervous complaints, as also of the gout. To which are added rules and directions now to preserve good health and long life.* 8vo, pp. 265. Birmingham.

MONRO, JAMES (1737). *Harveian Oration.* Pp. 26. London: George Strahan.

MONRO, JOHN (1757). *Harveian Oration.* Pp. 13. London: Gul. Russel.

MONRO, JOHN (1758). *Remarks on Dr. Battie's treatise on Madness.* 8vo, pp. 60. London.

NEALE, H. J. *Practical Dissertations on Nervous Complaints and other Diseases.* London, 1788, 8vo. Berlin, 1790, 8vo.

PARGETER, W. *Observations on Maniacal Disorders.* Reading, 1792, 8vo. Leipzig, 1793, 8vo.

PARGETER, W. (1795). *Formulae Medicamentorum Selectae.* London.

PARGETER, W. (1801). *A Sermon, etc.* Pp. 12.

PARSONS, J. *Human Physiognomy explained in the Croonian Lectures on Muscular Motion of the Year 1746.* 4to, pp. 86.

PAXTON, P. (1701). *Essay concerning the Body of Man, wherein its changes or diseases are considered and the operations of medicines observed.* 8vo. London.

PEART, E. (1798). *Physiology on an attempt to explain the functions and laws of the nervous system, the contraction of muscular fibres.* 8vo. London.

PERCIVAL, T. (1767). *Essays Medical and Experimental etc.* 8vo, pp. 238. London.

PERFECT, W. (1763). *An Elegy on a Storm which happened in West Kent, on the 19th of August 1763.*

PERFECT, W. (1766). *The Laurel Wreath.* 2 vols.

PERFECT, W. (1778) *Methods of Cure in Some Particular Cases of Insanity.* 8vo. London.

PERFECT, W. *Cases of Insanity, the Epilepsy, Hypochondriacal Affection, Hysteric Passion, and Nervous Disorders, Successfully Treated.* 2nd edition, with many additional cases, 8vo, pp. 217, Rochester, 1779. 8vo., pp. 345. Rochester, 1787.

PERFECT, W. (1781). *Ibid.* Pp. 217. London.

PERFECT, W. (1780). *Ibid.* Translated into German. 8vo. Leipzig.

PERFECT, W. *Select Cases in the Different Species of Insanity, Lunacy, or Madness, with the Modes of Practice as adopted in the Treatment of Each.* Rochester, 1787, 8vo. Ueberj. v. C. F. Michaelis, Leipzig, 1789, 8vo. 3rd edition under title of *Annals of Insanity,* 1793. Hann., 1804.

PERFECT, W. (1787). *Methods of Cure in some Cases of Insanity, Epilepsy, etc.* 8vo. Rochester.

PERFECT, W. *A Remarkable Case of Madness, with the Diet and Medicines used in the Cure.* 8vo, pp. 52. Rochester, 1791. Leipzig, 1794.

PERFECT, W. (1791). *Select Cases in the Different Species of Insanity, or Madness; with the Diet and Medicines used in the Cure.* London.

PERFECT, W. (1805). *Annals of Insanity: comprising a large selection of curious and interesting cases in the different species of insanity, lunacy, or madness, with the medical and moral treatment of each.* 4th edition, London. Printed for the author.

PERRY, C. (1723). *On the Causes and Nature of Madness. As also the natures and properties of opium and volatiles considered in a remonstrance to Dr. Herrm. Lafnau, on his behaviour touching a late case. To which is added a postscript.* 8vo. London.

PERRY, C. (1755). *A Mechanical Account and Explication of the Hysteric Passion under all its Various Symptoms and Appearances.* 8vo. London.

POMME, P. (1777). *On Hysterical and Hypochondriacal Diseases.* Translation from the fourth edition, with a preface by John Berkenhout. 8vo, pp. 357. London: P. Elmsley.

PRESCOTT, J. (1788). *An Account of the Rise and Present Establishment of the Lunatic Hospital in Manchester.*

PURCELL, J. *A Treatise of Vapours, or, Hysterick Fits. Containing an analytical proof of its causes, mechanical explanations of all its symptoms and accidents, according to the newest and most rational principles: together with its cure at large.* 12mo, pp. 150. London, 1702. 12mo, pp. 238. London, 1707.

ROBINSON, N. (1729). *A New System of the Spleen, Vapours, and Hypochondriack melancholy: wherein all the decays of the nerves, and lowness of the spirits, are mechanically accounted for. To which is subjoined, a discourse upon the nature, cause, and cure, of melancholy, madness, and lunacy. With a particular dissertation on the origin of the passions; the structure, mechanism and modulation of the nerves, necessary to produce sensation in animal bodies. To which is prefixed, a philosophical essay concerning the principles of thought, sensation, and reflection; and the manner how those noble endowments are disconcerted under the foregoing diseases.* 8vo, pp. 408. London.

ROWLEY, W. (1788). *A Treatise on Female, Nervous, Hysterical, Hypochondriacal, Bilious, Convulsive Diseases; Apoplexy and Palsy; with thoughts on Madness,*

Suicide, etc. In which the principal disorders are explained from anatomical facts, and the treatment formed on several new principles. 8vo, pp. 521. London, for C. Nourse, E. Newbery and T. Hookham.

ROWLEY, W. *Truth Vindicated or the Specific Differences of Mental Diseases.* 8vo. London, 1789. 8vo. Breslau, 1790.

RYMER, J. *A Tract upon Indigestion, and the Hypochondriac Disease, and upon the Atonic or Flying Gout; with the methods of cure by means of a new remedy of medicine; and directions for taking it in a variety of cases of nervous affections, muscular and vascular relaxation, broken constitutions, in malignant and putrid fevers.* 12mo, pp. 56. London, 1785. *Idem. With above fifty-six select cases, chiefly anomalous, of dyspepsy, hysteria, hypochondriasis, the inflammatory and atonic gout, vertigo, apoplexy, palsy.* 8vo, pp. 239. London, 1789.

SCOTT, J. (1780). *Histories of gouty, bilious and nervous cases, with the safe and easy means by which they were remedied, related by the patients themselves in sundry letters.* 8vo, pp. 24. London.

SIMSON, T. (1752). *An inquiring how far the vital and animal actions can be accounted to be independent of the brain.* In five essays, being the substance of the Chandos lectures for the year 1739, and some subsequent years. 8vo, pp. 270. Edinburgh.

SMITH, W. (1775). *An Apology to the Public for Practice in Hysterical Cases.* 8vo. London.

SMITH, H. (1794). *An Essay on the Nerves.* 8vo. London.

SMITH, W. (1768). *A dissertation upon the nerves, containing an account, 1. of the nature of man, 2. of the nature of brutes, 3. of the nature and connection of soul and body, 4. of the threefold life of man, 5. of the symptoms, causes and cure of all nervous diseases.* 8vo, pp. 302. London.

STEARNS, S. (1791). *The History of Animal Magnetism, revealed to the world, containing philosophical reflections on the publication of a pamphlet, entitled: A true and genuine discovery of animal electricity and magnetism; also an exhibition of the advantages and disadvantages that may arise in consequence of said publication; and many other curious observations never before published.* 8vo, pp. 58. London.

THOMSON, A. *An Inquiry into the Nature, Causes and Method of Cure of Nervous Disorders. In a letter to a friend.* 8vo, pp. 35. London, 1781, 1782, 1783, 1795. 2nd edition, 8vo, pp. 98. London, 1782. 4th edition. London, 1794.

THORNTON, R. J. (1796-97). *Medical Extracts on the Nature of Health, with practical observations, of the nervous and fibrous systems. By a friend to improvements.* London.

TURNER, D. (1726). *On the Force of the Mother's Imagination on the Foetus in Utero.* London.

TURNER, D. (1729). *An Answer to a Pamphlet on the Power of Imagination in Pregnant Women.* London.

UVEDALE, C. (1758). *The Construction of the Nerves and the Causes of Nervous Disorders practically explained.* 8vo, pp. 54. London.

VERE, J. (1778). *A Physical and Moral Enquiry into the Causes of that Internal Restlessness and Disorder in Man, which has been the Complaint of all Ages.* For B. White.

WALKER, S. (1796). *A Treatise on Nervous Diseases, in which are introduced some observations on the structure and functions of the nervous system; and such an investigation of the symptoms and causes of those diseases as may lead to a rational and successful method of cure.* 8vo, pp. 224. London.

WANLEY, N. (1788). *The Wonders of the Little World; or, a general history of man, in six books, displaying the various faculties, capacities, powers, and defects of the human body and mind, in several thousand most interesting relations of persons remarkable for bodily perfections or defects . . . or for the uncommon powers of weakness of the senses and affections, as the memory, sight, feeling, taste, smelling, etc. and of love and hatred, fear and anger, joy and grief, desire and hope, scorn and envy, etc. Together with accounts of the invention of arts, the advancement of science; surprising escapes from death and dangers; strange discoveries of long-concealed murders, and a vast variety of other matters equally curious. The whole collected from the writings of the most approved historians, philosophers, and physicians of all ages and countries, etc.* 4to, pp. 752, 6 pls. London.

WESLEY, J. (1747). *Primitive Physic.*

WHYTT, R. (1752). *Physiological Essays containing an enquiry into the causes which promote the circulation of the fluids in the very small vessels of the animals, with observations on the sensibility and irritability on the parts of man and other animals.* 12mo. Edinburgh.

WHYTT, R. *Physiological Essays, containing: I. An inquiry into the causes which promote the circulation of the fluids in the very small vessels of animals. II. Observations on the sensibility and irritability of the parts of men and other animals; occasioned by Dr. Haller's late treatise on these subjects.* Three editions with an appendix containing an answer to M. de Haller's remarks in the 4th volume of the *Memoires sur les parties sensibles et irritables.* 12mo, pp. 223. Edinburgh, 1755, 1761, 1766. 12mo. Gallia Par., 1759.

WHYTT, R. (1768). *The Works,* published by his son. 4to, 8vo, pp. 745, 15 ll, appendix (8 leaves). Edinburgh.

WHYTT, R. (1765). *Observations on the Nature, Causes, and Cure of those Disorders which have been Commonly called Nervous, Hypochondriac or Hysteric: To which are prefixed some Remarks on the Sympathy of the Nerves.* 1st edition, 2nd edition, 8vo, pp. 520, advertisement leaf, 7 ll. Edinburgh.

WHYTT, R. (1767). *Observations on the Nature, Causes, and Cure of those Disorders which have been Commonly called Nervous, Hypochondriac or Hysteric: To which are prefixed some Remarks on the Sympathy of the Nerves.* 8vo, 7 ll., advertisement leaf, 3rd edition, pp. xiii + 507. Edinburgh.

WILSON, A. (1777). *Medical Researches: being an enquiry into the nature and origin of hysterics in the female constitution, and into the distinction between that disease and hypochondriac or nervous disorders. Comprehending . . . Together with the substance of a discourse, proving that the motions of the blood and animal fluids do not depend on the impulses of the heart upon the blood, but must be referred to other causes, and particularly to an animal modification of that universal principle which is the common cause of all organisation, and of all organical motions in bodies. To which are added, four letters to Sir Jacob on the materiality, density and activity of light and on air.* 8vo, pp. 316. London.

ANON. (1772). *A Description of Bedlam with an Account of its Present Inhabitants both Male and Female. To which is subjoined an essay upon the nature causes and cure of madness.* 8vo. London.

ANON. (1727). *A Treatise on Diseases of the Head, Brain and Nerves: more especially of the palsy, apoplexy, lethargy, epilepsy, convulsions, frenzy, vertigo, megrim, inveterate headache etc. with directions for their thorough cure, and how these and many other deplorable nervous distempers may be prevented as well cured, and consequently many lives saved, by the medicine herein, in English prescribed without the least reserve. To which is subjoined, a discourse on the nature, real cause, and certain cure of melancholy in men and vapours in women, instructing persons how to cure themselves absolutely of those perplexing and pernicious disorders with safety, ease and expedition.* By a physician. 8vo, pp. 74. London.

ANON. (1735). *An Account of the Progress of an Epidemical Madness, in a letter to the President and Fellows of the College of Physicians.* 8vo. London.

ANON. (1749). *Reflections on ancient and modern musick with the application to the cure of diseases; to which is subjoined an essay to solve the question wherein consisted the difference of ancient musick from that of modern times.* 8vo. London.

ANON. (1783). *An Historical Account of the Origin, Progress and Present State of Bethlem Hospital.* 4to. London.

ANON. (1788). *An attempt to ascertain the causes of the King's present Illness with a new method of treating it, applicable to all who suffer in like manner, most humbly recommended by a dutiful subject.* 8vo. London.

ANON. (1788). *Report of the Lords Committees appointed to examine the Physicians who have attended His Majesty during his Illness, touching the present state of His Majesty.* 8vo. London.

ANON. (1788). *A Narrative of the extraordinary case of G. Lukings of Yetton, who was possessed of evil spirits for near 18 years.* 8vo. Bristol and London.

ANON. (1789). *Reflexions of the Consequences of His Majesty's Recovery from his late indisposition.* For G. G. J. & J. Robinson.

MANCHESTER ROYAL LUNATIC HOSPITAL, *in connection with the Royal Infirmary.* 4to. London, 1706.

THE LUNATIC WARD OF GUY'S HOSPITAL. 8vo. London, 1728.

PAMPHLET, Hoxton Asylum, England. 8vo. London, 1741.

PAMPHLET, Brooke House, Clapton (Dr. Monro's). 8vo. London, 1759.

MADHOUSES. *A report from the Committee appointed* (27th January 1763) *to enquire into the state of the Private Madhouses in the Kingdom. With the proceedings of the House thereon.* Published by Order of the House of Commons. For John Whiston. Fol. 1763.

MANCHESTER ROYAL LUNATIC HOSPITAL, at Cheadle. *Rules for the Government of the Lunatic Hospital and Asylum in Manchester.* 12mo, pp. 21. Manchester, 1791.

CHAPTER II

John Haslam, M.D.
1764–1844

THE eighteenth century saw a change in the professional status of those concerned with the care of lunatics. The "Keeper", whether layman or doctor, usually rough and uneducated, began to give way to the physician specializing in, and often writing about, mental disorder. William Battie, as we have seen, was one of the few psychiatrists ever to be made President of the Royal College of Physicians; whatever their drawbacks, the Monros were all educated men, and Thomas Arnold's book was considered worth translating into German. These pioneers were essentially men of their time; John Haslam, the subject of this essay, was born in 1764 and died in 1844 (Fig. 1). His career bestrides the two centuries, pointing both forwards and backwards, and providing an interesting contrast to our other two subjects, James Cowles Prichard, and John Conolly.

> One of the most successful practitioners, and able writers on this branch of medical practice (madness), is Dr. Haslam. His whole life has been devoted to the investigation of insanity; and having been connected for so many years with a large public and private establishment for the cure of this class of diseases, he is considered an oracle on the subject, and examined in all disputed cases of any consequence. This eminent "Mad Doctor", as he is peculiarly termed, is a very original thinker. His works are considered to be the most able productions which have appeared in this or any other country, on the subject of derangement of mind, and are largely quoted and read by all who are desirous of arriving at a correct knowledge of this important and interesting branch of Science. . . . Dr. Haslam is now in the decline of life. . . . In private life he is much esteemed. He possesses a kind benevolent disposition and is much beloved by a large circle of admiring friends and relations.

This extract is taken from the interesting *Physic & Physicians*: "A Medical Sketch Book exhibiting the Public and Private Life of the Most Celebrated Medical Men of Former Days; with Memoirs of Eminent Living London Physicians and Surgeons" written by Forbes Winslow, and published in 1839, when Haslam was 75. In Pinel's *Traité Medico–philosophique sur la Manie*, published in 1801, Haslam is

mentioned more frequently than any other English authorities save
Ferriar, and Pinel amplifies many of his own conclusions by quotations

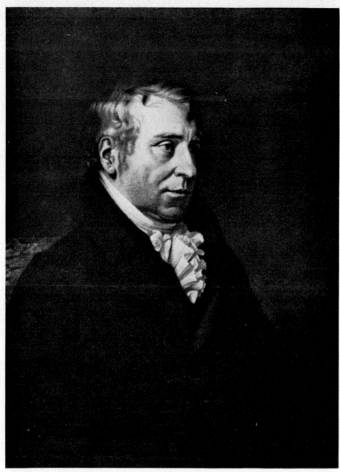

Fig. 1.   John Haslam, M.D., 1764–1844. Apothecary to Bethlem
1795–1816.

from Haslam. And yet Haslam was comparatively neglected by his
English contemporaries, and is spoken of in derogatory terms by Tuke
in his *History of the Insane in the British Isles* (1882), thus—"Haslam
wrote his *Observations on Madness* in 1798, and he was the author of

several other works, but, whatever their value and interest, we know but too well the condition of the patients in the asylum of which he was apothecary" (p. 142). "Mr. Haslam, the resident apothecary, ruled supreme. He was responsible for the dreadful condition in which the notorious Norris was discovered" (p. 152). "If Haslam may seem to have stumbled upon General Paralysis, we may well accord to French alienists the merit of having really discovered the disorder . . ." (p. 444). And when he died, Haslam's obituary in the *Lancet* of 27 July 1844 was so condescending and so misleading that it stands today as a reproach to its writer.

> The newspapers announce the decease of Dr. John Haslam, at his house in Lamb's Conduit Place, at the advanced age of 81. This well-known physician had retired from active practice for several years previous to his death. His labours in the cause of science exist in the form of a monograph on *Sound Mind* published in 1819, and a course of Lectures on the Intellectual Composition of Man, delivered before the Medical Society of London, in the session 1827–28, and published at that time in the *Lancet*. Dr. Haslam was an amusing companion, and his conversation abounded in anecdote, chiefly having reference to John Hunter, of whom he was an intimate friend, and for whom he had a very high respect. Dr. Haslam's writings can scarcely be called those of a man of genius, they exhibit however, a profound knowledge of his subject, and a deep train of philosophic thought.

Recently, however, Haslam's life and work has been re-assessed. Beginning with Arnold Pick, who in 1924 first drew attention to Haslam's original description of the simple dementing form of schizophrenia, Zelmanowits in 1953 continued the work of rehabilitation by pointing out that Haslam's pioneer accounts of obsessive–compulsive neurosis and of manic–depressive psychosis put him in the forefront of psychiatric nosologists. "It is with Haslam that the line of modern psychiatric writers begins, to whom credit is due for contributions which are the basis of our present-day nosological views regarding the group of manic–depressive psychoses." Although Haslam is credited with the discovery of General Paralysis of the Insane, doubt has been cast upon this by the present writer. It seems clear, therefore, that a more intensive re-appraisal of Haslam's life and work is needed.

STUDENT DAYS

John Haslam was born in London in 1764, his father also a John Haslam. Of his early years little is known, but

> after a period of apprenticeship I became a student of St. Bartholomew's Hospital, and afterwards House Surgeon. My medical knowledge was first derived from the lectures of Dr. G. Fordyce, and as a physician's pupil, from the hospital practice of Dr. David Pitcairn. Afterwards, I attended, for more than two years, the Medical and Chemical Lectures at Edinburgh; and during that time, was elected a President of the Royal Medical, Natural History, and Chemical Societies in that University. Subsequently I studied at Uppsala, in Sweden, and lastly, at Pembroke Hall, in the University of Cambridge.

The apothecary occupied the lowest rung on the medical ladder, although five years' apprenticeship, six months' attendance at hospitals, and an examination in the vulgar tongue, not only in pharmacy, but in medicine, anatomy and physiology were necessary, as compared with the physicians two years' residence at a regularly constituted university in any country, and three examinations taken in Latin. Three classes of students attended Bart's in the eighteenth century, the apprentices, the dressers and the pupils. Unfortunately I have been unable to trace Haslam's attendance at the hospital. His name does not appear in the journals relating to the Apothecary and his shop, and no records exist at this time concerning medical students.

Haslam's two mentors—Dr. George Fordyce and Dr. David Pitcairn—were both remarkable men of quite distinct temperaments. Fordyce (Fig. 2) had been one of Cullen's favourite pupils in Edinburgh before coming to London to study under William Hunter. In 1764 he began to lecture on the practice of physic and on materia medica, in addition to lecturing in chemistry, and soon became one of the most popular teachers in London. His courses lasted for nearly four months; he began his lectures at 7 a.m. and ended at 10 a.m., an hour being devoted to each of the three subjects—and the instruction took place six days a week. He had a remarkable memory, and although he is said to have read very little, he remembered all he read. He rendered much service to the College of Physicians, and was a man of convivial, albeit of somewhat eccentric nature. He ate only one meal a day— dining at Dolly's Chop-house at four o'clock, for his researches into comparative anatomy had convinced him that man generally ate more

G

than was good for him. Nevertheless, his meal was a substantial one. On the table

was placed a silver tankard full of strong ale, a bottle of port wine, and a

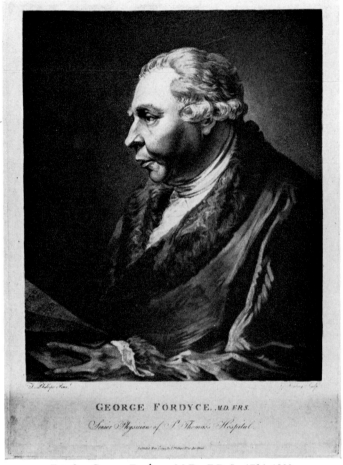

FIG. 2.   George Fordyce, M.D., F.R.S., 1736–1802.

measure containing a quarter of a pint of brandy. The moment the waiter announced him, the cook put a pound and a half of rump steak on the gridiron, and on the table some delicate trifle, as a bonne-bouche, to serve until the steak was ready. This was sometimes half a boiled chicken, sometimes a plate of fish. When he had eaten this, he took one glass of brandy, and then proceeded to devour his steak. When he had finished his meal, he took the remainder of his brandy, having during his dinner drank his tankard of ale, and afterwards a bottle of port. He thus daily spent an hour and a half of his time, and then returned to his house in Essex Street, to give his six o'clock lecture on chemistry.

He was not as successful in practice as in lecturing, spending little time with his patients, his appearance being unprepossessing and his intemperate habits unappealing. But he was probably the best lecturer of his time, and according to his friend, William Charles Wells (whom we shall meet later in this narrative), was more skilled in the sciences related to medicine than any of his fellow-physicians. Coming from Wells, this was high praise indeed.

David Pitcairn was a remarkable contrast, being one of the most beloved and popular physicians of his day. Tall, erect and handsome, his practice included patients from every rank of society; he spent much time with them, and often forgot his fee—"No Medical man, indeed, of his eminence in London, perhaps ever exercised his profession to such a degree gratuitously." In 1780 he was elected Physician to St. Bartholomew's Hospital, and he became a Censor, Goulstonian Lecturer and Harveian Orator at the College of Physicians. Although he was a most astute as well as a most learned physician, he published not a single line, but in dying from a previously unrecognized disease "the peculiar and melancholy privilege was reserved for him to enlighten his profession in the very act of dying". These are the two men whom Haslam singled out for mention. In some respects they illustrate two sides of Haslam's character, the convivial, somewhat hasty and eccentric character, which was to bring him so much trouble, and the essentially humane and kindly person who could, through his writings, be admired by Philippe Pinel.

In 1785 Haslam left Bart's and like so many keen young men of his day, travelled North to Edinburgh, then at the height of its fame as a medical school. Cullen had almost retired from clinical practice, his faculties being considerably diminished, although he still remained Professor of the "Institutes" of Physic. On his death in 1790 he was succeeded by Andrew Duncan the elder (1744–1824), with whom Haslam came into contact at the Royal Medical Society, and who had a special interest in insanity. Almost immediately on arriving in Edinburgh, Haslam joined the Society (10 December 1785) and soon became a prominent member. In 1786 he became one of its Junior Presidents. He delivered two dissertations to the Society, the texts of both being preserved in its archives, written in Haslam's own hand. The first was given in the session 1785–86, the subject being "In what manner are parts of the human body reproduced when they have been destroyed? Can the extensive reproduction of the lower animals be rationally accounted for?" Haslam obviously did not relish the subject, his first paragraph implying that he had been given a rather disagreeable task, had been too busy to devote sufficient time to the subject, and worst of all had been unable to obtain the necessary references—"the works of those authors who have treated professedly upon the subject he is unable to procure (particularly those of Spallanzani)". This does not speak highly for the library facilities available to the medical students. In spite of suggesting to the Society that he should speak on the theory of vomiting, upon which he had begun to make experiments, he had been prohibited from this "under a fine". Needless to say, a dissertation begun in this manner makes for little profundity or originality, and Haslam frequently apologizes for its "thinness". Indeed, he deals mostly with the process of inflammation and the recovery of parts of the body following injury or disease, leaving the question of the extensive reproduction of the lower animals severely alone.

His second dissertation was given in the Session of 1786–87 on the more conventional topic of *Lues Venera*, and Haslam was thoroughly at home with the subject. In view of the claims put forward by later writers that Haslam discovered General Paralysis of the Insane, the dissertation is worth careful scrutiny. It begins:

> S. H. a week after connection with a venereal woman, perceived a sore upon the prepuce which did not heal. In a few days a swelling in the groin came on. . . . Mr. President! There can be no doubt of the present case being *Lues Venerea*. In this paper we shall begin with chancre; and follow the disease in its progress to the constitution; examine some opinions respecting the constitutional form of the disease; and, lastly, give the method of cure.

Almost at once an interesting point arises—Haslam describes how the application of venereal matter to certain parts of the sound living body, under certain circumstances, will result in inflammation and ulceration. But not all parts are capable of

> receiving this poison. . . . As far as my limited enquiries have reached, the

brain has never been contaminated primarily, or in a secondary manner by venereal pus. To inquire into the cause of this would be hopeless. We can see nothing in its structure which should exempt it. It may be asked if any direct application of venereal pus were ever made to the brain? Of this I have heard from a gentleman who had the boldness to make the experiment; which, fortunately for the patient, failed—As to its secondary infection, I can speak with more confidence, having examined many venereal heads, without observing any disease in that organ; nor has any testimony furnished cases.

There the matter ends, for Haslam goes on to deal with mundane matters—the clinical development of the syphilitic infection, the appearance of the chancre, the ensuing glandular enlargement, and then a progress to "the constitution"—sore throat, skin rashes, ophthalmia, and bone disease. One of the most dreadful forms of the latter affected the internal tables of the skull.

Intense pain is first felt, this is succeeded by drowsiness; the disease continuing, the apoplectic stertor succeeds, and in a few days, the patient is killed. Upon examination there is found an inflammation and thickening of the bone pressing upon the brain.

So ends the clinical description. The last third of the dissertation deals with treatment, and Haslam gives a fair account of the contemporary therapeutic approach to syphilis.

These dissertations are Haslam's earliest available writings, and reveal something of the young man's mind—a strong disinclination to speculation, a tendency to express his views freely and somewhat aggressively, and an interest in the brain. Of his other clinical work at Edinburgh nothing is known, but he took an active part in a misunderstanding which occurred between the Managers of the Royal Infirmary and the students. The Managers had passed a somewhat hasty resolution regulating the hours of admission for the students attending the Infirmary, and censuring the general body of the students for the misconduct of the few. The students, also acting hastily, formed a body entitled "The Associated Students", elected Thomas Beddoes chairman, and published a pamphlet in connection with the dispute. The committee of "The Associated Students" which was appointed to submit a representation to the Managers of the Infirmary consisted of the chairman Thomas Beddoes, and nine students, eight of whom were members of the Society. Of these latter, James Mackintosh and John Haslam were the most active. From the style of his later writings it seems highly probable that the Narrative was written by Haslam. The twenty-four page pamphlet is entitled "A Narrative of some late injurious proceedings of the Managers of the Royal Infirmary against the Students of Medicine in the University of Edinburgh". It is written in an admirably lucid style, and many of the phrases are very characteristic of Haslam. Unfortunately, however, there is no direct evidence in the archives of the Royal Medical Society as to the identity of the author. The intervention of the Medical Faculty ended the misunderstanding satisfactorily, but the student organization continued for several years to maintain the rights of the students.

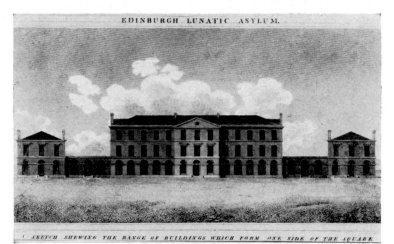

FIG. 3.   The Edinburgh Lunatic Asylum. Showing elevation. (*From an engraving in the Wellcome Historical Medical Museum.*)

Whilst at Edinburgh Haslam would have come into contact with Dr. Andrew Duncan, the founder of the Public Dispensary in West Richmond Street, and of the Edinburgh Asylum for the Insane, who later became Professor of the Institutes of Medicine. Dr. Duncan's interest in the treatment of the insane was aroused when, as a young practitioner, he was called to attend the poet Fergusson in the local madhouse. In 1792 he proposed the erection of a public lunatic asylum in Edinburgh, the idea having lain in his mind for many years. So many difficulties arose that not until 1807 was a Royal Charter granted under which a lunatic asylum was built at Morningside (Fig. 3). A year later Duncan received the Freedom of Edinburgh for his service to this foundation and to his dispensary. He was a very convivial man, in his youth being known as the "smiling boy", and his character for good nature was retained throughout his life. He was President of the Royal Medical Society in 1764, and five times afterwards, his fondness for the Society continuing until his death. He was its Treasurer for many years, and in 1786, the year of Haslam's presidency, was voted a gold medal for his services. Such a man could not fail to have influenced the young Haslam—also of a convivial nature and keenly interested in his profession.

Then occurs a gap in Haslam's life which I have been unable to fill. He himself tells us that he studied at Uppsala, but no record exists of his attendance at that famous University. He had a lifelong interest, however, in the "Northern Group of Languages", and his library contained a variety of works relating to Sweden. In this period he married, and for a time lived in Shoreditch, for his son Thomas, born 12 June 1790, was baptized at St. Leonard's, Shoreditch.

The next certain event in his life is his appointment as Apothecary to Bethlem in 1795.

APOTHECARY TO BETHLEM

He succeeded John Gozna, who had filled the post since 1772. Gozna left no writings, but over the twenty-three years of his connection with Bethlem he collected some of the first statistics of insanity. At his death his brother presented the manuscript to Dr. William Black, who published the figures in his book *Dissertation on Insanity*, which appeared in 1811. Gozna's colleague and friend, Bryan Crowther, the surgeon to Bethlem, also mentions that "Mr. Gozna informed me that of the patients who took the smallpox infection, the majority of such were restored to their sense". However, Crowther sadly confessed that he had been unable to confirm this impression statistically, much as he would have cherished the opportunity of transmitting his old friend's discovery to posterity.

Haslam remained Apothecary until his dismissal by the Governors in 1816. During this period Bethlem was in a phase of transition. The palatial building erected in Moorfields in 1676 was by now no more than an elegant hulk. Floors gaped, walls cracked, and the expanding city engulfed the once open fields surrounding the hospital. In 1801 the Hospital Committee decided that Bethlem should remove to another district and negotiations were begun which eventually resulted in the opening of the third Bethlem at St. George's Fields in 1815 (Fig. 4).

Although the hospital in Moorfields was showing signs of wear and tear, the remarkable Monro family, which supplied the Physicians to Bethlem for one hundred and twenty-five years, continued as steadfast as ever. During Haslam's service his physician was Dr. Thomas Monro (1759–1833), the connoisseur and patron of many British water colour

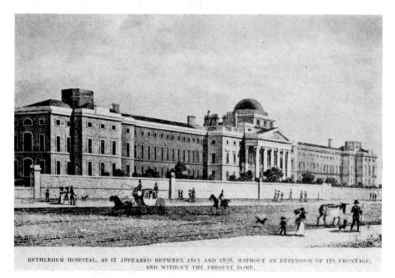

BETHLEHEM HOSPITAL, AS IT APPEARED BETWEEN 1815 AND 1838, WITHOUT AN EXTENSION OF ITS FRONTAGE, AND WITHOUT THE PRESENT DOME.

Fig. 4.   The Third Bethlem, opened 1815.

artists (Fig. 5). The surgeon was Bryan Crowther, whose publications included *Practical Observations on the Diseases of the Joints* and *Practical Remarks on Insanity*. A vivid picture of the working of the hospital, which at this time consisted of about 120 beds, is given in the minutes of evidence taken before the Committee appointed by the House of Commons to consider Provisions being made for the Better Regulation of Mad-houses in England. Haslam told this Committee in 1815 that he possessed extracts from records extending as far back as 1577. He attended the hospital "very regularly every day, frequently goes round, passes along the galleries, and if there is a patient he has a particular desire to see, he sees that person". Haslam had formerly lived in the hospital, but owing to part of the building being taken down had latterly lived at Islington. He came to the hospital at eleven o'clock, "stays half-an-hour, or sometimes longer than that", and had "never been absent from the hospital above three days, and then had leave of absence from the Treasurer". If any emergencies arose, Dr. Haslam was the only

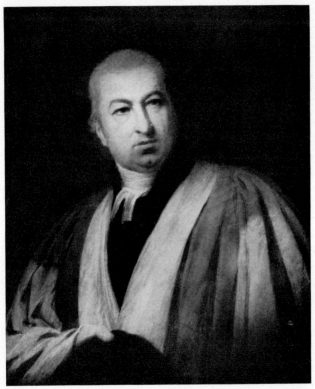

FIG. 5.   Thomas Monro, M.D., F.R.C.P., 1759–1833. Physician
to Bethlem 1792–1816.

person who might be called, but as the patients were locked in their cells every night, there were in fact no night calls. For these services he received £335 a year, whilst Dr. Monro, the Physician, whose orders he carried out, received £100 a year. Dr. Monro visited Bethlem three times a week, made enquiries about the state of the patients, but did not always make a tour of the wards. In general, patients were brought to see him in his private room, where he examined them both with regard to their mental as well as their physical complaints. His relation to Haslam was similar to that of consultant to registrar today, although he seems to have left the running of the hospital largely to Haslam. Medicine was given at particular times of the year, "in the months of May, June, July, August and September," said Dr. Monro, "we generally administer medicines, we do not in the winter season, because the house is so excessively cold that it is not thought proper". Bleeding, vomiting and purging were carried out on particular days of the week—bleeding during the months of May and June, followed by vomiting and purging—"that has been the practice invariably for years, long before my time, it was handed down to me by my father, and I do not know better practice". Bethlem did not, on the whole, deal with incurable patients; then, as now, patients were admitted for care and treatment; if adjudged to be incurable they were then transferred to other institutions, although exceptions, of course occurred. Two of these exceptions, John Tilly Matthews and James Norris, were to contribute largely to Haslam's eventual downfall and his dismissal from Bethlem.

For the 120 patients there were two female and three male keepers, with the result that a good deal of restraint was necessary in the form of chains, although Dr. Monro considered that chains and fetters were only fit for pauper lunatics, "if a gentleman was put into irons, he would not like it". Pauper lunatics could not afford to pay for the regular attendance which prevented them "doing mischief" and in Bethlem there were so few servants kept for this purpose that chains were the only way of restraining them. In Monro's own "private house" no chains were used. In addition to the physician and apothecary, there were two surgeons, Bryan Crowther—who was in a rather comparable position to Haslam, and the distinguished surgeon, William Lawrence, who acted as surgical consultant. The steward and matron, the last two important members of the staff, were both in their seventies.

Such is the setting in which Haslam carried out his work. Unfortunately for him, public interest in insanity, awakened by the recurrent madness of George III, was growing in intensity as the Reformist zeal of the time increased. The foundation of the Retreat, and the philanthropic work of other Quakers such as John Howard, stimulated yet more citizens to concern themselves with the public weal. One such was Edward Wakefield, a land agent. For many years he had been in the habit of visiting places where the insane were confined, both in the metropolis and in the provinces. In 1814 he first visited Bethlem, and as a result of this visit, and the agitation which had been going on for some time over the abuses discovered in the York Lunatic Asylum, a Select Committee was appointed by the House of Commons "to consider the Provisions being made for the better Regulations of madhouses in England". It began its work in 1815, and during its existence conducted the most thorough and minute investigation of its remit. Under the Chairmanship of Mr. George Rose, the Committee first met on May 1815 and proceeded to deal with the affairs of the York Lunatic Asylum, moving on next to Bethlem. Wakefield was called and told of his visits to the hospital—of seeing naked men and women patients chained by an arm or a leg to the wall, and most ominous for Haslam recounted his meeting with William Norris, a man of 55 who had been confined for fourteen years, nine of them shackled in such a way as to rouse Wakefield's indignation to fever point. Wakefield had a drawing made of Norris in his chains, and brought a number of Members of Parliament to see him.

Norris was an American by birth, and had served in either the British or American Army. When he was first admitted, according to Haslam, he appeared perfectly calm, and it was intended soon to discharge him, until he suddenly stabbed one of the keepers. Thenceforth his violence was so constant that in Haslam's opinion he was "the most malignant and the most mischievous lunatic I ever saw in my life, and he had been equally so, by his own confession, when he was in the army, and his back bore many records of the whip". He bit off a fellow-patient's finger, tried to kill another keeper with a shovel, and proved so recalcitrant that a special apparatus had to be devised in order to restrain him. It was this apparatus which so shocked Wakefield—even so, during his confinement Norris read many books, and played with his cat; he died of tuberculosis eight months after being released from his chains (Fig. 6).

JOHN TILLY MATTHEWS

Although Norris's plight provoked considerable hostility toward Bethlem, and more particularly toward Haslam, it was John Tilly Matthews who played the most decisive part in Haslam's career. In 1810 Haslam had published a most remarkable book, with an equally remarkable title. *Illustrations of Madness:* "Exhibiting a Singular Case of Insanity, And a No Less Remarkable Difference in Medical Opinions: Developing the Nature of Assailment, And The Manner of Working

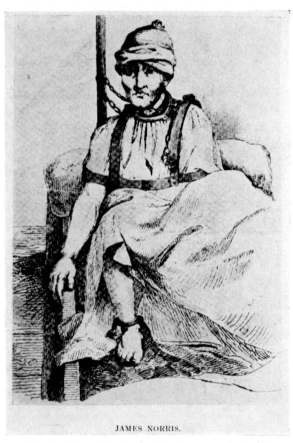

JAMES NORRIS.

FIG. 6.   James Norris, the American seaman, in his
restraining harness.

Events; with A Description of the Tortures Experienced by Bomb-Bursting, Lobster-Cracking, and Lengthening The Brain. Embellished with a Curious Plate. By John Haslam." This was, in effect, the history of John Tilly Matthews, a patient in Bethlem suffering from what would now be called paranoid schizophrenia. The book is the first adequate record of a particular type of mental illness to be published in English, and is a masterpiece of clinical description. Previous case reports had indeed been published, notably by Robinson, Perfect and Pargeter, but they were fragmentary and tedious to read.

Matthews had been admitted to Bethlem on 28 January 1797, but his relatives did not agree that he was mad, and almost at once instituted legal proceedings. These were unsuccessful, Matthews was committed to Bethlem, and in January 1798 was transferred to the "incurable" section of the hospital. In this situation he continued for many years; sometimes an automaton moved by the agency of persons known as Bill the King, Jack the Schoolmaster, or the Glove Lady, at other times by the Emperor of the Whole World. Matthews was a man of some education who had previously been a tea-broker in Leadenhall Street, and he was well able to deceive his family and visitors as to his true state of mind. In 1809 a further legal fracas occurred, two doctors employed by the relatives found Matthews sane, and his release was demanded. Haslam's comments are worth quoting.

> It had been the unvarying opinion of the medical officers of Bethlem Hospital, that Mr. Matthews had been insane from the period of his admission to the present time. Such opinion was not the result of casual investigation; but a conclusion deduced from daily observations during thirteen years. But aware of the fallibility of human judgment, and suspecting that copious experience which sheds the blessings of light upon others, might have kept them in the dark: perhaps startled at the powerful talents, extensive learning, and subtile penetration which had recorded in the face of day the sanity of a man whom they considered as an incurable lunatic: and flinching at an oath contradictory to such high testimony, the medical officers prudently referred the determination of the case to the constituted and best authorities in the kingdom.

For this purpose they assembled a consultation of eminent medical practitioners, who, after a deliberate examination of the patient's mind, decided that Matthews was insane. His relatives once more returned to the attack in 1815, and Haslam was closely questioned about Matthews by the Select Committee. By this time Matthews had been transferred, "for a change of air", to the care of a Mr. Fox, who kept a private house, London House, in Hackney. Half the fees were paid by Bethlem and half by his relatives. Here he soon made himself at home, and when the philanthropic visitors carried out their inspection, was acting as the advising manager on the conduct of the patients, showed them over the place, and told them the case of every patient. He died in 1814. Although he would have been delighted at Haslam's dismissal from Bethlem in 1816, he enjoyed several favours from him. He was taught engraving by one of Haslam's friends, and books and materials were provided for him by Haslam. Matthews' skill with the pen was remarkable, and there is in my possession a manuscript which he executed for Haslam. A handwritten note states that "He could imitate black letter type most beautifully, and I have seen in the possession of the late Sir Anthony Carlisle, a black letter book, a leaf of which having been lost, another was copied from a complete example by Matthews so well as to be indistinguishable from the original type." In addition he was a considerable draughtsman and submitted plans for the new hospital which was to be built. The Governors presented £30 to him as an acknowledgement of his skill and trouble, surely a remarkable tribute to their generosity in dealing with such a formidable trouble-maker as John Tilly Matthews. Haslam was alleged to have conceived a violent animosity toward him. When the patient argued, for instance, that he was being illegally detained, Haslam is said to have replied, "You dispute our authority, (with an oath). Sir, we will soon let you know what our authority is." The next day Matthews is supposed to have been put in irons. Again, when discussing Matthews' case in a coffee-house, Dr. Haslam was supposed to have stated that the man had no right to be in Bethlem. One of Matthews' relatives brought the matter up before the Committee of the hospital, saying "Mr. Haslam, on what grounds can you recommend to the Committee still to persevere in the keeping of Mr. Matthews, after your assertion in the City of London tavern, at such a time, that he was as well as you." Mr. Haslam made no reply to this.

Haslam was minutely questioned by the Select Committee on the care and treatment of both these men, and on his attitude to restraint in general. His replies were not calculated to placate the reformers, for his answers were somewhat arrogant, and in many respects even casual. He had a good opinion of himself, and stated that he was "so much regulated by my own experience, that I have not been disposed to listen to those who had less experience than myself". The thorny question of restraint was treated somewhat cavalierly, and Haslam stoutly maintained that the restraints used at Bethlem were for the patients' own good. To the end of his life he maintained that there was a definite place for restraint in the treatment of psychiatric patients. It is small wonder that Hack Tuke treated him so badly when he wrote that

> Mr. Haslam, the resident apothecary, ruled supreme. He was responsible for the dreadful condition in which the notorious Norris was discovered. "There is," says Sydney Smith, "much evasive testimony, to shift from himself the burden of this atrocious case; but his efforts tend rather to confirm than to shake the conviction which the evidence produces. . . . The conduct of Haslam with respect to several other patients was of a corresponding description; and in the case of a gentleman whose death was evidently accelerated by the severities he underwent, and of several other persons, there is abundant proof of cruelty. . . . It is in proof that a patient actually died through mere neglect, from the bursting of the intestines, overloaded for want of aperient medicine."

O'Donoghue, the chaplain to Bethlem, in his scholarly history of the hospital does not agree. After reading and re-reading the Minutes of Evidence he endorsed the opinion of one of the Governors of the Hospital in Haslam's time, who considered that Haslam had been "sacrificed to public clamour and party spirit". In fact, Haslam had proposed that two adjoining rooms should be set aside for Norris— one for a day-room, the other for his bed; nor did Haslam suggest the iron apparatus in which Norris was confined. Haslam had carried out the system approved by his Governors, introduced many reforms, and had only been absent from the weekly meetings of the sub-committee three times in twenty-one years.

At the close of the enquiry in 1815 Haslam's health had been drunk by the Governors, but soon, particularly after publication of the Report of the Select Committee, there was a change of heart. Bethlem had obviously not come off very creditably, and the House of Commons ominously expressed their desire that the Governors should carefully consider the Report before the annual re-election of the Medical Officers. As a result the Governors ordered "That the Evidence so communicated should be transmitted to each of them, to afford him an opportunity of offering such reasons in his justification as he may see expedient". Monro and Haslam made their reply in a joint paper which was printed and sent round to each of the Governors, under the title "Observations of the Physician and Apothecary of Bethlem Hospital upon the Evidence taken Before the Committee of the Hon. House of Commons For Regulating Mad-Houses". Both men set out dignified answers to the allegations made against them. Monro pointed out that after thirty years he was suddenly charged with undefined offences, and was thereby compelled to frame his own accusations in order to enter upon his defence. Wakefield, in a letter to the newspapers, had made specific charges against him, and in fact had forwarded copies of "his letter" to the Governors. The charges were that Monro had been wanting in humanity toward the patients, had pursued "a course of medical treatment indiscriminate in its application, cruel in itself, useless in my own opinion, and injurious in that of others", and lastly that he had been guilty of neglect in his attendance at the hospital and in the performance of his duties as the physician. These accusations Monro answered without rancour—pointing out that the imposing of restraint was, by the hospital regulations, expressly confided to the apothecary, and that he, Monro, did not question this trust, "or, on light grounds, to presume that the confidence had been abused". As for his treatment of insanity, that had been "handed down to me by my father, and I do not know any better practice".

Haslam's reply was couched in a similar vein, although it is apparent that he was by now regretting some of the things he had said, and the way he had behaved before the Select Committee. His examination by them was, he wrote

> a mode of examination to which I had not been accustomed, but in which, to the best of my judgement, my demeanour was most modest and respectful, to the high authority before which I stood. I often felt extremely pressed, but I sustained it with patience, nor was there a single moment in which I betrayed the slightest irritation.

He proceeds to refute their allegations about the ill-treatment of Norris and Matthews, quoting chapter and verse of his recommendations to the Bethlem Sub-Committee on Norris's care. Unfortunately, Haslam's remarks to the Select Committee on his surgical colleague Bryan Crowther had given rise to considerable adverse comment—for he had said that Crowther was "generally insane and mostly drunk. He was so insane as to have a strait-waistcoat." This had been the case for the last ten years of Crowther's life (and he had died only a month before Haslam gave evidence to the Select Committee). Haslam described to the Governors how Crowther had been for many years his intimate friend until he suffered a "paroxysm" which required restraint, and thenceforth

> the habitudes of his mind became gradually changed, and latterly he grew

suspicious of his former friends, and misinterpreted their motives—for imaginary injuries he was disposed to retaliate with a degree of virulence and severity, quite opposite to his former character. He imagined, for instance, that I had reviewed a book he published, and, notwithstanding every effort I made to convince him to the contrary, by letters and the

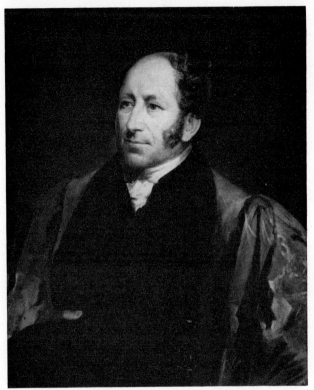

FIG. 7.   Edward Thomas Monro, 1790-1856

most friendly assurances, he continued to pursue me with the rankest hostility."

But the damage had been done, and Haslam was bitterly to regret his evidence before the Select Committee. The Governors did not accept their two doctors' explanations and neither was re-elected. It is of some interest that yet another Monro, however, became Physician to Bethlem, Edward Thomas, son of Thomas Monro (Fig. 7).

H

DISGRACE

At the age of 52 Haslam was cast adrift with no pension but, luckily, still with good friends. This bitter blow saddened Haslam's life, as can be seen from the dedication of one of his last publications to his daughter, which runs thus:

> My dearest Daughter. This Essay on Thought is appropriately dedicated to a lady of whom I am constantly thinking—whose dutiful conduct, and filial affection, have rendered a protracted life the subject of consolation, under all its contingent miseries.

He had forthwith applied for an M.D. from Marischal College, Aberdeen, being sponsored by William Charles Wells, and Alexander Peter Buchan. On 17 September 1816 he received his degree, a special note appearing after his name in the list of graduates, "The usual fortnight's delay dispensed with, Mr. Haslam having already acquired great celebrity by his medical productions." This refers to the regulation in force at the time that no M.D. degree should be granted till the Senatus had taken into consideration the character and qualifications of the candidate at two different meetings held at a fortnight's interval. Both his sponsors were remarkable men, and together with other of Haslam's friends will be referred to later. He set forthwith to establish himself as a physician in London. He experienced some difficulty in complying with the regulations of the College of Physicians, the "Gentlemen of Warwick Lane", to whom he scathingly refers in the introduction to *Illustrations of Madness*, and was only finally admitted a licentiate of the College on 12 April 1824, at the age of 60. The reason for this very late entry into the fold is obscure. But even in 1810, in his *Illustrations of Madness* he had written:

> It is true, a Doctor may be blind, deaf and dumb, stupid or mad, but still his diploma shields him from the imputation of ignorance. It has also not unfrequently occurred, that a man who has been dubbed a Doctor of Medicine at Leyden, Aberdeen, or St. Andrews, and whose Diploma sets forth his profound learning, accomplishments, and competence to practise on the lives of His Majesty's good and faithful subjects, has been found incapable of satisfying the gentlemen in Warwick Lane that he possessed the common rudiments of his profession, and has been by them accordingly rejected: so that learning in many instances appears to be local.

Perhaps this indicates some trouble Haslam had already had with the College, although I can find no evidence for this.

HASLAM'S LIBRARY

The catastrophe of 1816 must have had severe financial implications, for Haslam had to sell his library. Leigh and Sotheby's held a four-day sale of his books on 5 July 1816. The catalogue is of great interest, for it gives a vivid picture of the sources used by Haslam. There were 1167 items, the last two being a "handsome mahogany Bookcase 9 feet 3 inches high, 11 feet wide, 2 feet deep, in two heights with drawers and wardrobe at bottom, enclosed with mahogany doors, the upper part with fast doors", and lot 1167 "A Mahogany Ladder for ditto". The library consisted of "A Curious Collection of Books printed in black letter; Old English History, Tracts etc. relative to London, Facetiae; Old English Poetry and Plays; German, Dutch, Saxon and Northern Literature; Classics; Treatises on Languages; Voyages and Travels, etc. etc." There was one Caxton—Higden's (Ranulph) *Polycronicon*, printed by William Caxton, 1482. The books show the remarkable taste and learning of their owner, and even today the impact of his dismissal on Haslam can be felt by any book lover on reading through the list of volumes he had been forced to sell.

The medical books consisted of 79 items, written in English, German, Latin and French. The psychiatric works include Pinel, *Whytt on Nervous Disorders*, Tuke's *Description of the Retreat*, Cullen's *First Lines*, *Cox on Insanity*, Ferriar's *Medical Histories and Reflections*, *Auenbrugger on Mania Vicorium*, Tryon's *Medical Works*, Perfect's *Annals of Insanity*, Crichton's *Inquiry into the Nature and Origin of Mental Derangement*, Hill's *Essay on Insanity*, Arnold's *Observations on Insanity*, Pargeter's *Observations on Maniacal Disorders*, and Harper's *Treatise on Insanity*. These represent practically the total worthwhile English psychiatric works published during the eighteenth century apart from those of Dr. William Battie. It is not surprising that these are absent, for Battie had attacked Bethlem, and particularly the Monros, in his *Treatise on Madness* published in 1758. Nor however is John Monro's *Remarks on Dr. Battie's Treatise on Madness* present in the list.

The remaining medical volumes include works on anatomy, chemistry, neurology and general medicine. There are several reminders of Haslam's professional life—the *Memoirs of the Life of Thomas Beddoes* by J. E. Stocks, and a collection of tracts by Beddoes and by Watt recall his days at Edinburgh and the dispute between the Governors of the Infirmary and the students. Four volumes by the Buchans point to his friendship with Alexander Peter Buchan, the son of the better known Dr. William Buchan, whose *Domestic Medicine* went into more than a score of editions. A. P. Buchan was one of Haslam's sponsors for the M.D. he received from Marischal College in 1816. He had probably met Haslam whilst studying under the Hunters and Dr. George Fordyce, or at Edinburgh. The second sponsor, a far more distinguished man, was William Charles Wells, author of the well-known *An Essay on Dew*, but none of his works appears in Haslam's library. Wells was a man somewhat similar in nature to Haslam, devoted to his profession, a profound thinker, very warm hearted and generous, yet irascible and somewhat eccentric. In spite of attainments which Sir Benjamin Brodie considered placed him well above contemporary physicians, he was never a success in practice.

"OBSERVATIONS ON INSANITY, WITH PRACTICAL REMARKS ON THE DISEASE AND AN ACCOUNT OF THE MORBID APPEARANCES ON DISSECTION" 1798

Haslam's first book had appeared in 1798, and was entitled *Observations on Insanity*, "with Practical Remarks on the Disease and an Account of the Morbid Appearances on Dissection". It was an immediate success, a second edition appearing with the title changed to *Observations on Madness and Melancholy*, "including Practical Remarks on the disease, and an account of the morbid appearance on dissection". A German translation was published in 1800. Haslam's observations were widely quoted, particularly in works on Forensic Medicine, and his name became well known both in America and Europe. The reason is not far to seek, for the English psychiatric writings of the eighteenth century were either tedious, second hand, or anecdotal. Haslam had a remarkably easy style and a facility for clear thought and writing. His particular interest in etymology, shown by the large number of books in his library on this subject, led him to consider his language some-what more carefully than the average medical writer of this period, and he begins his first book by defining his terms. The first question he deals with is the then current division of mental disorders into mania and melancholy, to which he was strongly opposed. His experiences at Bethlem convinced him that they were *only phases of a single disorder*. He described the signs and symptoms encountered in both states more clearly than any previous writer. Then follow excellent descriptions of the types of memory defect which occur in psychiatric patients, and an account of schizophrenia which is of much historical significance. Both Pick and Zelmanowits have given Haslam priority in the recognition of the simple dementing form of schizophrenia—described in Haslam's own words as follows.

> Connected with loss of memory, there is a form of insanity which occurs in young persons; and, as far as these cases have been the subject of my observation, they have been more frequently noticed in females. Those whom I have seen, have been distinguished by prompt capacity and lively disposition: and in general have become the favourites of parents and tutors, by their facility in acquiring knowledge, and by a prematurity of attainment. This disorder commences about, or shortly after, the period of menstruation, and in many instances has been unconnected with hereditary taint; as far as could be ascertained by minute enquiry. The attack is almost imperceptible; some months usually elapse, before it becomes the subject of particular notice; and fond relatives are frequently deceived by the hope that it is only an abatement of excessive vivacity, conducing to a prudent reserve, and steadiness of character. A degree of apparent thoughtfulness and inactivity precede, together with a diminution of the ordinary curiosity, concerning that which is passing before them; and they therefore neglect those objects and pursuits which formerly proved sources of delight and instruction. The sensibility appears to be considerably blunted; they do not bear the same affection towards their parents and relations; they become unfeeling to kindness, and careless of reproof. To their companions they show a cold civility, but take no interest whatever in their concerns. If they read a book, they are unable to give any account of its contents: sometimes with steadfast eyes, they will dwell for an hour on one page, and then turn over a number in a few minutes. It is very difficult to persuade them to write, which most readily develops their state of mind: much time is consumed and little produced. The subject is repeatedly begun, but they seldom advance beyond a sentence or two; the orthography becomes puzzling, and by endeavouring to adjust the spelling, the subject vanishes. As their apathy increases they are negligent of their dress, and inattentive to personal cleanliness. Frequently they seem to experience transient impulses of passion, but these have no source in sentiment; the tears which trickle down at one time, are as unmeaning as the loud laugh which succeeds them; and it often happens that a momentary gust of anger, with its attendant invectives, ceases before the threat can be concluded. As the disorder increases, the urine and faeces are passed without restraint, and from the indolence which accompanies it, they generally become corpulent. Thus in the interval between

puberty and manhood, I have painfully witnessed this hopeless and degrading change, which in a short time has transformed the most promising and vigorous intellect into a slavering and bloated idiot.

Could there be a more concise account of what became known as dementia praecox?

Haslam next describes the appearances of the brain in thirty-seven autopsies performed at Bethlem, and it is on these clinico-pathological case histories that Haslam has been judged the discoverer of general paralysis of the insane. A close study of this section and of his other writings shows that this is almost certainly incorrect. Despite the brevity of the case reports, such is Haslam's clarity that the diagnosis can be made within the framework of present-day classification—alcoholics, melancholics, puerperal psychotics, and schizophrenics march through the pages. Case XV is the only example of what might be considered to be the clinical picture of general paralysis. It will be described fully when we come to review the early history of general paralysis. He concludes the essentially clinical part of his work by a description of three insane children. The first developed convulsions following vaccination, at the age of two and a half, and became demented—no doubt an example of post-vaccinal encephalitis. (One of the most refreshing aspects of Haslam's writings is the clarity of the clinical descriptions, and the resultant possibility of today making a clear-cut diagnosis.) The second was a high-grade defective, and the third was a child who, at the age of two, had become over-active, aggressive and destructive. In spite of much personal attention the child had continued to be distractible and violent—so that when Haslam examined him at the age of ten

> on the first interview I had with him, he contrived, after two or three minutes' acquaintance, to break a window and tear the frill of my shirt. He was an unrelenting foe to all china, glass, and crockery ware, whenever they came within his reach he shivered them instantly . . . to tear lace and destroy the finer textures of female ornament, seemed to gratify him exceedingly . . . the most singular part of his character was, that he appeared incapable of forming a friendship with any one: he felt no considerations for sex, and would as readily kick or bite a girl as a boy.

One of the most important sections of the book is Haslam's review of the statistics of Bethlem. From 1748 to 1794, a period of forty-six years, 4,832 women and 4,042 men had been admitted to the hospital.

Haslam analysed both the discharge rate for the two sexes and the prognosis with regard to age of onset and the duration of the disorder. He showed that mania is more apt to remit than melancholy, and that when frequent swings of mood occur, the prognosis is correspondingly poor. Epileptic deterioration, "religious madness", and the prognosis of "paralytic disorders" are all discussed. In passing he cannot refrain from a dig at the Rev. Francis Willis, and from an outburst against Methodism, to which he was obliged for "the supply of these numerous cases which has constituted my experience of this wretched calamity". One of Haslam's characteristics was his occasional lapse into a some-what coarse and biting comment on the subject at large—a character-istic which appeared in his evidence before the Select Committee, and which was to do him much harm. Another example occurs in the following passage from his statistical review—

Whether it be that we have more mad persons in England than in other countries, and thereby have derived a greater experience of this calamity; or, whether the greater number of receptacles we possess for the insane, and the emoluments which have resulted from this species of farming, have led persons to speculate more particularly on the nature and treat-ment of this affection, may be difficult to determine. Dr. Pinel[1] allows the reputation we have acquired; but, with a laudable curiosity, is desirous to understand how we became possessed of it (Fig. 8).

"Is it," he says, "from a peculiar national pride, and to display their superiority over other nations, that the English boast of their ability in curing madness by moral remedies; and at the same time conceal the cunning of this art with an impenetrable veil? or, on the contrary, may not that which we attribute to a subtile policy, be merely the effect of circum-stances; and, is it not necessary to distinguish the steps of the English empirics from the methods of treatment adopted in their public hospitals?

"Whatever solutions may be given to these questions, yet, after fifteen years' diligent enquiry, in order to ascertain some of the leading features of this method, from the reports of travellers; the accounts published of such establishments; the notices concerning their public and private receptacles, which are to be found in the different journals, or in the works of their medical writers, I can affirm, that I have never been able to dis-cover any development of this English secret for the treatment of insanity, though all concur in the ability of their management. Speaking of Dr. Willis,[2] it is said, that sweetness and affability seem to dwell upon his

[1] *Traité Médico-Philosophique sur l'Aliénation Mentale*, 8vo. Paris, An. 9, p. 47.
[2] The late Reverend Dr. Willis.

countenance; but its character changes the moment he looks on a patient: the whole of his features suddenly assume a different aspect, which enforces respect and attention from the insane. His penetrating eye appears to

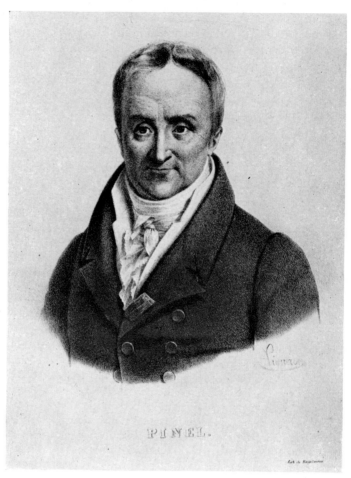

FIG. 8.   Philippe Pinel, 1745–1826.

search into their hearts, and arrest their thoughts as they arise. Thus he establishes a dominion, which is afterwards employed as a principal agent of cure. But, where is the elucidation of these general principles to be sought; and, in what manner are they to be applied according to the character, varieties, and intensity of madness? Is the work of Dr. Arnold otherwise remarkable than as a burdensome compilation, or a multiplication of scholastic divisions, more calculated to retard than advance the progress of Science? Does Dr. Harper, who announces in his preface, that he has quitted the beaten track, fulfil his promise in the course of his work? and is his section on mental indications any thing but a prolix commentary on the doctrines of the ancients? The adventurous spirit of Dr. Crichton, may justly excite admiration, who has published two volumes on maniacal and melancholic affections, merely on the authority of some observations drained from a German Journal; together with ingenious dissertations on the doctrines of modern physiologists, and a view of the moral and physical effects of the human passions. Finally, can a mere advertisement of Dr. Fowler's establishment for the insane in Scotland, throw any light on the particular management of such persons, although it profess the purest and most dignified humanity, successfully operating on the moral treatment of madness?"

Dr. Pinel is deserving of considerable credit for directing the attention of medical men to this very important point of the moral management of the insane. I have also heard much of this fascinating power which the mad doctor is said to possess over the wayward lunatic; but, from all I have observed amongst the eminent practitioners of the present day, who exercise this department of the profession, I am led to suspect, that, although this influence may have been formerly possessed, and even to the extent attributed to the late reverend doctor, it ought now to be lamented among the artes deperditae. Could the attention of lunatics be fixed, and could they be reduced to obedience, by

> Strong impression and strange powers which lie
> Within the magic circle of the eye,

all other kinds of restraint would be superfluous and unnecessarily severe. But the fact is notoriously otherwise. Whenever the doctor visits a violent or mischievous maniac, however controlling his physiognomy, such patient is always secured by the straight waistcoat; and it is, moreover, thought expedient to afford him the society of one or more keepers.

It has, on some occasions, occurred to me to meet with gentlemen who have imagined themselves eminently gifted with this awful imposition of the eye, but the result has never been satisfactory; for, although I have entertained the fullest confidence of any relation, which such gentlemen might afterwards communicate concerning the success of the experiment, I have never been able to persuade them to practise this rare talent tête-à-tête with a furious lunatic.

However Dr. Pinel may be satisfied of our superiority in this respect, it is but decorous to return the compliment, and if any influence were to be gained over maniacal patients by assumed importance, protracted staring, or a mimicry of fierceness, I verily believe that such pantomime would be much better performed in Paris than in London.

As might be expected from a man with so much practical experience of insanity, Haslam's account of the management of patients is excellently drawn. First

> he who pretends to regulate the conduct of such patients, should first have learned the management of himself. It should be the great object of the superintendent to gain the confidence of the patient, and to awaken in him respect and obedience; but it will readily be seen, that such confidence, obedience and respect can only be procured by superiority of talents, discipline of temper, and dignity of manner,

—all fundamentals of pyschiatric practice. Haslam continues—"by gentleness of manner and kindness of treatment, I have seldom failed to obtain the confidence and conciliate the esteem of insane persons". So much for the evil man portrayed by Tuke, this man who for fourteen years had been "daily in the habit of visiting a very considerable number of madmen, and of mixing indiscriminately among them, without ever having received a blow or personal insult".

His last chapter is concerned with therapy, which ranges from bleeding to cold bathing. He devised an instrument for forced feeding which enabled the keeper to carry out each feed without knocking out a tooth, but apart from this invention, Haslam's therapeusis is undistinguished (Fig. 9). Indeed, the reader is left with the impression that medicine had little to offer the lunatic, moral management being of far greater importance.

The *Observations* is a most outstanding piece of work, surpassing in merit any previous publication both in England or on the continent. The works of previous English psychiatrists—most of whom were represented in Haslam's library—were based on Celsus, Paulus Aeginatus or Cullen. Haslam's book stands alone in its clarity and in the excellence of the clinical descriptions, based as they were on a daily and intimate acquaintance with mental disorder.

His next publication was *Illustrations of Madness*, which appeared in 1810, and to which reference has already been made. Then came a gap until he was dismissed from office. The catastrophe proved a spur to his pen, for he published four books in the period 1816–1820. The first was entitled *Considerations on the Moral Management of Insane Persons* and appeared in 1817.

"THE MORAL MANAGEMENT OF
INSANE PERSONS" (1817)

The outcry of the non-restraint school and the parliamentary enquiries had made "moral management" an issue of the day, and no subject could have been more topical. Haslam wastes no time in stating his view that some form of restraint is necessary during the active phase

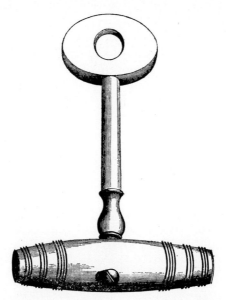

FIG. 9.   "In those cases, where patients have been obstinately bent on starving themselves, or where they have become determined to resist the introduction of remedies calculated for their relief, I have always been enabled to convey both into their stomachs, at any time, and in any quantity that might be necessary, by the employment of an instrument, of which the figure and dimensions are here given." (Reduced by one-half.)

of both the manic and depressive illnesses. "It is in the passive state of both forms of this disease where moral discipline can be most effectually administered." He then passes on to consider confinement, coercion, keepers, "the distribution of insane persons into classes", diminished sensibility of the insane, involuntary passage of faeces and urine, forcing of food and medicine, and the occupation and amusement of the insane. In other words, his book is concerned with the practical management of mental patients. He points out that some form of restraint is necessary to prevent certain types of patients from injuring themselves or others. Restraint may actually contribute to the cure of insanity at times as a practical example of that self-control which forms so large a part of mental action. His remarks on the keepers, or as we would call them today the mental nurses, strike a modern note, for he laments the poor status and working conditions of these much-maligned individuals. The dangerous and thankless tasks they undertook as often as not rendered them more liable to abuse than to gratitude. He suggests that a pension scheme should be started, and that a very careful supervision, indeed education, should be undertaken by the physician under whom they work. Details of the general medical care of lunatics include careful attention to bowels and bladder, adequate feeding and the provision of work and relaxation. In all, the book is a fair and judicious statement of the care of lunatics at that time. Like so many moderate opinions, it was to be overshadowed by the enthusiasms and over-statements of the non-restraint school of psychiatrists.

"MEDICAL JURISPRUDENCE AS IT RELATES TO INSANITY ACCORDING TO THE LAW OF ENGLAND" (1817)

This, his next book, was second only in importance to his *Observations on Insanity*. It is the first work on forensic psychiatry in English.

English law had not recognized insanity as a defence until the beginning of the fourteenth century, the influence of demonology successfully militating against any rational treatment of the insane. Fitzherbert, writing early in the sixteenth century, did not consider insanity as a defence at law, although he wrote,

> He who is of unsound Memory, hath not any Manner of Discretion; for if he kill a Man, it shall not be Felony, nor Murder, nor he shall not forfeit his lands or goods for the same, because it appeareth that he hath not Discretion; for if he had Discretion he should be hanged for the Same, as an Infant who is of the age of Discretion, who committeth Murder or Felony, shall be hanged for the Same.

Fitzherbert did not state exactly what he meant by "Discretion". Lord Hale (1609–1676) was the first to distinguish between "total insanity", excusing criminal responsibility, and partial insanity, which did not. He laid down that

> the moon hath a great influence in all diseases of the brain, especially in this kind of dementis: such persons, commonly in the full and change of the moon, especially about the equinoxes and summer solstice, are usually at the higher of their distemper—but such persons as have their lucid intervals (which ordinarily happens between the full and change of the moon) in such intervals have usually at least a competent use of reason.

The common law, as expounded by Blackstone, recognized two types of psychiatric patients, "the idiot, or natural fool", and the lunatic, or *non compos mentis*, who by disease, grief or other accident had lost the use of reason. Moreover—a lunatic

> is indeed properly one that hath lucid intervals; sometimes enjoying his senses, and sometimes not, and that frequently depending upon the change of the moon. But, under the general name of *non compos mentis* are comprised not only lunatics, but persons under frenzies, or who lose their intellects by disease; those that grow deaf, dumb, and blind, not being born so; or such, in short as are judged by the court of chancery incapable of conducting their own affairs.

Judged by the state of psychiatric knowledge at that time, the law was sound, and reflected the current medical opinions. However, the madness of George III, and the attempt made to kill the King in 1800, awakened public interest in the legal aspects of insanity (Fig. 10). At Hatfield's trial a new principle was introduced into law by Lord Erskine, a brilliant criminal lawyer defending the accused. In his address to the jury, he stressed that "Delusion, therefore, where there is no frenzy or raving madness, is the true character of insanity". In later life Erskine considered that the delusion must be connected with the act if it is to be admitted as a defence.

As a result of Hatfield's trial, a new Act was passed through Parliament—"The Insane Offenders Act". Previously when a prisoner had been acquitted on the grounds of insanity, owing to lack of suitable provision for the care of the criminally insane, he was often set free. This Act laid down that a criminal lunatic should be "detained during His Majesty's pleasure", but as the Act had been passed so hurriedly, there was no place of detention for such persons. The Governors of Bethlem were approached, but not until 1816 was a ward set aside for the "criminal lunatics". Here, incidentally, they remained until Broadmoor was completed and ready for occupation in 1863. In fact, even

before 1816 many criminal lunatics found their way to Bethlem—
Hatfield lived there for forty-nine years. Walsh, a naval mutineer, and
Barnett, who had attempted to shoot Miss Frances Kelly, a popular
actress of the day with whom Charles Lamb had fallen in love, were
also inhabitants of Bethlem for many years.

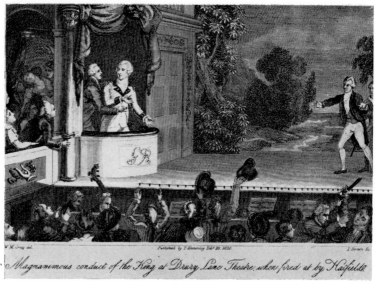

FIG. 10.   The attempted assassination of George III at Drury Lane
in 1800 by James Hatfield.

The medical men connected with Bethlem were therefore excellently
situated for a study of medico–legal problems. Haslam opened his
book by remarking that

> The consideration, that in our own language, no work existed on the
> subject of Medical Jurisprudence, as it relates solely to Insanity, urged me
> to the present performance. . . . The following sheets are addressed to the
> readers of different pursuits, law and medicine,

and he is quick to stress that his intention is certainly not to encroach
on the lawyers' province. Rather is his purpose to portray for the
lawyer a clear picture of "the general phenomena of disordered intellect, and the criteria of insanity", and for the doctor, to give an
account of what is likely to be expected of him when giving evidence

as to mental state. Somewhat bitterly, owing to his own chastening experience before the Select Committee of the House of Commons, he writes that he had also intended to submit to the public "the consideration of insanity in a political view", in order to emphasize the need for a bill to protect the insane, and

> as insanity is a disease, by the unanimous concurrence of physicians, most certainly to be remedied at the commencement of the attack; it ought to be a leading object with those who possess the power to legislate, to afford every facility to the medical attendant, that he may have early access to the treatment of this malady.

This enterprise was unfortunately never accomplished.

Haslam recognized at once that the obscure and difficult terminology of psychiatry had little place in a Court of Law.

> The technical language of the learned professions is commonly enveloped in mysterious obscurity:—persons for the most part acquire names without investigating their force and legitimate import; and currently employ them rather from habit than comprehension: it has therefore been my anxious endeavour to scrutinize words of important meaning, and to convey the manifestations of mind and the symptoms of disease, by expressions generally understood, and emancipated from the thraldom of professional nomenclature.

The medical man must realize that he has to convince the jury of the accused's insanity, he "has not to palm on the court the trash of medical hypothesis as the apology for crime". Above all he must be able to defend his opinion under cross-examination. The physician comes to court not merely to give his opinion but to explain it, and to give his reasons for it. The lamentable behaviour of psychiatrists in the witness-box today would not be so frequent a spectacle if these simple facts were complied with. The judge must be impressed, and the jury convinced by the doctors evidence; it must always be remembered that they are lay people. Haslam, too, realized that it was important to consider the state of "popular feeling and intelligence concerning madness" among the generality of persons. Lay concepts of insanity were then, as they are now, not very easily removed or altered, and were mostly derived from stage or literary madmen, or from visits to Bethlem. "To impress ordinary persons with the existence of insanity, some prominent and strongly marked features are absolutely required."

Delusional insanity, or melancholia, are particularly difficult to understand, and to explain them in simple language will be a most important function for the doctor in court. But then what of the very important questions of good and evil, right and wrong, which prosecuting counsel invariably raises?

> If it should be presumed that any medical practitioner is able to penetrate into the recesses of a lunatic's mind, at the moment he committed an outrage; to view the internal play of obtruding thoughts, and contending motives—and to depose that he knew the Good and Evil, Right and Wrong he was about to commit, it must be confessed that such knowledge is beyond the limits of our attainment.

It is sufficient for the doctor to state that the accused's mind is deranged, and that his insanity will be sufficient to account for those actions which, in a sound mind, would be deemed criminal. As for the rationality of lunatics, Haslam realized how easy it is for the lay or inexperienced observer to be confused on this topic—few are mad in every aspect of their being, but none the less "the map of his mind will point out that the smallest rivulet flows into the great stream of his derangement". A radical perversion of the intellect is the basis of this delusional insanity, and the psychiatrist must demonstrate this to the jury in such a manner as to convince them that here in court is a man bereft of reason.

Then again there are some cases of sudden paroxysmal bouts of fury accompanied by a retrospective amnesia which are important legally. Whatever their provenance, the altered state of consciousness during these paroxysms is sufficient to render a person immune from the legal consequences of his actions during such periods. Haslam described the case of a very powerful man, in his youth subject to epileptic attacks and to intervals of sullen abstraction which increased after the epileptic fits had subsided. He became suddenly "furious, and during the transports of his disorder destroyed two children and a woman; for this act there appeared to be no motive". During many years of confinement in Bethlem Haslam had constant opportunities of seeing him and questioning him. The patient always persisted that he had no recollection whatever of his act. The many paroxysms Haslam witnessed were always accompanied by an amnesia, and although the man was blooded during one paroxysm, he had no memory of this, or of the people then about him. Haslam is certainly the first to have drawn

attention to the importance of this type of epilepsy in relation to crime
and responsibility.

The second part of his treatise is devoted to consideration of "that
morbid condition of intellect which requires the interposition of the
law to protect the person and property of the party so affected". Again
Haslam stresses the importance of the jury, and the necessity of the
jury system in view of the conflicting opinions expressed by medical
gentlemen who have devoted their lives to the study of insanity.
Haslam would have had little time for the panel of experts. Similarly,
he condemns the lawyers who introduce phrases such as "unsound
mind", without clearly defining them; there can be only three states
of the human mind: "Sound Mind, Insanity, and Idiotcy". Different
degrees of these states, of course exist, but the law ought clearly to
recognize these three mental states and nothing more. The snags and
pitfalls inherent in the assessment of sound mind, insanity or idiocy
are then explored, Haslam defining his terms and giving a succinct
account of the problems. He devotes a little attention to the hoary
problem of the "lucid interval". According to the legal interpretation
of lunacy, a person in a "lucid interval" would be fully responsible
for his acts. But Haslam pointed out that the term "interval" had not
been defined, and was extremely indefinite. Moreover, "as a constant
observer of this disease for more than twenty-five years, I cannot
affirm that the lunatics with whom I have had daily intercourse, have
manifested these alternations of insanity and reason". They may at
times become quieter or more tranquil and less inclined to talk, but
their distempered notions remain. The volume ends somewhat
abruptly, with a short account of testamentary capacity to which little
could be added today. Haslam insists throughout on frequent examinations of the patient, enquiry into family history, and a particular
note of the patient's writings. The lucid, sensible, modest and yet
knowledgeable way in which the book was written led to its immediate
acceptance as an authority.

The first book in English of any magnitude or value with regard to
forensic medicine had appeared in 1816. *An Epitome of Juridical or
Forensic Medicine; for the use of Medical Men, Coroners, and Barristers*, was
written by George Edward Male, a Physician to the General Hospital,
Birmingham. The section on Insanity is almost entirely based on
Haslam's *Observations on Insanity* and on his *Illustrations of Madness*.
The next important date in forensic medicine is 1823, when two books

I

appeared, one in America, written by Theodric Romeyn Beck, entitled *Elements of Medical Jurisprudence*, and a three-volume work
published in London, *Medical Jurisprudence*, by J. A. Paris, M.D., and
J. S. M. Fonblanque, Barrister-at-Law. Haslam is extensively quoted in
both books, Beck's chapter on insanity in particular being largely
derived from Haslam's works. It is strange, therefore, that Prichard
makes no mention of the *Medical Jurisprudence* in his book *On the
Different Forms of Insanity in Relation to Jurisprudence*, which appeared in
1843. But Prichard was a xenophil and practically every reference he
quotes is either French, German or American. He did scant justice to
Haslam, who was still active, and although by now 80 had read a paper
before the Society for Improving the Condition of the Insane in the
same year. The title of this paper shows that the legal problems of
insanity still interested him—"An Attempt to Institute the Correct
Discrimination Between Crime and Insanity". Haslam suggested that
it might be desirable to send patients or delinquents before trial to
Bethlem Hospital, "where the state of their minds might be accurately
ascertained, and veraciously reported". For this purpose a section of
Bethlem would be set aside, and the courts would then have the
advantage of carefully considered and disinterested opinion. In the
same year the famous Five Questions were put to the Fifteen Judges of
England, and as a result the McNaghten Rules were formulated. In
spite of what Haslam had so clearly written in 1817 on Good and Evil,
Right and Wrong, the concept of defect of reason, and of right and
wrong prevails.

Haslam's book, as we have seen, gained wide acceptance. His tract
on Medical Jurisprudence was reprinted in a compendium published
in America in 1819 by Thomas Cooper, M.D., Professor of Chemistry
and Mineralogy in the University of Pennsylvania, which had a wide
circulation. *Cooper's Tracts* included Haslam's work, *Farr's Elements
of Medical Jurisprudence*, *Dease's Remarks on Medical Jurisprudence*, and
Male's Epitome. In spite of, or perhaps because of this, Haslam's study
did not reach another edition, but in a rare tract in my possession,
published in 1823 when Haslam was 59, he returned to the attack.
Entitled "A letter to the Right Honourable the Lord Chancellor on
the Nature and Interpretation of Unsoundness of Mind and Imbecility
o1Intellect", he re-iterates several of the points he made in his original
work. The occasion for this pamphlet was the Commission held to
enquire into Lord Portsmouth's sanity in 1822, and a previous Com-

mission in 1814. Some eminent physicians had testified that his lordship was sane, others that he was insane, and the Lord Chancellor had delivered a judgment which aroused Haslam's indignation, largely because it conflicted with the opinions he had expressed in his book on *Sound Mind*. This seems to have been somewhat of a favourite with him; published in 1819 it was to be his last important work.

"SOUND MIND; OR, CONTRIBUTIONS TO THE NATURAL HISTORY AND PHYSIOLOGY OF THE HUMAN INTELLECT" (1819)

The method was analytic

> the mind of every rational person may be considered as an elaboratory, wherein he may conduct psychological experiments; he is enabled to analyse his own acquirement, and if he be sufficiently attentive, he may note its formation and progress in his children; and thus trace the accumulation of knowledge, from the dawn of infancy to the meridian of manhood.

Starting from a simple consideration of perception and its relation to consciousness which he regards as "the knowledge we possess of our own personal identity", Haslam leads on to memory, for perception and consciousness, without the adjunct of memory, are by themselves inefficient and useless. Memory shows two very curious phenomena; first, many of the transactions of childhood appear to be wholly obliterated, and second, they may be "accidentally revived by our being placed in the situation which originally gave them birth". These preliminary pages are then followed by a longer passage on Speech, Language, and the Hand. Haslam points out how greatly man has advanced by the possession of his hand with its powerful thumb, and how important is the connection between speech and the hand. He uses his concept of the body image to illustrate how many standards of measurement have been derived from the human body, and how geographical terms too have a root in the terms of anatomy. In the section on language Haslam demonstrates his knowledge of what he calls "the Northern Group of Languages". As the sale of his library showed, etymology ranked high amongst his interests, and he criticizes Dr. Johnson for several mistaken or false derivations which are given in the famous dictionary. He repeats his view that "all the terms which designate the faculties and operations of our minds, are of physical origin, as well as those which characterize the thinking or immaterial principle itself".

Will or Volition is the next subject. He proceeds to discuss the development of will "from the dawn to the meridian"; the baby, "that helpless mass of animation", at first appears to have no voluntary control, but as perception grows, so likewise does volition. With language "our perceptions become doubly aimed, and impress the memory with additional effect: the employment of the term as the representative of the object, recalls the original perception, and thus invests the mental phantasm with a local habitation and a name". Thus our earliest recollections are never anterior to a certain progress in the art of speech. Man is gifted with few instincts, and these appear to decline as his reason advances. This relative freedom from instinctual dominance arises as a result of his acquisition of "will", and is the reason why man has attained his present stature. Man is the architect of his own mind, animals, although wonderfully composed, lack the qualities of reflection and of language. In man, the act of thought or reflection stems directly from perceptions.

MINOR WORKS

In 1818 there appeared his apologia, "A Letter to the Governors of Bethlem Hospital". He explains that "considering the uncertainty of life, until I had communicated some opinions on professional subjects which had long occupied my reflections" he had delayed the publication of his narrative. The lapse of time had given him scope for reflection and enabled him to present his address to the Governors in a manner free from rancour. But his duty to himself, to his children, and to the medical profession required that a true account of his dismissal be presented to the public. In the following 58 pages he proceeds to give a good account of himself, and to show quite conclusively how unjustly he had been treated, "sacrificed to public clamour and party spirit", and cast adrift without a pension, whilst the late hospital porter, "a shattered victim of gin and paralysis, basks in the sunshine of a pension". James Tilly Matthews figures prominently as Haslam's evil genius. It was he who furnished the Parliamentary Committee with a manuscript the contents of which formed the basis of the cross-examination of Haslam and of the other servants of Bethlem. Matthews had often threatened to make his manuscript public and, "pluming himself on the retaliation he could make for the supposed injuries he had received, he read to me the greater part of it". Haslam admits that here he made a fundamental mistake when he

> conceived that its circulation ought not to be prevented, on the presumption, that there existed in the judgment of those who passed for persons of sound mind, a sufficient disrelish for absurdity, to enable them to discriminate the transactions of daylight, from the materials of a dream.

In fact the document was to be Haslam's downfall, for there seems to have been sufficient truth in it concerning the mismanagement of Bethlem. Although there is no suspicion from any material I have read of any incompetence by Haslam, Haslam himself in this "Letter to the Governors" provides a dreadful indictment of Bethlem during the time he was Apothecary. The surgeon often drunk, the matron careless, the keepers profligate, gin sodden and venal, and the steward incompetent! Haslam claimed that he was powerless to act, the authority residing with the Governors, but there is no evidence that he tried to remedy such glaring abuses. He was essentially a clinician, and the gulf between clinical practice and administration can at times be impossible to bestride.

At the age of 71, Haslam published a pamphlet "On the Nature of Thought, or the Act of Thinking and its connexion with a perspicuous sentence", in which he repeats some of the arguments he put forward in *Sound Mind*. The tenor of the argument is now more religious, frequent reference being made to the "Supreme Artificer", but there is very little difference in its main theme. Thought is effected by the selection and arrangement of words, each of which has a definite meaning, and is capable of being used in a variety of combinations. The act of thinking Haslam considers "becomes unfolded in the progressive formation of a perspicuous sentence".

In 1843, when he was 79, Haslam read his last three papers before the Society for Improving the Condition of the Insane. This Society had been founded by Sir Alexander Morison and the Earl of Shaftesbury in 1842, most probably as a reaction to the extreme "non-restraint" school. The more conservative psychiatrists wished to show that psychiatry was not all "non-restraint", and the society numbered, among its medical members, Haslam, Monro, Sutherland and Burrows. Prizes for essays, and premiums for meritorious service by attendants were offered in an endeavour to improve the status of both psychiatry and mental nursing. The papers Haslam presented were "On Restraint and Coercion", "An Attempt to Institute the Correct Discrimination between Crime and Insanity" and "On the Increase of Insanity, with an Endeavour to detect the Causes of its Multiplication".

In the first essay he returns to his views on the necessity for some type of restraint; in the second he pleads that criminals be examined before their trial by a psychiatrist, preferably at Bethlem Hospital, so that the state of their minds could be accurately assessed. Having got into his stride, the old hard-hitting Haslam re-appears for a moment when he writes of the "pretence and imposture of non-restraint". In his last essay, he attempts to discover the reason for the increase in insanity—rejecting intemperance, or political causes, and maintaining that it is because patients are discharged from hospital too soon.

> If these persons are prematurely liberated under the presumption that they are cured, both women and men return to their husbands and wives, fully competent to transmit this disease to the offspring that may ensue from the more frequent intercourse that naturally results, and from the same causes those who are single require but little persuasion to the altar.

Throughout his career Haslam had been impressed by the genetic aspects of mental disorder, and although he was not in a position to investigate the subject fully, he had always expressed his belief in the importance of what is now called eugenics. Born into the great era of the gentleman, Haslam was no doubt somewhat autocratic, and indeed arrogant, and in these three essays this spirit reasserts itself, and he has a last, dying fling at the new-fangled school of psychiatrists, gentler and more liberal than those of his day. These were his last works, for the next year, in July 1844, he died.

SKETCHES IN BEDLAM

In 1823 there appeared a curious publication *Sketches in Bedlam*: "or characteristic traits of insanity, as displayed in the cases of one hundred and forty patients of both sexes, now, or recently, confined in New Bethlem". The author went under the title of "a Constant Observer", and it was quite obvious that he was, or had been very recently, on the staff of the hospital. The tone of the book is coarse, the disclosure of individual case histories unethical, so that it was small wonder that the Governors were outraged. To obtain an injunction would no doubt promote the sale of the book, as the Governors had bitterly experienced in 1817 when dealing with William Lawrence's book *Physiology, Zoology, and Natural History of Man*. At a special meeting at Bridewell on 16 July, and at Bethlem on 19 July, the Governors recorded their displeasure.

> Resolved that the publication entitled *Sketches in Bedlam* contains statements of the cases of several patients, the greater part of which are false and erroneous: that such statements are drawn up in almost every instance with unfeeling levity, in many cases with considerable inhumanity and in most with gross indecency; that the information conveyed to the public of the private history of the patients and their relatives, together with copies of their suppressed letters presents an abuse of confidence in some quarter: that the several statements of the cases of the criminal patients, both as to the crimes with which they are charged, and also as to their deportment in the hospital, are detailed in an equally offensive way: in addition to which there appeared printed various extracts from the hospital visiting book with the signatures of the persons making such entries; and the committee is of opinion, on the whole, that the work in question is disgraceful to the writer, and disgusting to the reader, displaying an inexcusable violation of the confidences of the governors in some person, who is, or has been, under their employ, and manifesting the most unkind and improper feeling towards the unhappy patients and their friends in making the public parties to their private history, their mental affliction, and their personal infirmities.

The calumny spread around that the "Constant Observer" was John Haslam. In the library of the Maudsley Hospital is John Conolly's copy of the book, with a note made in pencil by Conolly that Dr. Hood, physician to Bethlem from 1852 to 1862, believed that Haslam was the author. The story has persisted—certainly amongst booksellers—to the present day.

O'Donoghue "puzzled over the secret of the authorship" for many years, until he came across the records of the two meetings at Bridewell and Bethlem. In these "Dr. Wright, the resident apothecary, stated that a "late keeper, James Smyth" had "verbally and by letter" avowed himself the author of the book. He refused, however, to produce the letter which (as he alleged) he had received from Smyth, and he declared that he had kept no copy of the letter which he professed to have sent in reply to the former attendant. The suspicions of the committee had by this time been thoroughly aroused, and they made an effort to secure a personal interview with Smyth, to ascertain if he

was the "Constant Observer": Smyth, however, "respectfully declined
to attend". O'Donoghue, who was a most careful historian, considered
that he had solved the problem, and that Haslam, of whom he writes
affectionately, was not the author. Examination of the handwriting of
a dedication from the author of *Sketches in Bedlam* by a handwriting
expert shows that Haslam's writing was quite different, and the suggestion which I put forward in a previous publication that Haslam was in
fact the author of this book must therefore be disregarded in the light
of the later handwriting analysis.[1] But the secret of the writer's identity
still remains hidden.

HASLAM AND THE DISCOVERY OF GENERAL PARALYSIS

Numerous writers have stated that Haslam "discovered" General
Paralysis of the Insane. Bucknill and Tuke in 1879 wrote, "it would
appear that [although] Haslam first described the disease, [he] did not
name it. Calmeil who followed the English Psychologist gave it a
name and got the honour of the discovery." Tuke in 1882 wrote, "If
Haslam may seem to have stumbled upon General Paralysis, we may
well accord to French alienists the merit of having really discovered
the disorder which, in our department, is the most fascinating, as it has
formed the most prominent object of the research during the last forty
years." Robertson, writing in 1922, awarded the palm to Haslam, a
view with which Zilboorg concurred.

On what are these statements based? Zelmanowits in 1953 cited the
precise pages of Haslam's books where a description of the disease
could be found.

> The description first appeared in the *Observations on Insanity* 1798, on
> page 120. . . . In the second edition of this work, published in 1809 and
> re-christened *Observations on Madness and Melancholy* it is found enlarged,
> beginning on p. 259. The expansive form of the disease is here described

---

[1] An analysis of known specimens of Haslam's handwriting has been compared with a dedication inscription on a copy of *Sketches in Bedlam*, formerly
the property of John Conolly and now in the library of the Institute of
Psychiatry, London. Mr. E. C. Williams, a handwriting expert and examiner
of questioned documents, has listed twelve points of distinctive dissimilarity,
and concludes that "it is highly improbable that the two scripts are written by
the same person".

for the first time. The report of a case identifiable as that of general
paralysis of the insane appears on p. 64 in the first and on p. 115 in the
second edition. It includes post-mortem findings.

Let us see what these extracts consist of. In the 1809 edition, the
general description occurs in a chapter headed "Probable Event of the
Disease" in modern terminology—the prognosis of the illness—

> Paralytic affections are a much more frequent cause of insanity than has
> been commonly supposed, and they are also a very common effect of
> madness; more maniacs die of hemiplegia and apoplexy than from any
> other disease. In those affected from this cause, we are, on enquiry, enabled
> to trace a sudden affection, or fit, to have proceeded the disease. These
> patients usually bear marks of such affection, independently of their in-
> sanity; the speech is impeded, and the mouth drawn aside; an arm, or leg,
> is more or less deprived of its capability of being moved by the will: and
> in most of them the memory is particularly impaired. Persons thus dis-
> ordered are in general not at all sensible of being so affected. When so
> feeble, as scarcely to be able to stand, they commonly say that they feel
> perfectly strong, and capable of great exertion. However pitiable these
> objects may be to the feeling spectator, yet it is fortunate for the condition
> of the sufferer, that his pride and pretensions are usually exalted in pro-
> portion to the degradation of the calamity which afflicts him. None of
> these patients have received any benefit in the hospital; and from the
> enquiries I have been able to make at the private mad-houses, where they
> have been afterwards confined, it has appeared, that they have either died
> suddenly, from apoplexy, or have repeated fits, from the effects of which
> they have sunk into a stupid state, and gradually dwindled away (p. 259).

The case report—one out of 37 cases described by Haslam is as follows:

Case XV. Observations on Insanity

J. A. a man, forty-two years of age, was first admitted into the house on
June 27, 1795. His disease came on suddenly whilst he was working in a
garden, on a very hot day, without any covering to his head. He had some
years before travelled with a gentleman over a great part of Europe: his
ideas ran particularly on what he had seen abroad; sometimes he conceived
himself the king of Denmark, at other times the king of France. Although
naturally dull and wanting common education, he professed himself a
master of all the dead and living languages; but his most intimate acquaintance was with the old French: and he was persuaded he had some faint
recollection of coming over to this country with William the Conqueror.
His temper was very irritable, and he was disposed to quarrel with every
body about him. After he had continued ten months in the hospital, he

became tranquil, relinquished his absurdities, and was discharged well in June 1796. He went into the country with his wife to settle some domestic affairs, and in about six weeks afterwards relapsed. He was re-admitted into the hospital August 13th.

He now evidently had paralytic affection; his speech was inarticulate, and his mouth drawn aside. He shortly became stupid, his legs swelled, and afterwards ulcerated: at length his appetite failed; he became emaciated, and died December 27th, of the same year. The head was opened twenty hours after death. There was a greater quantity of water between the different membranes of the brain than has ever occurred to me. The *tunica arachnoidea* was generally opake and very much thickened: the pia matter was loaded with blood, and the veins of that membrane were particularly enlarged. On the forepart of the right hemisphere of the brain, when stripped of its membranes, there was a blotch of a brown colour, several shades darker than the rest of the cortical substance; the ventricles were much enlarged, and contained, by estimation, at least six ounces of water. The veins in these cavities were particularly turgid. The consistence of the brain was firmer than usual.

Haslam certainly made no differentiation between this case and the remainder of the patients in his group. Although the description is that of a cortical atrophy, it is difficult to maintain, short of special pleading, that this is an easily recognizable picture of the macroscopic anatomy of general paralysis. Calmeil in his *De la Paralysie considérée chez les Aliénes* (1826) and Esquirol in his *Maladies Mentales* (1838) do not mention Haslam in the context of paralysis and mental disorder. Calmeil's study was however a particularly penetrating survey of the problem of paralysis in mental disorder, and it was he who coined the expression "general paralysis of the insane". To Bayle, however, belongs the real credit for the discovery. In 1822 he published his *Recherche sur l'arachnite chronique*, in which he put forward the view that the condition was a single disease entity. He continued to work on the problem, and in 1826 published his *Traité des maladies du cerveau et de ses membranes*. In this book he developed his previous views, and in fact established that the illness was characterized by a definite group of signs and symptoms, with a definite course and outcome. It is difficult to maintain that Haslam, by virtue of the extracts quoted above, can be regarded as the discoverer of general paralysis, nor indeed, did he ever lay claim to that distinction.

More controversy raged over the relationship of paralysis and mental disorder during the first half of the nineteenth century than over any other mental illness. The storm and fury was largely confined to France, but it is none the less strange how little this controversy was reflected in the writings of English psychiatrists of the time. Haslam was interested in French literature, whilst Prichard and Conolly was Francophil to an excessive degree. The recent scholarly paper by Hare has done much to clarify the position. He writes

> Although *dementia paralytica* presents (or did present, when it first became prevalent) a very striking clinical picture, yet there is no clear description of it and certainly no evidence that it was at all common until the Parisian outbreak described by Esquirol, Georget, Bayle and Calmeil. The hypothesis of a mutant strain of spirochaete spreading by venereal infection from a centre somewhere in Northern France would largely explain the varying times at which *dementia paralytica* was recognized in different countries and the variations in prevalence and sex ratio reported in these countries during the years after its first recognition.

Hare's thorough study must be consulted by all who are interested in the history of psychiatry—it corroborates the view I have put forward that Haslam cannot be seriously considered as the discoverer of General Paralysis.

SOCIAL ACTIVITIES

Haslam's friends and enemies were legion. He was a well-known figure in literary as well as medical circles. William Jerdan, the energetic editor of the *Literary Gazette*, writes in his autobiography that

> Dr. Haslam was a great gun for several years. Himself an original, and with a tinge of that eccentricity which seems frequently to have accrued from scientific devotedness to the medical treatment of insanity, and mingling much with insane patients; he was an astute and yet lively writer, with a vein of good humoured satire, which tickled everybody and hurt nobody. A series of clever papers, called "The Barleycorn Club", were from him, and principally by him.
>
> Haslam himself was very droll and entertaining in society, he had one literary patient to whom he was much attached—a Mr. R.—but the best jest with regard to whom was that during the half of the twelvemonths he was usually out of restraint he was absolutely employed to read the manuscripts and pronounce his judgement on the expediency or inexpediency of publishing productions submitted by numerous writers to one of the most extensive houses in the trade.

Of his medical friends, he is said to have been an acquaintance of
John Hunter—for in his obituary notice in the *Lancet* is a statement
that his conversation "abounded in anecdote, chiefly having reference
to John Hunter, of whom he was an intimate friend, and for whom he

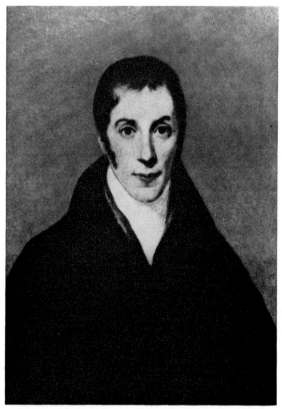

Fɪɢ. 11.   Sir Alexander Morison, 1779–1866. (*From the portrait by Milburn.*)

had a very high respect". It seems unlikely that he had been any other
than a student under Hunter. Mr. Le Fanu has informed me that there
is no record of Hunter's friendship with Haslam and indeed as Hunter
died in 1793, when Haslam was only 29, a close friendship seems improbable. Haslam's sponsors for his M.D. were A. P. Buchan and
William Charles Wells—both of whom he had probably met whilst
studying in Edinburgh. Both had also studied under the Hunters and

Dr. George Fordyce, and it again seems likely that Haslam had met them in these classes. Later in life Haslam was an intimate of Sir Alexander Morison, the founder of the well-known Morison Lecture

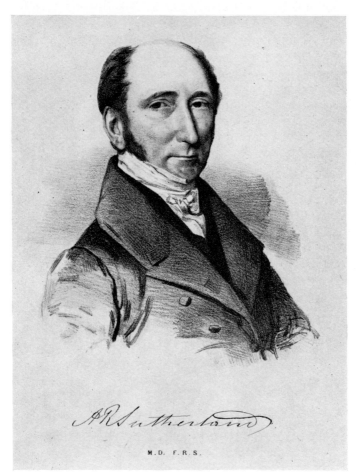

M.D. F.R.S.

FIG. 12.   Alexander Robert Sutherland, 1782–1861. Physician to St. Luke's.

at the University of Edinburgh (Fig. 11). Morison was Physician to Bethlem from 1835 to 1853 and his diaries are now in the library of the Royal College of Physicians of Edinburgh. From these diaries it emerges that Morison's most intimate friends in London were Dr. Sutherland of St. Luke's (Fig. 12), and John Haslam. Morison had inaugurated a course of Lectures on Mental Diseases, and at the first lecture, given at the Argyll Rooms on 9 February 1826, those present included Haslam, Willis, Burrows and MacGregor. Spurzheim, the phrenologist, and Dr. MacMichael, the author of the *Gold Headed Cane*, attended later lectures. After Haslam's death Morison attested to his signature to some document, and their friendship was clearly a happy one, for when Morison founded the Society for Improving the Conditions of the Insane in 1842, Haslam was one of the first to read a scientific paper before its members.

In addition to his psychiatric acquaintances, Haslam moved freely amongst a wider circle of literary friends. He was an intimate of William Kitchiner, M.D., the eccentric writer of the first really practical cookery book. A private income of £2,000 a year allowed Kitchiner to entertain lavishly, and his luncheons and dinners were memorable occasions. "To the former only intimate friends, like Charles Kemble the actor, Incledon the singer, and Dr. John Haslam the medical writer, were invited." Kitchiner was a prolific writer, and published books ranging from his *Aspicius Redivivus, or the Cooks Oracle* to *The Economy of the Eyes*. Haslam and Kitchiner were also friendly with William Jerdan, editor of the *Literary Gazette* for thirty-three years. Jerdan's aim was "to praise heartily and censure mildly" and he gathered around him a distinguished group of writers, including Crabbe, Miss Mitford and Thomas Campbell. Haslam was a popular member of this literary group, and wrote for the *Literary Gazette* for several years. In legal circles also Haslam was in demand as an expert witness and appeared in many cases.

From 1827 to 1829 he was President of the Medical Society of London, an honour showing how well his reputation had been re-established. Haslam's portrait had been painted in 1812 by George Dawe, A.R.A., and was engraved by Henry Dawe. It was exhibited at the Royal Academy in 1831, and depicts a man of strong features, with a firm lip and chin, but withal of a benign and humorous aspect. Unfortunately no trace yet exists of the original painting.

Of his family life, little is known. His wife was Sarah, and she gave him at least three sons and one daughter. One son, John, was a surgeon in the Royal Navy, and wrote an interesting account of a voyage to New South Wales in a convict ship.

The 23-page pamphlet is entitled "Convict Ships: A Narrative of a Voyage to New South Wales in the Year 1816 in the Ship *Mariner*, describing the nature of the accommodations, stores, diet etc. Together with an Account of the Medical Treatment and Religious Superintendence of these Unfortunate Persons."

Young Haslam considered that it was first proper to state that he was a Surgeon in the Royal Navy, and had "derived some experience from the exercise of my professional duties in the service of my country". On 6 April 1816 he was appointed Surgeon to the ship *Mariner*, 446 tons, hired for the conveyance of 146 convicts to New South Wales. With careful attention to hygiene very little sickness occurred on the voyage, and 146 live convicts landed at Port Jackson on 16 October. The most interesting part of the pamphlet deals with Haslam's "moral survey of this depraved assembly". Numerous Bibles and prayer books had been provided, and Haslam read the service performed in the Church of England every sabbath day "with appropriate exhortations to repentance". Even in the middle of a storm off the Cape of Good Hope, when the vessel was in danger of foundering, Haslam found this "a favourable opportunity to impress the minds of the convicts with a due sense of their awful situation" and exhorted them to spend the short time that probably remained in prayer and repentance. Unfortunately he was met only by a "roar of blasphemy" and a licentious song. One young man alone appeared to be influenced by Haslam, serving as clerk during divine service, reading the Scriptures, and behaving generally in an exemplary manner during the voyage. Unfortunately, once arrived in Australia, he was soon detected "picking the pocket of an inhabitant, whom curiosity had induced to become a spectator" of the inspection of the convicts. Sadder, but wiser, Haslam reached Port Jackson, having failed to produce any moral reformation amongst "these desperate outcasts", his attempts at what he called "moral therapeutics" having failed.

Little is known of the other children. Another son, Thomas Haslam, was born in 1790 and became an Ensign in the Honourable East India Company's Army (Bengal) in 1810. He was promoted Captain in the 25th Native Infantry in 1824 and died in 1832 at Barrackpore. All three sons were educated at the Merchant Taylors' School.

Haslam died in 1844. A search for his Will, for his portrait in oils, and for any of his descendants has been unrewarding, although I have travelled as far afield as Chicago in trace of his portrait. Many gaps remain to be filled. The period between his leaving Edinburgh and his appointment to Bethlem is a blank; his career in practice following his dismissal from Bethlem and details of his family life are all lacking.

HASLAM'S PLACE IN PSYCHIATRY

Haslam has been unduly neglected by the medical historian, although Arnold Pick and, more recently, Zelmanowits have recognized his merits. The rise of the professional psychiatrist, beginning with Battie, and to some extent the Monros, is well illustrated in his career. Lacking the qualification of physician until late in life, the use he made of his opportunities must arouse our admiration. In 1955 I expressed the view that Haslam "was by far the most original and discerning writer on psychiatry in the period 1798 to 1828", and the years that have passed have done nothing to alter this opinion. He left original descriptions of the simple dementing form of schizophrenia, of obsessional neurosis, and of manic–depressive illness. His was the first contribution in English on forensic psychiatry, his the most concise and lucid exposition of the moral management of the insane, in France, Germany and America his contributions were acknowledged. Pinel, in his *Traité Médico–philosophique sur la Manie*, published in 1801, mentions Haslam more frequently than any psychiatrist other than Ferriar. Although Pinel is somewhat sarcastic in his references to England, he shows a considerable respect for Haslam, and amplifies many of his own conclusions by quotations from Haslam. Although this is not the place for a detailed comparison of the two men, their lives illustrate the abyss separating success and failure. Pinel appears to posterity as the greatest psychiatrist of the period. With revolutionary fervour, and a dramatic gesture, he cast off the chains of the lunatics in the Bicêtre, but a study of his writings shows that in effect this was indeed largely a gesture. His book abounds in references to restraint and coercion, and his practice differed in few respects from that of Haslam. It is an interesting comment on fame that Haslam, a far more original and discerning writer, was to be dismissed from his post and his memory allowed to lapse into obscurity, whilst Pinel was to go from success to success and his name to become a household word in psychiatry. Both men were leaders of psychiatric thought in their time, but for solid intellectual merit a study of Haslam's work will leave little doubt as to which of them has left more to posterity.

What are the reasons for Haslam's comparative obscurity? The hostility towards him shown by the rising school of "non-restraint", headed by Tuke, Gardiner Hill and Conolly, and the xenophilic zeal of Prichard have no doubt played their part. Haslam's personality, however, seems to provide the real reason—his disgrace, his biting comments on contemporary psychiatrists, his "die-hard" attitude toward the reformers, and no doubt his very real talent must have made him a difficult man to deal with. As a young man at Edinburgh he had shown his aggressive nature and his readiness to notice a slight. The proud and harsh old man may have been convivial in his literary circle, but he was poles apart from the younger psychiatrists. His opinions were to be disregarded and forgotten as this new generation grew up. Unlike Conolly, he was out of joint with the times, and he suffered accordingly. But his mind was as profound and logical as Conolly's was superficial and emotional—it is his writings which assure him an important place in the history of psychiatry.

BIBLIOGRAPHY

A Catalogue of the Entire Library of John Haslam, Esq. London: Leigh & Sotheby, 1816.

ANON. (1785). *A Narrative of some Late Injurious Proceedings of the Managers of the Royal Infirmary.* 24 Pp. Edinburgh.

ANON. (1839). *Physic & Physicians. A Medical Sketch Book.* Vol. 1, pp. 360. London: Longman, Orme, Brown & Co.

BECK, T. R. (1829). *Elements of Medical Jurisprudence.* 3rd edition, pp. 640. London: Longman.

BLACKHALL-MORISON, A. "Sir Alexander Morison, M.D." Unpublished monograph.

CALMEIL, L. F. (1826). *De la Paralysie considérée chez les Aliénes.* Pp. 446. Paris: Chez J-B. Baillière.

COX, J. M. (1804). *Practical Observations on Insanity.* Pp. 166. London: C. & R. Baldwin.

CRICHTON, A. (1798). *An Inquiry into the Nature and Origin of Mental Derangement,* pp. 407, 455. London: T. Cadell, Jr., & W. Davies.

CROWTHER, B. (1808). *Practical Observations on the Disease of the Joints, commonly called White Swelling.* Pp. 295. London: J. Callow.

CROWTHER, B. (1811). *Practical Remarks on Insanity.* Pp. 130. London: Underwood, Black, Gilbert & Hodges.

ESQUIROL, E. (1838). *Des Maladies Mentales, Considérées sous les Rapports Médical, Hygiénique et Médico-légal.* 2 vols., pp. 393, 380. Paris: Chez J-B. Baillière.

K

Dictionary of National Biography, vol. 25, p. 107. London: Smith Elder & Co., 1891.

The Gentleman's Magazine, 1844, n.s. **22**, 322.

GRAY, J. (1952). *A History of the Royal Medical Society*. Pp. 355. Edinburgh: Edinburgh University Press.

HARE, E. H. (1959). "The Origin and Spread of Dementia Paralytica." *J. Ment. Sci.*, **105**, 594.

HASLAM, J. (1798). *Observations on Insanity, with Practical Remarks on the Disease, and an account of the Morbid Appearances on Dissection*. Pp. 147. London: F. & C. Rivington.

HASLAM, J. (1809). *Observations on Madness and Melancholy, including practical remarks on those diseases; together with cases: and an account of the morbid appearance on dissection*. The 2nd edition, considerably enlarged, Pp. 345. London: J. Callow.

HASLAM, J. (1810). *Illustrations of Madness: exhibiting a singular case of insanity, and a no less remarkable difference in medical opinions: developing the nature of assailment, and the manner of working events; with a description of the tortures experienced by bomb-bursting, lobster-cracking, and lengthening the brain.* Pp. 81. London: G. Hayden.

HASLAM, J. (1816). *Observations of the Physician and Apothecary of Bethlem Hospital, upon the evidence taken before the Committee of the Hon. House of Commons for Regulating Mad-Houses.* Pp. 55. London: H. Bryer.

HASLAM, J. (1817). *Considerations on the Moral Management of Insane Persons.* Pp. 80. London: R. Hunter.

HASLAM, J. (1817). *Medical Jurisprudence, as it relates to insanity, according to the law of England.* Pp. 150. London: C. Hunter.

HASLAM, J. (1818). *A Letter to the Governors of Bethlem Hospital, containing an account of their management of that institution for the last twenty years; elucidated by original letters and authentic documents; with a correct narrative of the confinement of James Norris, by order of their subcommittee; and interesting observations on the parliamentary proceedings.* Pp. 58. London: Taylor & Hessey.

HASLAM, J. (1819). *Sound Mind; or, contributions to the natural history and physiology of the human intellect.* Pp. 192. London: Longman, Hurst, Rees, Orme & Brown.

HASLAM, J. (1823). *A Letter to the Right Honourable the Lord Chancellor, on the nature and interpretation of unsoundness of mind, and imbecility of intellect.* Pp. 32. London: R. Hunter.

HASLAM, J. (1827-28). "Lectures on the intellectual composition of man." *Lancet*, **1**, 38, 71, 119, 207, 288, 335.

HASLAM, J. (1835). *On the nature of thought, or the act of thinking, and its connexion with a perspicuous sentence.* Pp. 42. London: Longman, Rees, Orme, Brown, Green & Longman.

HASLAM, J. (1850). *Selection of papers and prize essays on subjects connected with insanity*. Read Before the Society For Improving the Conditions of the Insane. Pp. 200. London: published by the Society.

HILL, B. (1952). "Mrs. Beeton's predecessor. William Kitchiner, M.D. (*c.* 1775-1827)." *Practitioner*, **168**, 624-27.

JERDAN, W. (1853). *The Autobiography of William Jerdan*. 4 vols., pp. 279. London: Hall, Virtue & Co.

Lancet, 1844, **1**, 571.

LAWRENCE, W. (1819). *Lectures on Physiology, Zoology, and the Natural History of Man*. Pp. 579. London: J. Callow

LEIGH, D. (1954). "John Haslam, M.D. A pioneer of forensic psychiatry." *Brit. J. Delinquency*, **4**, 201-206.

Literary Gazette, 1844, p. 484. London: Robson, Levey, and Franklyn.

NICOL, W. D. (1956). "General Paralysis of the Insane." *Brit. J. Vener. Dis.*, **32**, 9.

O'DONOGHUE, E. G. (1914). *The Story of Bethlem Hospital*. Pp. 427. London: T. Fisher Unwin.

PARGETER, W. (1792). *Observations on Maniacal Disorders*. Pp. 140. Reading: printed for the Author.

PERFECT, W. (1794). *Annals of Insanity*. Pp. 412. London: Chalmers.

ROBERTSON, G. M. (1922). "The discovery of general paralysis." Address to Royal Medical Society of Edinburgh.

ROBINSON, N. (1729). *A New System of the Spleen, Vapours, and Hypochondriack Melancholy*. Pp. 408. London: Bettesworth, Innys & Rivington.

SHARPE, J. B. (1815). *Report together with the minutes of evidence and an appendix of papers from the Committee appointed to consider of Provision being made for the Better Regulation of Madhouses in England*. Pp. 399. London: Baldwin, Craddock & Joy.

TUKE, D. H. (1882). *Chapters in the History of the Insane in the British Isles*. Pp. 548. London: Kegan Paul, Trench & Co.

ZELMANOWITS, J. (1953). "A historical note on the simple dementing form of schizophrenia." *Proc. Roy. Soc. Med.*, **46**, 931-33.

ZILBOORG, G. (1941). *A History of Medical Psychology*. Pp. 686. New York: W .W. Norton & Co. Inc.

CHAPTER III

James Cowles Prichard, M.D., F.R.S.
1786–1848

JAMES COWLES PRICHARD (Fig. 1) has been sadly neglected by the medical historian. His concept of moral insanity, although based on faulty premises, exercised an important influence on psychiatric thought in England during the latter part of the nineteenth century. He is considered by some psychiatrists to have been a pioneer in the description and recognition of psychopathy. He played a decisive part in the introduction of French psychiatry to Great Britain, and was perhaps the first proponent of the idea that modern psychiatry began with Pinel, and was essentially a French creation. His life was one of enormous industry, for his psychiatric work, important as it is, was dwarfed by his monumental contributions to anthropology, ethnology and philology. His working days were passed as a busy general physician to the Bristol Infirmary, attending out-patients, visiting private patients, and at the same time contriving to be one of the founders of Bristol College, and of the Bristol Literary and Philosophical Society, in addition to fulfilling a host of other obligations. It is no exaggeration to call this many-sided man an intellectual giant, or as Thomas Hodgkin wrote in his quaint Victorian manner "a superior individual". His life and work provide an interesting contrast to those of both John Haslam and John Conolly.

HIS CAREER

James Cowles Prichard, the eldest son of Thomas and Mary Prichard, was born on 11 February 1786 at Ross, in Herefordshire, where his family had lived for several generations. His parents were members of the Society of Friends, his great-grandfather Edward Prichard having been imprisoned on account of his religious beliefs in 1684. Thomas Prichard was a cultivated man of great poetical imagination, somewhat prosaically engaged in commercial life with a firm of iron and tin-plate merchants in Bristol. In 1793, when aged 7, Prichard was sent to a school in Bristol for a short time, but soon returned to the family bosom where his studies, under a series of tutors, were supervised by his father. He was taught French by an émigré called de Rosemond,

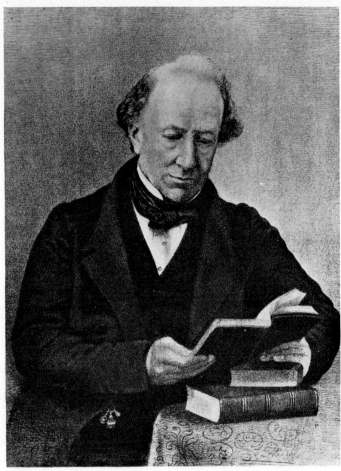

FIG. 1. James Cowles Prichard, M.D., F.R.S., 1786–1848.

Spanish and Italian by Signor Mordenti, "who called himself a Roman", and Latin and Arithmetic by an Irishman named John Barnes.

It formed part of his father's plan early to introduce a practical acquaintance with French as well as English, and for this purpose it was his practice to devote most evenings to reading English from a French book, often from *Rollin's History*. He then required his children to give in French what he had said in English. Familiarity with French, and a taste for history, were thus imparted together. The boy became fond of tracing the genealogies of kings of the most remote historic times, and living in a cosmopolitan port such as Bristol, he employed himself in finding out and examining the specimens of the natives of different countries who came as seamen to the city, occasionally bringing a foreigner to his father's house. His familiarity with Spanish and Modern Greek was in part attributable to this cause.

Prichard was often forced to leave his books in order to have "needful recreation and exercise; yet when he joined his companions in the playground, he entered into their sports with as much animation as the idlest and gayest". His facility for languages was quite remarkable, and he delighted in accosting seafaring men in Bristol in their own tongue. He is said on one occasion to have spoken to a Greek sailor in Romaic, and the man was so delighted that he caught the boy-linguist in his arms, and kissed him heartily. This interest in foreigners and in language was to remain the dominant theme of his life work.

He appears to have had an early inclination toward medicine, which his father did not encourage, as he desired his son "should retain the primitive simplicity and orthodoxy of genuine Quakerism which he feared the study of medicine would contaminate". The boy got his wish however, and at 17 attended lectures under a Dr. Thomas Pole, in Bristol. Dr. Thomas Pole, an American, and a member of the Society of Friends, gave scientific lectures to mixed audiences at his house in St. James's Square, Bristol. These discourses covered a wide range of subjects; indeed, the learned Quaker might almost be said to have constituted himself "Professor of Things in General". His course, which he entitled "The Economy of Nature", included Surgery, Botany, Chemistry, Physics, the use of the Globes, Midwifery, Optics and Astronomy. His fees were four guineas for the whole course, or two shillings and sixpence for single lectures.

In the summer of 1802 Prichard moved to Staines, where he lived with Mr. Tothill, partner of the Dr. Pope who subsequently became a physician to George III. Both Tothill and Pope were Friends, and Prichard is said to have pursued his studies assiduously under their care. In September 1804 he attended St. Thomas's Hospital, and then went to Edinburgh in September 1805, where he was a medical student until he took his M.D. after three years of hard study. At Edinburgh he first began to gather together his ideas on the varieties of the human race. Among his fellow-students the most distinguished were Arnould, Estlin and Hancock, and they continued to be his intimate friends for the remainder of his life. Arnould later wrote of these student days:

> From the year 1807 we were very much together, and from that time, during our stay in Edinburgh, the history of his book is the history of his life, for it was the continual occupation of his mind. In our daily walks it was always uppermost: a shade of complexion—a singularity of physiognomy—a peculiarity of form—would always introduce the one absorbing object. In the crowd and in solitude it was ever present with him. I well remember when one evening we were wending our way amidst the mountains in the neighbourhood of Loch Katrine, not so much frequented then as it has been since the *Lady of the Lake* appeared: it was near the going down of the sun, when, amidst the wildest scenery, we saw a Highlander on a distant crag, standing out clear and distinct, and seemingly magnified to a large size, and his huge shadow stretching out towards us. The effect for my friend was magical: fatigue was felt no longer, and he at once resumed all his powers of mind and body, and poured out a most splendid dissertation on the history of the Celtic nations—the dark, fearful, gloomy, and savage rites of the Druids—and conjured up the horrors we should have endured, if in those earlier times we had been lonely wanderers in that remote district, and beguiled the weariness of the way till we reached our place of rest at night.
>
> His favourite topic was a frequent subject of discussion in a private debating society called the Azygotic. It consisted of six members, Charles and Patrick Mackenzie, Hampden, Estlin, Prichard and Arnould. We met at each other's houses one evening in the week for literary, scientific, and philosophical discussion. On the night of Prichard's paper, which was the basis of his thesis for his doctor's degree, we had a very long, animated and interesting debate.

This thesis, which was much longer and more elaborate and learned than such compositions usually are, showed the direction in which his studies were already tending—it was called "De Generis Humani Varietate". It was eventually to become his five-volume *magnum opus*, *Researches into the Physical History of Man*. He corresponded with his father on the subject of his investigations, who not only took a lively interest in the enquiry but expressed his desire that his son would maintain the orthodox side of the question with respect to the unity of the species "Man".

Having completed his curriculum and taken his degree in Edinburgh, Prichard passed a year at Trinity College, Cambridge; "the superior liberality of that University allowing Dissenters the privilege of study- ing, though not of graduating there". He probably studied mathe- matics and theology, and whilst at Cambridge made a decisive step, renouncing the Society of Friends and entering the Church of England. This change enabled him to enter as a student at the University of Oxford, where he first resided at St. John's and afterwards at Trinity College, of which he was a gentleman commoner. He took no degree. The reasons for his separation from the Society of Friends are not clear, but the change must have upset his old father considerably. He returned to Bristol shortly afterwards in 1810, at the age of 24, and set up in practice.

HIS PRACTICE

In 1812 he was appointed physician to St. Peter's—a hospital con- taining a number of patients suffering from mental and nervous dis- orders. 1816 saw his election as Physician to the Bristol Infirmary, and as we might expect, his work on the wards was, it is said, "marked by the learning, skill and energy which characterized all he did". The patients thought otherwise, for a doggerel rhyme by one of them tells how

> Dr. Prichard do appear
> With his attendance and his care
> He fills his patients full of sorrow
> You must be bled today and cupped tomorrow.

They had some reason to be full of sorrow, for he not only bled and purged them freely, but he was fond of applying blisters, setons and other strong counter-irritants (Figs. 2 and 3).

In his medical practice he believed in and acted on the prevalent idea of that time; namely, that inflammation, usually depending on a plethoric state of the system, was the cause of almost all diseases, and he acted on his convictions, giving remedies in full doses, and following up the antiphlogistic treatment in the most active way. His son, Augustin Prichard, in his reminiscences, describes a day's work as his father's dresser.

> . . . and when the coincidence occurred that my father and Dr. Riley, then the junior physician, very French and fresh from Paris and Broussais,

saw their out-patients on the same day (for there were no assistant physicians or surgeons then), the work of the dresser was almost more than the length of the day would allow him to get through; and this will

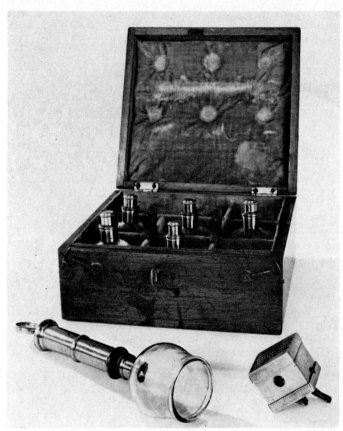

FIG. 2. Cupping and scarifying set. (*From the author's collection*, 1840.)

be recognized when I say that I have had to bleed as many as forty out-patients in one day, and after that had to bleed and cup the in-patients in the wards for whom the physicians had prescribed it, to spread my dressings and dress my patients, and to attend to the not infrequent summons of the old low-toned casualty bell. My father originated the plan of making the long issue in the scalp in brain diseases; and although a strong remedy, it was sometimes undoubtedly the means of saving life. A cut was rapidly made with a sharp scalpel, through the thickness of the scalp from just above the occipital protuberance to the edge of the hair in front, and filled with a string of peas, which soon set up the needed suppuration as counter-irritation to the morbid process going on within the skull. We had, in addition, not infrequently to insert setons, or make an issue in the arm or elsewhere by incision or caustic.

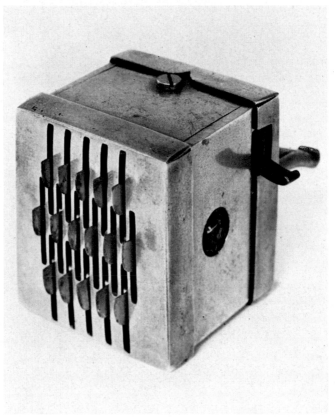

Fig. 3.   Scarifier. (*From the author's collection, c.* 1840.)

It was many years before his practice amounted to anything; not until he had published the first edition of the *Physical History of Man*, which had no real reference to his own profession, did work begin to flow in to him. Eventually he had a very considerable private practice, purely as a physician on consultations. He never encroached, his son maintains, upon the domain of the surgeon, although an extraordinary affair took place in 1826, which reflects a controversy current at the time. Like other physicians, he "magnified his office" and took a firm stand on matters of etiquette. The physicians were at that period attempting to set themselves up as a distinct class of practitioner, differing from the surgeons in their functions. On 13 January 1826 Dr. David Davies, a member of the College of Physicians in London and a busy Bristol practitioner, asked Prichard to meet him in consultation. Prichard refused—stating that Dr. Davies was attending the patient as a physician, although he was a surgeon on the staff of St. Peter's Hospital—this was contrary to customary modes of proceeding. This refusal started an avalanche of indignant letters from Dr. Davies, quoting Acts of Parliament, historical figures in medicine, and even Frenchmen, that a physician is perfectly entitled to act as a surgeon. He went so far as to maintain that legally Dr. Prichard had no authority to practise as a physician—and to cap it all, published the correspondence and his comments in a pamphlet for all Bristol to read. Prichard seems to have treated the affair with some indifference, having taken his original stand on the consultation, and nothing further is heard of Dr. Davies.

As a practitioner of medicine Prichard was remarkable for decision on the character of the disease, and for promptness and energy in the application of remedies. Boldness was his keynote. He took notes on his patients in the Infirmary in short, terse Latin sentences in his case book, and whenever he travelled usually had books piled on the seat of his carriage.

He took an active part in the social and intellectual life of Bristol (Fig.4). In the large old oak drawing-room of the Red Lodge, Prichard's home, many clever and learned men used to meet for two or three hours of intellectual conversation.

> The most intelligent and literary men among the inhabitants of this city, the masters of the old Bristol College, and as on account of his book on the Physical History of Man my father's name was held in as much, if not more, esteem on the Continent than in England, any celebrity that was passing through or temporarily resident, formed the company invited according to the custom of the time to drink tea: they came about eight o'clock and dispersed soon after ten, and it was a matter sometimes of great interest, even to us boys, to be present.

He was a founder of Bristol College, of the Bristol Literary and Philosophical Society and President of the Medical Library. His

𝕭𝖗𝖎𝖘𝖙𝖔𝖑 𝕴𝖓𝖘𝖙𝖎𝖙𝖚𝖙𝖎𝖔𝖓.

THREE LECTURES

ON

EGYPTIAN MUMMIES, EGYPTIAN ANTIQUITIES,

AND THE

ROSETTA STONE,

ARE ABOUT TO BE DELIVERED,

FOR THE BENEFIT OF THE INSTITUTION,

BY

J. C. PRICHARD, M.D., F.R.S., &c.

AND

G. T. CLARK, Esq.

This Course has been undertaken in consequence of the liberal offer of a Gentleman to allow a splendid Egyptian Mummy belonging to him, to be opened for the purposes of scientific information, and for the benefit of the Institution.   Other Specimens will be brought from the Museum.

———o———

First Lecture .... MONDAY, March 31st ⎫
Second......................... WEDNESDAY, April 2nd ⎬ At Half-past Seven o'clock in the Evening.
Third .... FRIDAY,   — 4th ⎭

Subscription to the Course, 7s. 6d.—Single Ticket, 3s.

Every Member of the Institution, subscribing to the Course, is entitled to a Set of Privilege Tickets, transferable to any one of his Family residing with him, to a Lady, or a Minor.

Subscribers to the Course may have Tickets to admit Minors at 4s.

☞ Tickets to be had at the Institution.

———o———

During the Month of April will be commenced a Course of Ten Lectures on GEOLOGY, by SAMUEL WORSLEY, Esq.; also in aid of the Funds of the Institution.

Printed at the Bristol Mirror Office by John Taylor.

FIG. 4.   Advertisement of lectures given on Egyptology by J. C. Prichard.

marriage to Miss Estlin, sister of his old friend, seems to have been a happy one, and they had ten children; one of them, Augustin Prichard, becoming a distinguished surgeon to the Bristol Infirmary and the author of two entertaining books of reminiscences.

Many religious notables, Quakers, Baptists and Anglicans, figured as his patients and friends, probably because in the phrases of his friend Thomas Hodgkin

> High moral and religious principle, an affectionate disposition, an instinctive sentiment of delicacy, propriety, and consideration of the feelings of others, and a retiring modesty and simplicity of deportment, as much distinguished and endeared him in the domestic and social relations of life, as his literary and scientific attainments elevated him to the eminence he held in public estimation; he furnished, indeed, a bright example of the scholar, the gentleman and the Christian.

A great friend, and godfather to many of his children was The Rev. John Eden, Vicar of St. Nicholas Church, Bristol. He was a very learned man, and published a metrical version of the Psalms of David in a quarto volume; he was also a clever artist, and was a member of a society which met in its members' houses for an evening's drawing and painting; leaving, according to their rules, all the evening's results behind them. He had made Prichard promise on his death to take some means to be sure that he was really dead, having a great fear lest he should be buried alive. Bishop Monk, the first Bishop of the United Sees of Gloucester and Bristol, John Foster, the great Baptist divine, and members of the Quaker community were numbered amongst Prichard's friends and patients. He also frequently met Southey and Coleridge.

Of the medical fraternity, his group of friends included James Addington Symonds, Thomas Hodgkin, William Lawrence, Hack Tuke and Dr. Alexander Tweedie. Honours fell thick upon him. He was an F.R.S., a Corresponding Member of the National Institute of France, and of the French Academy of Medicine, and Statistical Society, and a President of the Ethnological Society. In 1835 the University of Oxford conferred on him the degree of Doctor of Medicine by diploma. In that year the Provincial Medical and Surgical Association held its anniversary in Oxford, under the Presidency of the Regius Professor of Medicine, Dr. Kidd. Prichard had been appointed to deliver the annual address, and his diploma was handed to him by the President on the occasion. He was also a Corresponding

Member of the Academy of Natural Sciences of Philadelphia, the American Philosophical Society, the Oriental Society of America, the Ethnological Society of New York, the Scientific Academy of Siena, and other bodies, as well as a Member of the Royal Irish Academy.

In 1845 he left Bristol for London, having been appointed Her Majesty's Commissioner in Lunacy, resigning the office of Physician to the Bristol Infirmary which he had held for more than twenty-six years. Prior to the Gordon-Ashley Act of 1828, the care of the insane had been under the surveillance of five Fellows of the College of Physicians, who did not always carry out their duties satisfactorily. That Act replaced them by fifteen Metropolitan Commissioners in Lunacy, charged with the supervision of lunatics in the Metropolitan area only. In 1842 an important step forward occurred when it was decreed that provincial Houses were to be visited by the Metropolitan Commissioners, and a memorable report was published by them in 1844 on the state of asylums in England and Wales. This led to the Act of 1845 which provided for the appointment of new Commissioners in Lunacy—presumably Prichard was one of them.

He was not to remain long in his new office, for whilst on one of his official tours he was taken ill at Salisbury, and died shortly afterwards at his home in London, on 23 December 1848, the doctors in attendance being baffled by his illness, the fever being of "a rheumatic and gouty character, and terminating his life, after much suffering, by pericarditis and extensive suppuration in the knee-joint". Two outstanding tributes to him were written by his friends, John Addington Symonds, and Thomas Hodgkin.

Symonds described him as rather below middle height in stature and of rather slight make.

> He had light hair and grey eyes, which, though somewhat small, were of singularly intelligent expression. The form of his head was very fine; broad and prominent in the forehead, lofty and capacious in the crown. The countenance, to the most superficial observer, betokened deep thoughtfulness, with something of reserve and shyness, but blended with true kindliness. His voice was rather weak and low, but very distinct in articulation. His manners and deportment were simple and unaffected;— and in general company he evidently spoke with effort or even reluctance, unless upon subjects of business or of scientific and literary interest.
>
> It was wonderful how much he contrived to accomplish, even while engaged in his large private practice. This was in part owing to his power

and habit of employing small fragments of his time. His knowledge was so completely under his command, and his faculties were in such constant exercise, that he could immediately return to an argument or a train of thought, undistracted by any recent interruption. He made time also by his habit of early rising, which gave him three or four hours before the business of the day commenced. Whatever he undertook, he devoted the whole energy of his mind to its completion. He used to say that he experienced what John Wesley used to feel when a student at Oxford, "the lust for finishing".

Symonds writes—

All men of powerful minds have strong memories, for memory is the feeder of the other faculties; even if originally robust, these must pine and languish unless maintained by the nutriment which the former supplies. But Dr. Prichard's memory was above the average, even for one of his general mental caliber. His perceptions were by no means defective in acuteness, yet it was not by acute observation that he was particularly distinguished; nor though his judgment was sound and accurate, should I say that this faculty was so prominent as to be singled from the rest as one of his characteristics. Had he been engaged in the legal profession, I think he would have shone particularly in collecting and methodically arranging, and in luminously and eloquently stating an immense mass of evidence bearing upon a particular point; not, however, in the spirit of a mere advocate or partisan, but as one whose mind, magnetized by a particular idea, attracted and assimilated to itself every thing that could give support to that idea. It was not a mind to produce a mere agglomeration of facts and notions, but one that impregnated, informed, and organized them all into one living whole. Yet, had he been placed on the bench, I think he would not have been remarkable for mere judicial qualities, such as made Tenterden and Eldon so eminent. Comprehensiveness, rather than subtlety, was the character of his understanding. In conversation he showed his preference to broad decided views, rather than to the fine-drawn distinctions, the hair-splittings of metaphysical analysis. Yet in his writings it will not appear that his mind was warped by a foregone conclusion. Few compositions give one a stronger impression of fairness and equity in weighing evidence.

Fancy and imagination were not prominent faculties in Dr. Prichard. He was never at a loss for a suitable illustration to enrich his style, which was affluent as well as terse and vigorous. Yet there was not that conscious enjoyment in the pursuit of analogies and likenesses, which belongs to men in whom the faculties I have adverted to are strongly marked. And correspondently with this, I think that he had no decided aesthetical tendency, no such sensibility to the beautiful as would lead him to dwell on the enjoyments of poetry and the fine arts; though he was too much of a scholar, and in every way too well informed, not to be able to converse on these subjects. A powerful memory, and a strong philosophical bias, by which I mean the disposition to trace events to their causes, and to classify phenomena under general laws, together with an astonishing capability of undergoing mental labour, will, I think, be found to have been the most distinguishing traits of Dr. Prichard's understanding.

Ten years before his death he had been described by Professor Gibson of Philadelphia in very similar terms.

Dr. Prichard is about fifty years of age, is a short, compact, close-made man, with bluish-grey eyes, large and prominent features, and expression uncommonly mild, open, and benevolent; so much so, that almost any one would naturally inquire who he was. His hair is thin and scattering, and so white as to make him look older than he is, whereas, in former days, it was light chestnut, and so remarkably thick, bushy, and upright, as to form one of his striking characteristics. In dress he is singularly plain, simple, and unostentatious, and, if in drab attire, might pass readily for a Quaker. Starchiness and formality, however, make no ingredient in his composition. On the contrary, he is very cheerful, sociable, frank, easy and unpretending in his discourse and manner, and has so much modesty, artlessness, and child-like simplicity about him, that no one would be prepared to say, upon slight acquaintance, that he was anything more than an ordinary, sensible, well-disposed man, however much they might be pleased, which they would not fail to be, with his benign and agreeable countenance. But it is impossible to be in his company long, and to hear him talk on any subject, without being strongly impressed with the depth and originality of his views, his sterling good sense and wisdom, his profound and varied information, his clear and luminous conceptions, his ardent and unbounded love of science, his extreme liberality towards every nation under the sun, his entire freedom from envy or jealousy of any description, and from professional rivalry and bitterness, his singleness of purpose, his goodness of heart, and his reverence for all the duties that belong to a Christian, an accountable being, and a man.

So much for the man and his career.

PSYCHIATRIC WRITINGS

His works are concerned with four subjects, ethnology, philology, psychiatry and literature. He is certainly one of the giants of ethnology, and his studies of language are quite remarkable. In fact his psychiatric

writings, whilst our chief concern here, are dwarfed by his anthropo-
logical and philological works. None the less, let us deal first with
Prichard as a psychiatrist—particularly with his three books *A Treatise
on Diseases of the Nervous System* published in 1822, *A Treatise on
Insanity* published in 1835, and the *Different Forms of Insanity in Relation
to Jurisprudence* first published in 1842, and appearing in a second edition
in 1847. These publications must be seen against the background of
contemporary psychiatry from the time he set up in practice in 1810
until his death in 1848. In England, John Haslam, Sir Alexander
Morison, Powell, Sir Alexander Crichton, George Man Burrows,
John Conolly and Hack Tuke were perhaps the leading members of
the profession. In France, Pinel died in 1826, Georget in 1828, Esquirol
in 1848, Ferrus in 1861 and Falret in 1870. In Germany, Jacobi (1775–
1858), Friedreich (1796–1862) and Griesinger (1817–1868) were the
chief exponents of psychiatry. Prichard's psychiatric thought was
greatly affected by French concepts, first and foremost by those of
Pinel, who in his turn had been much influenced by English writers
of the late eighteenth century such as Perfect, Ferriar and Haslam.
Esquirol, to whom Prichard dedicated his *Treatise on Insanity*, was
second only in importance to Pinel. These influences pervade Prichard's
work, and may be traced most clearly by an individual consideration
of his books.

"A TREATISE ON DISEASES OF THE
NERVOUS SYSTEM" (1822)

Prichard's first book, *A Treatise on Diseases of the Nervous System*, is
a curious work. Considering Prichard's enormous erudition the bibliography is patchy, the most frequently quoted author being Ferriar of
Manchester, whilst of the French, Pinel, Sauvages, Bichat, Martinet
and Lorry are the only writers he mentions. The book is largely a
collection of cases, with an attempt at a broad classification which
owes most to Sauvages, the French nosographer, and to Pinel. Pinel
had thought that the primary seat of disease in cases of insanity lay in
the region of the stomach and intestines, and Prichard accordingly
divided his cases into uterine, enteric, hepatic and organic classes. The
Frenchman had written that he had "attended at thirty-six dissections
in the hospital of Bicêtre, and I can declare that I have never met with
any other appearances within the cavity of the cranium than are

L

observable on opening the bodies of persons who have died of *apoplexy*, *epilepsy*, *nervous fevers* and *convulsions*". "From such data, what light can be thrown on the subject of insanity?" asks Pinel. Prichard disagreed with this opinion for he considered that vascular factors were pre-eminent in the pathology of mental and nervous diseases, and that inflammation, whether primary or secondary, was responsible for the mental changes. Consequently, Prichard was a great advocate of bleeding, and the blood ran freely on his visiting days at the Bristol Infirmary. He was a strong organicist and felt that disease of the brain or "nervous fabrick" would eventually be found to underly the functional psychoses.

He writes:

> I am fully convinced that the pathology of these diseases is at present so imperfect, that we can scarcely regard one supposition on this subject as more probable than another. It is difficult to imagine how all the phaenomena of diseased brain can arise from affections of the primae viae, without the intervention of local disease in the cerebral structure itself: but it is equally unknown to us how disorders of the digestive functions should induce such local diseases. In considering this subject, it is necessary to discard all preconceived opinions, and to collect simply the inferences from facts.
>
> I am however persuaded, on surveying the facts which have fallen under my own observation, that among those cases of nervous or cerebral disease, which are consequent upon irregularities in the natural or vital functions, a great majority will be found to depend upon actual disease, and often organic disease in the brain, or some other part of the nervous fabrick, which, though in the first instance a secondary affection, becomes in the sequal a morbid cause of no less real existence, and often not less difficult of cure, than those diseases which primarily affect the brain itself. This, if I am not mistaken is the general conclusion we must adopt: and those instances before alluded to, in which the functions of the nervous system are deranged, while the structure itself is free from disease, must be regarded as exceptions to a general observation.

Strangely enough, however, he took exception to the strongly "organic" bias of Gall and Spurzheim, quoting one of their cases only to pour scorn on their opinions.

> Dr. Gall, in his work on Craniology, has mentioned some pathological observations, tending to evince the dependence of various active as well as intellectual powers on the brain, its organization and condition. Some

of these refer particularly to the propensities. I shall cite his account of one incident, which is adduced with this view, in which a disorder of the propensities is stated to have followed an injury of the head.

The accident happened to a boy in Copenhagen, who until his fourteenth and fifteenth years gave but very little promise of future abilities. At this epoch, however, he fell over a staircase from the fourth storey; and subsequently to the fall he displayed great intellectual acuteness. Nor was this the only change. Nobody was previously aware of any bad qualities in his disposition, but after this accident he displayed a depraved moral character, which eventually proved the cause of his ruin.

A relation of this kind proves nothing. That an individual at the age of this youth should begin to display the influence of powerful passions on his mind, is nothing extraordinary. If stories of this kind gain credit, the College of Surgeons may expect one day to march in triumph and take possession of the vacant seats of the criminal judges; and we shall proceed forthwith to apply the trepan where now the halter and gibbet are thought most applicable.

His views were to change a great deal over the next twenty years, for he could hardly have failed to include this case in his group of Moral Insanities if he had been considering it in 1842. His views on nosology were also to change with experience, and his somewhat idealistic statement that etiological classification was the only system of any practical advantage came to be modified over the years.

The main interest of the book in the development of Prichard's thought lies in his discussion of Pinel's concept of *manie sans délire*; that is, madness without any lesion of the understanding. In view of his later description of moral insanity, generally regarded as Prichard's most important contribution to psychiatry his first, tentative approach to the concept demands full consideration. Under the heading of Disease of the Active Powers, he writes:

> I must allow that there is a common persuasion among physicians that such a disease exists. It is even described by M. Pinel, one of the best practical authors on the subject of madness; who has adduced cases, which he regards as decided examples of this character. This species of disease is termed, by M. Pinel, "mania without delirium;" that is, madness without any lesion of the understanding. The victims of this dreadful malady display a propensity to violent paroxysms of rage, which exerts itself upon every person indiscriminately who happens to come their way.
>
> Notwithstanding the authority of general opinion and, what is of more consequence, the testimony of such a writer as M. Pinel, I cannot persuade

myself of the accuracy of the reports on which the existence of this
disease rests. That a human being, in the possession of a clear understanding, having, therefore, a correct apprehension of social relations, of his
own interest, and what he owes to others, should be suddenly transported
by a paroxysm of rage, without any incitement in what seems to be
universally and necessarily connected with the movements of anger, I
mean an apprehension of real or unreal injury or offence, would be a
phaenomenon quite at variance with the known laws of human nature.
A passion or emotion taking place in the mind, implies an impression or
idea adequate to call it forth. An emotion without corresponding impression on the understanding, is like a volition without a motive, or like
an effect without a cause.

It may be replied that this remark is well founded, in so far as it relates
to a sound mind, but that madness subverts, or throws into confusion, the
processes of the mind.

It must be allowed that the mental phaenomena take place, under
disease of the brain, in a different manner from that of the healthy state.
Still, however, the same laws govern these operations, though their action
is disturbed and thrown out of its usual course. But such a phaenomenon
as that of a man rushing with eagerness to commit the most atrocious
murders, under that influence of ungovernable fury, without any impression on his mind, that is calculated to excite anger, even without any
fancied ground of offence against his unfortunate victim, cannot be
imagined to result from the operation of any natural causes. Such a maniac
must be literally possessed by a daemon: his action is not that of a human
being, however insane. Yet M. Pinel describes this as the proceeding of a
man, who, in the common sense of words, must be called sane, as being in
full possession of his intellectual faculties.

I am convinced that experience will not support this representation. All
the atrocious murders committed by lunatics have been perpetrated under
some hallucinations. A hundred celebrated instances of such commissions
on historical record, will occur to every reader. Such facts are allowed on
all hands to be extremely rare, and hence the probability increases of an
incorrect report.

I believe the true explanation of these phaenomena to be the following.
The individuals who are the supposed subjects of this affection, are, in their
ordinary state, free from any maniacal illusion, and are hence supposed
to have an undisturbed possession of their intellectual faculties: but they
fall at certain periods under the influence of some sudden hallucination,
which excites their rage to a vehement degree, and gives rise to atrocious
attempts. Perhaps this sometimes amounts to nothing more than a vague
and undefined impression of some grievous injury or affront, inflicted

upon them by the person against whom their malice is directed. It often happens that the imaginary cause of anger is studiously concealed; and hence the opinion may have taken its rise, that the paroxysm of rage has arisen independently of any such impression.[1]

I may observe, that in all these instances of madness, which have been represented to me as examples of disorder affecting the active principles, without lesion of the understanding, I have discovered, on adequate inquiry, that the case was in reality otherwise. After minutely interrogating such patients, I have traced some latent impression, which has sufficiently accounted for the change observed in the feelings or affections.

It has often been observed that insanity reverses the whole moral character, that the habits and propensities undergo a complete revolution; that the temper becomes completely altered; but even in cases which verify this statement, a disorder of the understanding or some prevalent illusion, often gives rise to the peculiar tendency. The habits are also very much under the influence of the internal sensations which arise from the state of the natural functions, and the impression they give to the temper and spirits. When the stomach is oppressed by imperfect digestion, and all the secretions are performed with difficulty, a constant irritation is thence excited in the system, which occasions peevishness, fretfulness, and low spirits, in a person accounted sane, and gives a moody and discontented turn to his thoughts: the same causes acting on an insane person determine the complexion of his hallucinations. Thus we find melancholic patients, for the most part, dyspeptic: a fact from which the very term of hypochondriasis had its origin. On the other hand, when all the internal functions go on easily and prosperously, a general sense of animal enjoyment, a perpetual state of comfortable and pleasurable feeling arises, by which a cheerful flow of spirits is promoted. This state is liable to interruption in every instance of disease; but, as far as it exists, it determines in a great measure the natural temper, and has a great influence on the general habits.

I have at different times seen a number of maniacal patients, whose disorder has appeared, on a superficial view, to consist in a deranged state of the pathemata, or feelings. In all these cases, after an accurate examination, I have discovered some morbid bias of the understanding, some hallucination, more or less strongly marked, which has been sufficient to

---

[1] It must have been observed by every medical person, who has the care of lunatics, that they sometimes acquire the habit of concealing their impressions, particularly if frequently questioned respecting them, and that it requires some art and address to bring them to the subject without putting them on their guard.

account for the phaenomena. This species of disease generally appears in
occasional paroxysms: during the intervals the patient is tolerably sane,
and, if questioned at these times, he will exhibit no disorder of the understanding; but when the attack of his disease comes on, he is found to be
under the influence of some illusion.

It has been remarked, that this occasional recurrence of violent paroxysms is the particular form which madness assumes when combined
with epilepsy. I have seen several instances that were by no means in
accord with this observation.

These views were again to alter substantially over the next twelve
years, and his final description of Moral Insanity shows all the marks
of careful reappraisal of Pinel's work.

Some of the case histories show the type of practice to be found in a
large port such as Bristol. Cases such as that of Trusty Halsted perhaps
shed some light on Prichard's lifelong support of the Abolition of
Slavery.

Traumatic Cases

TRUSTY HALSTED, a negro sailor, aged twenty years.

He is a slave; and about four years ago his owner, or some other white
man, in a fit of anger, struck a blow on his head with a hammer. The
extent of the mischief occasioned by the blow was not ascertained, but he
soon after became subject to epileptic fits, and partially hemiplegiac on
his left side.

He was admitted into the Hospital as a patient of Dr. Wells, who
ordered him to have a blister, and perpetual drain at the nape of the neck,
and to take cathartic mixture.

The head being examined, it appeared probable that some injury of the
skull had been the consequence of the blow received; and accordingly
the operation of trepanning was performed. A piece of the cranium being
removed, a fragment of the interior table was found to have been forced
inwards upon the brain, and penetrating to the depth of the eighth part
of an inch.

An epileptic fit took place while he was under the operation, and the
same disorder assailed him occasionally as long as he remained in the
Hospital, though it appeared somewhat mitigated. He was taken away by
his owner, and obliged to go to sea before the wound was healed. It is
probable that some considerable disorganization had been induced in the
encephalon, by the long continued compression, and, perhaps, by the
irritation occasioned by a sharp fragment of bone forced in upon the dura
matter.

Although praised by Esquirol and translated into German, the book has little originality, and is reminiscent of the works of William Perfect, whom Pinel had so greatly admired. It appears as if Prichard was setting down his case notes in print with some connecting but tentative theoretical links, but as yet showing little evidence of any profundity of thought. This is in no way to derogate Prichard, for at this period he was engaged in writing some of his most original and brilliant ethnological and philological work.

"A TREATISE ON INSANITY AND OTHER DISORDERS AFFECTING THE MIND" (1835)

Prichard's friends John Conolly and Alexander Tweedie were two of the three principal editors of the *Cyclopaedia of Practical Medicine*—a joint production of sixty-seven of "the most eminent *Practical Physicians* of Great Britain and Ireland", to which Prichard contributed articles on Delirium, Hypochondriasis, Insanity, Somnambulism and Animal Magnetism, Soundness and Unsoundness of Mind, and Temperament. As a result he became convinced that

> although many excellent treatises exist on various matters connected with mental derangement in the English, French and German languages, there is yet not one work extant in either of them which exhibits the *present state* of knowledge and opinion on the whole subject of diseases affecting the mind.

To a man of Prichard's encyclopaedic bent this was a challenge after his own heart and he accordingly embarked on his *Treatise on Insanity*, which was eventually published in 1835.

Here a remarkable transformation has occurred. The book is compact, well-documented and the theoretical structure and arguments sound and closely argued. French influence is dominant, and we become more familiar with the Maison Royale de Charenton, the Bicêtre and the Salpêtrière than with Bethlem and St. Luke's. The dedication is to Esquirol (Fig. 5),

> the most distinguished writer of his age on the subjects which I have endeavoured to investigate. May I thus be allowed to connect with my work a name which will be handed down to posterity as that of one who, by elucidating the causes of the most severe of temporal calamities, and the means of its alleviation, has deserved the gratitude of mankind.

Prichard divided insanity into four groups, all of which are derived from French psychiatric concepts. Firstly, moral insanity, by which he meant

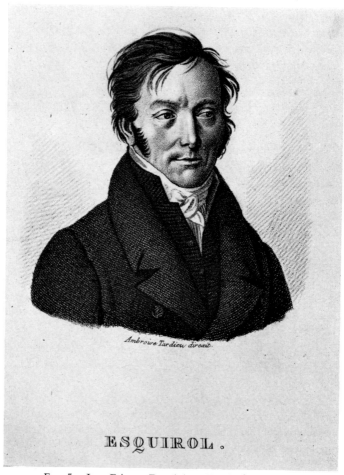

FIG. 5.   Jean Etienne Dominique Esquirol, 1772–1850.

madness, consisting in a morbid perversion of the natural feelings, affections, inclinations, temper, habits, moral dispositions, and natural impulses, without any remarkable disorder or defect of the interest or knowing and reasoning faculties, and particularly without any insane illusion or hallucinations.

The three following modifications of the disease may be termed *Intellectual Insanity* in contradistinctions to the preceding form, they are severally:

2. *Monomania*, or partial insanity, in which the understanding is partially disordered or under the influence of some particular illusion, referring to one subject, and involving one train of ideas, while the intellectual powers appear, when exercised on other subjects, to be in a great measure unimpaired.

3. *Mania*, or raving madness, in which the understanding is generally deranged; the reasoning faculty, if not lost, is confused and disturbed in its exercise; the mind is in a state of morbid excitement, and the individual talks absurdly on every subject to which his thoughts are momentarily directed.

4. *Incoherence*, or dementia. By some persons it may be thought scarcely correct to term this a form of insanity, as it has been generally considered as a result and sequel of that disease. In some instances, however, mental derangement has nearly this character from the commencement, or at least assumes it at a very early period. I am therefore justified in stating it, after Pinel, to be a fourth and distinct form of madness. It is thus characterised by that justly celebrated writer:

Rapid succession or uninterrupted alternation of insulated ideas, and evanescent and unconnected emotions, continually repeated acts of extravagance; complete forgetfulness of every previous state; diminished sensibility to external impressions; abolition of the faculty of judgement; perpetual activity.

The origin of these concepts is of such importance as to require quotation in full. First as to the moral insanities, Pinel had already described cases of *emportement maniaque sans délire*, and Prichard begins by quoting the following cases from the *Traité sur l'aliénation mentale*.

An only son of a weak and indulgent mother gave himself up habitually to the gratification of every caprice and passion of which an untutored and violent temper was susceptible. The impetuosity of his disposition increased with his years. The money with which he was lavishly supplied removed every obstacle to the indulgence of his wild desires. Every instance of opposition or resistance roused him to acts of fury. He assaulted his adversary with the audacity of a savage; sought to reign by force, and was perpetually embroiled in disputes and quarrels. If a dog, a horse, or any other animal offended him, he instantly put it to death. If he ever went to a fête or any other public meeting, he was sure to excite such tumults and quarrels as terminated in actual pugilistic rencontres, and he generally left the scene with a bloody nose. This wayward youth, however, when unmoved by passion, possessed a perfectly sound judgement. When he became of age, he succeeded to the possession of an extensive domain. He proved himself fully competent to the management of his estate, as well as the discharge of his relative duties, and he ever distinguished himself by acts of beneficence and compassion. Wounds, lawsuits, and pecuniary compensations, were generally the consequences of his unhappy propensity to quarrel, but an act of notoriety put an end of his career of violence. Enraged with a woman who had used offensive language to him, he threw her into a well. Prosecution was commenced against him; and on the deposition of a great many witnesses, who gave evidence to his furious deportment, he was condemned to perpetual confinement in Bicêtre.[1]

Prichard continues:

The following remarks by M. Esquirol, expressed as they appear to have been without the design of supporting any system or theory, prove that the writer was led by his ample experience to adopt an opinion similar to that of Pinel. He regards at least the perverted state of the moral feelings as not less essential to insanity than that of the intellectual faculties, and even as furnishing in some instances the whole manifestation of the disorder.

The insane conceive an aversion for those persons who are most dear to them, revile them, ill-treat them, anxiously shun them, in consequence of their mistrust, their suspicions, and their fears. Predjudiced against everything, they are afraid of everything. A few appear to form an exception to this general rule, in preserving a sort of affection for their relatives and friends; but this feeling of attachment, which is sometimes excessive, subsists without confidence in those persons who before the attack of disease had been the directors of the thoughts and actions of the patient. A Melancholic, who is devotedly attached to his wife, is deaf to her counsels and advice. A son would sacrifice his life for his father, but will not make the slightest attempt, in compliance with the entreaties of the latter, to overcome the morbid impression which occasions him so much grief.

"This moral alienation is so constant," says M. Esquirol, "that it appears to me to be the proper characteristic of mental derangement. There are madmen in whom it is difficult to discover any hallucination, but there are none in whom the passions and moral affections are not disordered, perverted or destroyed. I have in this particular met with no exceptions."

"A return to the proper and natural state of the moral affections," says the same writer, "the desire of seeing once more children and friends; the

---

[1] *Traité Médico-Philosophique sur L'aliénation mentale*, 2nd edition, Paris 1809, p. 156.

tears of sensibility; the wish manifested by the individual to open his heart and return into the bosom of his family, to resume his former habits, afford a certain indication of cure, while the contrary dispositions had been a mark of approaching insanity, or the symptom of a threatened relapse. This is not the case when there is merely a disappearance of the hallucination, which then only is a certain sign of convalescence, when the patients return to their natural and original affections."

Georget, too,

has described a morbid state of the feelings and active principles of the mind, or of the propensities and habits, as a particular modification of madness . . . individuals predisposed to mental disease by a faulty educa-tion or by previous attacks, have often continued for a long time, or perhaps even during their whole lives, to attract observation by caprices in their deportment, by something eccentric in their manner and habits of life, by an ill-regulated fondness for pursuits of the fancy, and the mere productions of the imagination, combined with a sinking in-aptitude in the study of the exact sciences. The last-mentioned particular will scarcely be sufficient to excite a suspicion of madness in this country, whatever may be the cause in France. These persons are noted for singular-ity of opinion, of conduct for transitory fits of intelligence, or sallies of wit, which are too strongly contrasted with their habitual state of nullity or monotony; for a levity in thoughts, a weakness in judgement, a want of connexion in their attempts at reasoning. Some individuals are pre-sumptious, desirous of undertaking every thing and capable of applying themselves to nothing; others are extravagant and mobile in the utmost degree in their opinions and sentiments, many are susceptible, irritable, choleric, and passionate; some are governed by pride and haughtiness without bound; a few are subject to vague anxieties or to panic terrors.

Prichard considered that one of the most striking types of moral insanity is distinguished by an unusual prevalence of angry and malicious feelings, which arise without provocation or any of the ordinary excitements.

All the examples of madness without delirium reported by Pinel belong to this class of disorders. On this account the cases described by Pinel failed for a long time to produce conviction of my mind, as to the existence of what he terms *manie sans délire* or *folie raisonnante*. I am now persuaded that he was correct in his opinion, and I have even been led to generalise his statement. M. Esquirol has assured me that his impression on this subject was similar. He considered Pinel's cases as inconclusive, and for a time was disposed to entertain strong doubts as to the existence of insanity without intellectual error or delusion. M. Esquirol has expressed his conviction of the reality of this form of mental derangement.

Prichard quotes several examples of moral insanity, of which the following three illustrate the variety of disorders embraced under the term.

Case 1.—A. B., a gentleman remarkable for the warmth of his affections, and the amiable simplicity of his character, possessed of great intellectual capacity, strong powers of reasoning, and a lively imagination, married a lady of high mental endowments, and who was long well known in the literary world. He was devotedly attached to her, but entertained the greatest jealousy lest the world should suppose that, in consequence of her talents, she exercised an undue influence over his judgement, or dictated his compositions. He accordingly set out with a determination of never consulting her, or yielding to her influence, and was always careful, when engaged in writing, that she should be ignorant of the subject which occupied his thoughts. His wife has been often heard to lament that want of sympathy and union of mind which are so desirable in married life. This peculiarity, however, in the husband so much increased, that in after years the most trifling proposition on her part was canvassed and discussed by every kind of argument. In the meantime he acquired strange peculiarities of habits. His love of order, or placing things in what he considered order or regularity, was remarkable. He was continually putting chairs, etc. in their places; and if articles of ladies' work or books were left upon a table, he would take an opportunity unobserved of putting them in order, generally spreading the work smooth, and putting the other articles in rows. He would steal into rooms belonging to other persons for the purpose of arranging the various articles. So much time did he consume in trifles, placing and replacing, and running from one room to another, that he was rarely dressed by dinner-time, and often apologised for dining in his dressing-gown, when it was well known that he had done nothing the whole morning but dress. And he would often take a walk in a winter's evening with a lanthorn, because he had not been able to get ready earlier in the day. He would run up and down the garden a certain number of times, rinsing his mouth with water, and spitting alternately on one side and then on the other in regular succession. He employed a good deal of time in rolling-up little pieces of writing-paper which he used for cleaning his nose. In short his peculiarities were innumerable, but he concealed them as much as possible from the observation of his wife, whom he knew to be vexed at his habits, and to whom he always behaved with the most respectful and affectionate attention, although she could not influence him in the slightest degree. He would, however, occasionally break through these habits; as on Sundays, though he rose early for the purpose, he was always ready to perform service at a chapel a mile and a half distant from his house. It was a mystery to his intimate friends when and how he prepared these services. It did not at all surprise those who were best acquainted with his peculiarities, to hear that in a short time he became notoriously insane. He fancied his wife's affections were alienated from him, continually affirming that it was quite impossible she could have any regard for a person who had rendered himself so contemptible. He committed several acts of violence, argued vehemently in favour of suicide, and was shortly afterwards found drowned in a canal near his house. It must not be omitted that this individual derived a predisposition to madness by hereditary transmission: his father had been insane.

Case 2.—The second case is one which had likewise for a considerable period the character of moral insanity, and degenerated into, or assumed that of monomania. The details which I relate are such as I collected from the friends of the individual, and from his own communications.

C. D., a gentleman about thirty years of age, has laboured for several years under symptoms of moral insanity. He has been long dejected in spirits and morose in temper, dissatisfied with himself, and suspicious of all that surrounded him. He was capricious and unsteady in his pursuits, frequently engaging in some new study in the most sanguine manner, and soon abandoning it in despair of making any progress, though possessed of good talents and considerable acquirements of knowledge. He passed the requisite period of time at one of the universities, but could not be prevailed upon to go in for his degree, either through timidity and want of resolution, or, as it was conjectured by his friends, from a morbid apprehension that the examiners would not deal fairly with him, and award him the station to which he aspired and believed himself entitled. He applied himself afterwards to the study of medicine, and then to that of metaphysics, and speedily relinquished both. He frequently changed his residence, but soon began to fancy himself the object of dislike to every person in the house of which he became the inmate. His peculiarities appearing to increase, he was visited by two physicians who were desired to investigate the nature of his case. On being questioned narrowly as to the ground of the persuasion expressed by him, that he was disliked by the family with which he then resided, he replied that he heard whispers uttered in distant apartments of the house indicative of malevolence and abhorrence. An observation was made to him that it was impossible for sounds so uttered to be heard by him. He then asked if the sense of hearing could not, by some physical change in the organ, be occasionally so increased in intensity as to become capable of affording distinct perception at an unusual distance, as the eyes of mariners are well known to be accommodated by long effort to very distant vision. This was the only instance of what might be termed hallucination discovered in the case after a minute scrutiny. It seemed to be a late suggestion. The individual had been for years labouring under a gradually increasing moral insanity. His judgement had become at length perverted by the intensity of his morbid feelings, and admitted as real an erroneous impression, suggested by his fancy, which happened to be in harmony with his feelings, and served to account for them.

Case 3.—This case was strictly one of moral insanity for some years after its commencement, and it maintained that character throughout its duration, except that at one period, under great excitement, the patient began to display signs of an approach of monomania, in the groundless suspicions which she expressed respecting persons who were about her. These symptoms, however, continued but for a very short time, and have never recurred. At the period when this individual came under my observation, her disorder had precisely the character of moral insanity.

E. F.—is a maiden lady, aged about forty-eight, of short stature, and somewhat deformed. "Her natural disposition was steady and industrious; she accomplished her undertakings by dint of application rather than by energetic or sudden efforts. She was constant rather than ardent in her attachments, free from resentment, never the subject of lively emotions; a great respecter of truth, just and very exact in all that she said or did. Her charitable acts were commensurate with her means, deliberate, and the result of principle rather than arising from the mere impulse of compassionate feeling. She was cautious and reserved in her communications, and scarcely if ever formed any familiar and particular intimacies with young persons of her own sex. Being debarred by her infirmities from associating with the young and active, she seemed more like an adult member of the family than a child. She was very clever in arithmetic and in all matters of business, and was fond of regulating and controlling the little affairs of those who formed the domestic circle surrounding her. Young persons and servants, finding that they derived advantage from her advice, generally gave her an opportunity of gratifying her inclination. Her dress, which was always plain and in good taste, was to her an object of greater attention than it often is to persons of fashion."

In March 1822 she was attacked by severe inflammation in the lungs, attended by expectoration of bloody mucus. This was the first time in her life when it was necessary to confine her to bed. She submitted with great reluctance to the restrictions that were needful for her recovery, and would not be persuaded, until she had heard the opinion of an old friend of her family, who is a medical practitioner, that the means adopted were proper and required by her case. She was then, however, in a great

measure reconciled, and after seven or eight weeks was so far recovered
as to bear a removal into her native county. At this period nobody believed that she would survive another winter. Her restoration to her usual
state of health was very slow, and her sister, who was her constant companion, perceived with sorrow that her temper was now much changed.
She appeared restless, always wishing to go somewhere, or to do something to which she was unequal; becoming unjustly irritated when she
could not urge her sister, whose health and spirits were declining, to fall
in with her ideas, and occasionally giving way to reproaches which were
keenly felt. She tried every method of persuasion to induce her sister to
go to the neighbourhood of London, though for the preservation of her
life the latter had been obliged to give up the custom of spending the
winter there, and the attempt was considered dangerous to her. Every
inducement, every argument was suggested to promote this favourite
object; other towns were too warm and too cold, too hilly, too much
intersected with water, too foggy. In 1827 she determined to go without
her sister to H—, near London. She went, and from her letters her sister
perceived that she was living in a state of excitement far surpassing that of
her former habits; paying short visits to friends in the surrounding villages,
going out in the common short stages, without so much regard to weather
as was usual to her even in the summer; receiving small parties at home,
attending a very crowded church, writing a great many letters, etc. etc.
She used to write to her sister in rather a boastful style, frequently mentioning her good health and high spirits, as if to justify her choice of a
residence near the metropolis. When the sisters met during the summer
at their house in —shire, her high spirits were gone, she looked more aged
than the time elapsed would have led any one to expect, took less interest
in her garden, appeared exhausted, and, without contributing her share
to the conversation, used frequently to sleep in her chair. She lay much in
bed, nursed herself up, and in October when again to H—, as much agog
as ever. Another winter passed much as the preceding one had done. She
spoke much again of her high spirits, visited much, was observed to be
unusually liberal in her presents to most of her acquaintances. A second
summer of inertness was succeeded by a winter at H—. She was now
weak, indisposed for visiting, and, in fact, so much worse as to be unable
to follow her inclinations. In the Spring of 1840 she had an attack of the
same nature as that in 1822, but not so severe or lasting. In the summer
she was nearly as before, and quite as eager to resume her plans, as
enthusiastic in her commendations of every body and every thing at H—.

About this time some riots took place in London, and more were
apprehended. She now expressed herself as apprehensive that "very awful
times were at hand", wrote frequent letters to her sister full of indecision,

and expressive of distrust in her servants, her host, and his family. A friend
who called upon her "was shocked to find her in so low a way". He
thought her unfit to be alone, and she was unwilling to adopt any plan for
leaving her lodgings, or having any one with her. She said she should be
happy with her sister, and knew that she should be taken care of by the
latter, but dreaded becoming a burden to her and making her ill; yet
feared that if she did not go to her sister, "some one would put her where
no one would know, and cause her to sign papers which she ought not to
sign". She was evidently apprehensive of being sent to a lunatic asylum.
She thought her host was a writer of "Swing Letters",[1] and dreaded that
he might fill the house with combustibles, and blow it up with her in it.
A medical man who was taken to see her, said that she was in a state of
great mental excitement, and ought to be taken to her sister as soon as possible. The frost was severe when she was escorted to her sister, who was then
settled at Bristol, yet she took no cold, experienced no injury from fatigue,
and lost that feeling of terror to which she had for some time been subject.
Since she has been with her sister, she has been increasingly obstinate,
suspicious, undecided, restless, parsimonious even to meanness, indisposed
to any employment bodily or mental, except as far as relates to a most
troublesome interference with the most minute actions of others. Could
she have her own way, she would control the food, dress, and employment of everyone near her. She has become negligent in dress, and comparatively dirty in her habits, yet has an insatiable desire for new clothes,
which she never finds the right time to wear. She is constantly predicting
her utter ruin, is sure she will not have money enough to live until such
and such a time; knows that enough will not be found to pay Dr. ——;
knows he will not let any one of so shabby an appearance be long in his
house; does not know where she shall go when he is tired of her; thinks
that "it is the devil that makes her behave as she does"; that her heart
is hardened to do what she ought not to do;" "she is like the man spoken
of in the Gospel, who could not be bound even with fetters". She sees
people look at her; hopes they don't think she drinks too much; is quite
sure she never did. These impressions are continually varying; but no
sooner is her mind tranquillized on one subject that another source of
disquietude arises, so that she exhausts every person who is long with her.
Her bodily health is better than it was for years previous to her mental
derangement. A constitutional asthma, to which she has been subject from
the age of six or seven years, has nearly subsided, and the habitual profuse

---

[1] It may hereafter require to be explained that, about the period above
mentioned, the threatening letters of incendiaries in various parts of the
country frequently bore the signature of Swing.

expectoration has considerably diminished. She wears less clothing and appears less sensible to cold or damp than heretofore.

I had several interviews with the subject of the foregoing relation, during some of which she gave replies to a variety of questions referring to the past and actual state of her health, both bodily and mental. No impression could be traced in her mind that bore the character of insane hallucination. The circumstance most observable in her condition was a perpetual disposition to find fault with every action, even the most trivial, that was witnessed by her. When asked if she was not aware of this propensity, she seemed to give an unwilling affirmative to the question, and she was plainly aware of the fact, for on the inquiry being made whether the habit had only existed of late years, or had been a part of her natural character, she steadily averred that such was not her natural disposition, "that she was formerly very different".

What Prichard meant, of course, by moral cause was emotional disturbance, as is clearly shown in the following extract and by the tables which follow.

Experience itself has led many to the conclusion that moral causes are mainly influential in the development of diseases of the mind. No writer has maintained this opinion to a greater extent than M. Georget. "The observations," says M. Georget, "which I have had it in my power to make, the more numerous ones which I have compared in authors, have convinced me, that among 100 lunatics, 95 at least have become such from the influence of affections and of moral commotions: it is an observation become almost proverbial in the hospital—the Salpêtrière,—'qu'on perd la tête par les révolutions d'esprit'." The first question that M. Pinel puts to a new patient who still preserves some remains of intelligence is, Have you undergone any vexation or disappointment? Seldom is the reply in the negative. "It is," continues the same writer, "in the age in which the mind is most susceptible of strong feelings, in which the passions are excited by the strongest interests, that madness is principally displayed. Children, calm and without anxiety, incapable of long and extensive combinations of thought, not yet initiated into the troubles of life, and old men, whom now the vanishing illusions of their preceding age, and their increasing physical and moral weakness render indifferent as to events, are but rarely affected. The same remark applies to persons who in their constitution approach to the character of children or of old Men."

Esquirol drew up a table listing the influence of emotion and of physical agents in the production of insanity in females of the lower classes admitted to the Salpêtrière.

M

TABLE 1

Cases produced by moral causes In the Salpêtrière during the years 1811 and 1812		Physical Causes In the Salpêtrière during the years 1811 and 1812	
Domestic grief	105	Hereditary predisposition	105
Disappointment in love	46	Convulsions suffered by the mother during pregnancy	11
Political events	14	Epilepsy	11
Fanaticism	8	Irregularities in menstruation	55
Fright	38	Consequence of parturition	52
Jealousy	18	Critical period	27
Anger	16	Advanced age	60
Poverty, reverses of fortune	77	Coup de soleil	12
Offended self-love	1	Blows or falls on the head	14
Disappointed ambition	—	Fever	13
Excess in study	—	Syphilis	8
Misanthropy	—	Mercury	14
		Intestinal worms	4
		Apoplexy	60
Sum	323	Sum	446

A similar analysis was carried out on

the cases in The Maison Royale de Charenton, which is appropriated to persons of a higher rank in society than those who are remitted to other hospitals near Paris. The following table contains the results of three years observation.

TABLE 2

Moral causes		Physical causes	
Domestic griefs	89	Hereditary predisposition	93
Excessive study and watching	8	Masturbation	23
Reverses of fortune	20	Libertinism	24
Passion for gaming	2	Use of mercury	16
Jealousy	13	Abuse of wine	64
Disappointments in love	21	Insolation	7
Injured self-love	6	Effect of carbonic acid gas	2
Fright	7	Suppressions of habitual evacuations	13
"Dévotion exaltée"	18	Consequence of parturition	10
Excess of joy	1	Blows on the head	4
Reading romances	7		
Total	192	Total	256

Of political events, a particular moral cause, Prichard again quotes Esquirol.

> The influence of our political misfortunes has been so great, says the same writer, "that I could illustrate the history of our revolution from the taking of the Bastille to the last appearance of Bonaparte, by describing in a series the cases of lunatics, whose mental derangement was in connection with the succession of events." Political disturbances, like the mental impressions which give rise to insanity, are among the exciting causes. They set the predisposing influences in operation, and bring out some particular character of madness; but this impress, even if general, is still only temporary. At the destruction of the old monarchy many persons became mad through fright and the loss of their property. "When the Pope came to France, religious maniacs were very numerous. When Bonaparte made kings, there were many kings and queens in the madhouses. At the time of the invasion of France by foreign troops, terror threw many into derangement. The Germans had experienced the same effects at the era of our irruptions into their country."

Having been brought up in a Quaker household and later converted to Anglicanism, and having friends of different religious beliefs, Prichard's views on the relationship of religion and insanity are of some interest. He obtains Jacobi's support for his view that the number of persons who become insane through the influence of religious hopes and fears is much less considerable than generally supposed. Cases do occur under the influence of strong emotions produced by vehement preaching—on this account Falret linked Methodism with the frequency of suicide in England, an opinion Prichard considered unjust, certainly in contemporary England. Catholic writers had maintained that Protestant institutions were more favourable to the development of insanity than Catholic institutions—Prichard brings forward figures to show this is not the case.

> Religious insanity so termed is a disorder from which the Society of Friends are in a great measure exempt. With respect to the more general question, whether insanity of any kind prevails among the Quakers to a great or comparatively small extent, those writers who have touched upon the subject have been divided in opinion. Dr. Haslam says that insanity is very rare among the members of that society. Dr. Burrows thinks it very frequent among them, and he accounts for the fact by another supposition, viz. that their marriages are confined to the families of their own society, and therefore within a very limited circle. With

respect to the first point, which only is relevant, to my present purpose, Mr. Tuke has furnished me with some data which are highly interesting. He says that the number of inmates of the Retreat who are members of the religious Society of Friends has of late years been usually about 64. The total number of Friends in England and Scotland does not, as he believes, exceed 22,000 or 23,000. The mean of these sums divided by the number of patients actually in the Retreat gives $2\frac{3}{4}$, or somewhat less than 3 in a 1,000, which is a very high proportion, and considerably exceeding that which is supposed to obtain in the general population of this and other countries.

But there are considerations which render it difficult to believe that such a comparative result is correct, and which seem to lead us almost inevitably to an opposite conclusion, or at least show that some other considerations must be introduced in order to explain facts which turn out so contrary to all expectations from the known circumstances of the case.

All in all, Prichard was disposed to regard true religious madness as comparatively rare, and the result of strong emotion aroused in a religious setting—he realized that a religious content in an illness did not imply that religion was the cause of that illness.

In spite of the importance Prichard assigned to moral causes, he nevertheless considered madness as an idiopathic disease of the brain, a view upheld by the French. The Germans came in for some criticisms. Heinroth and Jacobi maintained that madness was a disease of the mind, an opinion which "although it has been abandoned by most enlightened physicians in England, is still prevalent among the public". Pinel's idea of a "sympathetic cerebral disease", with a kind of "sanguineous organism" suffusing the brain and so producing derangement of nervous function was still very much to Prichard's liking, and he spoke warmly of bleeding in the treatment of insanity. He recognized however that

the instances of mental disorder which leave the greatest doubt with respect to the presence of disease in the brain are those of moral insanity, or disorder affecting merely the moral character, the propensities, habits, temper, and feelings, without involving any notable lesion of the understanding. The complaint is often brought on by moral causes alone; it lasts for a time, and disappears, without the aid of physical remedies, through the effect of time, and by the influence of circumstances which act upon the mind alone.

None the less—by using analogy, comparison with known cases of cerebral disorder, and by the use of Pinel's "sympathetic" concept, Prichard was able to adhere to his phlogistic theory of madness.

For the rest Prichard gives adequate descriptions of mania, senile dementia, and a good survey of "general paralysis complicated with insanity". He makes no mention of syphilis here although the occurrence of the condition in association with "libertinism" is remarked upon. Treatment, both physical and moral, is discussed, and the book ends with a long section on Mesmerism, and a smaller one on phrenology. Apart from the introduction of the Moral Insanities, the book is a competent piece of early-Victorian writing somewhat reminiscent of George Man Burrows' *Statistics of Insanity*. It shows, however, a very great dependence on, and admiration for, French psychiatry, and the only English writers Prichard mentions are Cox, Haslam, Ferriar, Willis, Powell, Crichton, Burrows, Darwin, Perfect and Hallaran.

"ON THE DIFFERENT FORMS OF INSANITY IN RELATION TO JURISPRUDENCE" (1842)

This attitude is still to be seen in his next book *On the Different Forms of Insanity in Relation to Jurisprudence*, "Designed for the use of Persons concerned in legal Questions regarding Unsoundness of Mind", published in 1842 and 1847. He tried to avoid all technicalities and all use of medical terms not absolutely necessary, so that the book could be understood by the lawyers. Much of the psychiatric content is derived from his *Treatise on Insanity*—the importance of the book lies in the legal implications of Prichard's ideas.

He begins with a general review of the legal aspects of insanity from the standpoint of English law. There is a chapter on the prevalent idea that insanity is equivalent to delusion. Locke said, "Madmen put wrong ideas together, and so make wrong propositions, but argue and reason right for them", and seems to have led astray Dr. Battie, who considered that "deluded imagination constituted insanity". Prichard then gives Erskine's views, and concludes:

> It seems on the whole to be the settled doctrine of English Courts at present, that there cannot be insanity without delusion, or as it is otherwise

expressed by physicians, without illusion or hallucination, that is, without some particular erroneous conviction impressed upon the understanding, the affected person being otherwise in possession of the full and undisturbed use of his mental faculties. This is the doctrine of partial insanity, so that a man is supposed to be mad on one point, and sane on every other particular; a state in itself most incredible.

Prichard maintains

that mental derangement, in almost every case, not only involves a disordered exercise of the intellectual faculties, but extends even farther than the understanding, and implicates more remarkably the moral affections, the temper, the feelings and propensities; that it affects, in reality, the moral character even more decidedly than the understanding. I shall lay before my readers the proof of this assertion. . . .

He again attaches much importance to moral insanity, although it is often difficult to be certain whether natural peculiarity or eccentricity of character underly the manifestations of the disorder. Then follow descriptions of the chief forms of insanity, which we have already noted in his *Treatise*. There is a discussion of homicide and suicide, pyromania and kleptomania—sections on responsibility, lucid intervals, idiotism and imbecility, and lastly, fatuity or dementia.

The existence of moral insanity is palpable and easily recognised only in those instances in which it comes on, as it often does, after some strongly marked disorder affecting the brain and the general state of health, such as a slight attack of paralysis, and when it displays a state of mind strikingly different from the previous, and habitual or natural character of the individual. If a person of quiet and sedate temper, little subject to strong emotions, becomes excitable, violent, impetuous, thoughtless, and extravagant to such a degree as to surprise his friends and relatives, a suspicion is often produced that this change may depend upon a disordered state of mind. There are many individuals who are subject to alternate fits of excitement and depression; the contrast renders the peculiarities of such persons apparent.

There are many individuals living at large and not entirely separated from society, who are affected, in a certain degree, with this modification of insanity. An attentive observer will often recognise something remarkable in their manners and habits, which may lead him to entertain doubts as to their entire sanity, and circumstances are sometimes discovered on inquiry, which add strength to this suspicion. In many instances it has been found that an hereditary tendency to madness has existed in the family, or that several relatives of the person affected have laboured under other diseases of the brain. The individual himself has been discovered to have suffered, in a former period of life, an attack of madness of a decided character. His temper and disposition are found to have undergone a change; to be not what they were previously to a certain time; he has become an altered man, and the difference has, perhaps, been noted from the period when he sustained some reverse of fortune, which deeply affected him, or the loss of some beloved relative. In other instances an alteration in the character of the individual has ensued immediately on some severe shock which his bodily constitution has undergone. This has been either a disorder affecting the head, a slight attack of paralysis, or some febrile or inflammatory complaint, which has produced a perceptible change in the habitual state of his constitution. In some cases, the alteration in temper and habits has been gradual and imperceptible, and it seems only to have consisted in an exaltation and increase of peculiarities, which were always more or less natural and habitual. . . .

When I was engaged in writing the treatise to which I have already referred (*Treatise on Insanity*), Moral Insanity was a new term; the disease which I intended to describe under that name, had not been previously recognised, and I visited many lunatic asylums both in England and on the Continent, for the purpose of obtaining information, and made inquiries of many physicians who had the most ample opportunities of observing phenomena of insanity, in order to collect their opinion as to the real existence of the affection which I have thus designated. From Dr. Hitch, superintendent of the County Asylum, at Gloucester, I received the following communication on this subject, which, as it is of great consequence to establish the existence of Moral Insanity to the full conviction of my readers, I shall cite the words of the writer:

"I could easily furnish a great number of instances coinciding with your description of Moral Insanity! We have recognised them here for a very considerable time, and term individuals so affected, 'insane in conduct and not in ideas,' a distinction which has often led us into a difficulty of explanation, and a still greater difficulty of producing conviction, when justifying our detention of a patient, who has made a plausible and very reasonable tale to the visiting magistrates. Your discrimination of this disease, from intellectual insanity, and the further separation of the latter from actual madness, or mania, has much gratified me; it accords with my own observations, and tends to support a belief which I have long indulged, that many who have been convicted of crimes ought to have been pronounced insane."

The cases he used to illustrate his thesis are a very heterogeneous collection, including a manic depressive country magistrate, an alcoholic squire, a child with a probable childhood schizophrenia, manics, and individuals showing a personality change following cerebral disorder. He ends with a little note—

> Many of the most singular characters in history noted for capricious and erratic behaviour, and furnishing to their habits and course of action a sort of exception to the general laws of human conduct, are probably susceptible of this explanation. Such instances occur in the Singular Christina of Sweden, in the Russian Emperor Paul, and in Frederick the Second of Prussia.

The essential feature of this moral insanity seems to be a moral perversion, without any illusion or the belief in any unreal or imaginary fact. Eccentricity or "natural singularity of character" are in fact nearly allied to insanity and at times legal interference may be necessary. Delusion is certainly not an essential feature of madness.

Monomania or partial insanity is equivalent to delusional insanity in law, but Prichard shows how absurd is this concept of partial insanity, "Nothing, indeed, can be more remote from the truth than the opinion that madmen of this description have their whole disorder centred in, and restricted to, one delusive idea." True monomaniacs are extremely rare. Prichard then goes on to describe delusional insanity, referring particularly to Esquirol who had made a particular study of the subject. Unfortunately the quotation he takes from Esquirol refers to both manic–depressive illness and to schizophrenia, with no distinction being made between the two conditions. There is a little footnote which is amusing, and somewhat out of character for the usually serious and sober Prichard.

"A monomaniac who fancied himself possessed of great riches, once asked me if he should give me a sum of money. He sat down and wrote a cheque, pay Dr. Prichard £1000 and charge on God's bankers." As to the question of responsibility, Prichard agreed with Georget that "partial insanity or monomania excludes the idea of criminality or culpability, and takes away from the affected person all responsibility for his action, whatever may be the nature and extent of the illusions under which he may labour."

Another important medico–legal concept to which Prichard turned his attention is that of the "irresistible impulse". English Law has persistently refused to recognize this plea in the absence of the criteria for unsoundness of mind laid down under the McNaghten Rules. One of the pre-occupations of French alienists at this period was forensic psychiatry, particularly in relation to responsibility and the cause of crime. Raymond de Saussure, in his paper on "The Influence of the Concept of Monomania on French Medico-Legal Psychiatry from 1828-1840", has pointed out that before Esquirol, individuals who had committed crimes or misdemeanours were considered mentally ill only if they were in a state of actual delirium or dementia. With the advent of monomania any criminal act could be looked upon as a mental disorder—as an example of instinctive monomania, a condition in which the patient is drawn away from his accustomed behaviour to the commission of acts which neither reason nor sentiment determine, which conscience rebukes and which the will has no longer the power to control. The actions are involuntary, instinctive, irresistible. Prichard agreed with this concept, and described an instinctive madness in which

> the will is occasionally under the influence of an impulse, which suddenly drives the person affected to the perpetration of acts of the most revolting kind, to the commission of which he has no motive. The impulse is accompanied by consciousness; but it is in some instances irresistible; some individuals who have felt the approach of this disorder have been known to take precautions against themselves; they have warned, for example, their neighbours and relatives to escape from within their reach till the paroxysm should have subsided.
>
> There is scarcely an act in the catalogue of human crimes which has not been imitated, if we may so speak, to this disease. Homicides, infanticides, suicides of the most fearful description have been committed under its influence.

Arson, irresistible lying and cheating are also found. To Pinel we owe the recognition of this form of madness which he called *Emportement maniaque sans Délire*. It is difficult to distinguish between instinctive madness and moral insanity diagnostically, and Prichard did not make it clear whether instinctive madness was to be considered as one of the members of the group of moral insanities. In any case, what is important is the change which had taken place in Prichard's opinions over the twenty years since the publication of his first book on psychiatry. Crime has become linked irrevocably with mental disorder—with the delusional states for long accepted as relevant by the lawyers, and with the new entities, the moral insanities and instinctive madness. This is one of Prichard's major contributions to the development of psychiatric thought in Great Britain.

PRICHARD'S POSITION IN PSYCHIATRY

In most psychiatric textbooks and in *Zilboorg's History of Psychiatry*, Prichard's name is linked with the first description of those states ultimately to be given the title of psychopathic. His moral insanity and moral imbecility, although passing into clinical desuetude, became enshrined in legal terms under the Mental Deficiency Act of 1913—although "moral imbecility" became "moral defective" in the later 1927 Act. Moral insanity was a perennial topic for discussion until the end of the nineteenth century.

For instance, in 1891 the Medico–Psychological Association met in Bristol, and Hack Tuke chose this occasion to deliver an address on Prichard and on J. A. Symonds, a Bristol physician who was a close friend of Prichard. When it was published later in the year he added two articles, one on moral insanity, a paper he had read in 1884 to the Section of Psychology of the British Medical Association meeting in Belfast, and the second read in 1885 on a case of congenital moral defect. Tuke's essay shows how strongly entrenched were Prichard's ideas—for Tuke still used the term moral in two senses, implying either anti-social behaviour, or disturbed emotion. Thus melancholia was classed amongst the moral insanities—as were sexual perversions, sadism, behaviour disorders of children, and syndromes following brain damage. The second essay is of some interest, Tuke describing a case of *mania sanguinis*, and recounting examples of blood drinking, and the murderer's delight in warm blood—very reminiscent of Haigh's account of his crimes.

In his *Dictionary of Psychological Medicine*, published the following year, Hack Tuke accepted Prichard's definition of moral insanity. He pointed out that a great difference of opinion existed as to its situation as an entity, and mentioned the varieties of cases where a "moral disorder" is the predominant feature, quoting Herbert Spencer and Hughling Jackson in support of the concept, and giving a useful bibliography, derived from French, German and Italian sources.

Henry Maudsley, in his *Responsibility in Mental Disease* published in 1897, devoted thirteen pages to moral insanity. "This is a form of mental alienation," he writes, "which has so much the look of vice or crime that many persons regard it as an unfounded medical invention. —Judges have repeatedly denounced it from the bench as 'a most dangerous medical doctrine', 'a dangerous innovation', which in the interests of society should be reprobated." Maudsley differed from the judges, however—and pronounced himself strongly in favour of Prichard. In the main he adopted Prichard's views—including in this group what we would today call psychopathic personalities, manic-depressives, epileptics and mental defectives. "Assuredly moral insanity is disorder of mind produced by disorder of brain—Can we doubt that moral insanity is a form of derangement as genuine as any other form of mental derangement." Maudsley only paraphrased Prichard, and alas, his thinking on the subject was just as muddled, confusing cause with effect, and effect with cause.

However, in the textbooks of the later nineteenth century moral insanity no longer occupies a prominent place. Bevan Lewis, Clouston and Bianchi, for instance, hardly mention it—there is a very modern ring about their approach, clearly under Kraepelin's influence. Sir David Henderson gives an excellent brief account of the historical development of the concept of psychopathy as we know it today; this does not concern us here. Rather are we concerned with how Prichard came to distinguish his group of moral insanities, and the reasons for the uncritical acceptance of this somewhat heterogeneous group of cases by outstanding psychiatrists in England, France, Germany and Italy as a homogenous disorder. The reason may lie in the use of the word "moral". Alexander Walk believes that it was generally used in the broad sense of "psychological", as opposed to physical, and was in fact a Gallicism, "for up to the translation of Pinel's work treatment other than medicinal is always called 'management', but after 1806 we hear of 'moral management' and 'moral treatment'; up to about 1840, however, severe and mild methods are described indiscriminately under this heading; it is only later that some authors claim to use 'moral treatment', as *opposed* to coercion". Prichard, however, used the term moral in two senses—in its ethical meaning, and also as the equivalent of emotion. To a man of his upbringing and background the two meanings were closely linked—"moral" meant conformity to existing standards of social behaviour, and control of those emotions which might, if unleashed, produce both personal catastrophe and national convulsion such as France had seen. French influence domin-ated Prichard's psychiatric thought. His ethnological and philological works abound in references from many sources and are copiously annotated, whereas his psychiatric books are almost entirely French derivatives. British psychiatry of the eighteenth century was in advance of French or Continental psychiatry, and it remains somewhat puzzling as to why so learned and well-read a man as Prichard, should have so neglected his forerunners. The impact of the French Revolution on a Quaker later turned Anglican may partly explain this, together with his early love of French, and the direction which French psychiatry took during his lifetime.

Prichard's views eminently suited the cultural atmosphere of the time, the emphasis on "morality", and the whole aura of Victorian life being favourable to a concept such as that of moral insanity. Although Prichard died in 1848 he is essentially a Victorian figure, far removed from the rough and tumble of the eighteenth century—a great and inseparable gulf divides him from John Haslam, who had died only four years earlier. In 1843 the McNaghten Rules were formulated, and the fifteen Judges certainly took no account of Prichard's views; perhaps an eminently sound decision, considering the many untenable propositions put forward by Prichard in support of his concepts. British psychiatry was largely concerned with the more humane treatment of lunatics, and Hack Tuke devotes only one and three-quarter pages to Prichard in his 548 page volume *Chapters on the History of the Insane in the British Isles*. Semelaigne in his book on Pinel makes no mention of the importance English psychiatry had for Pinel, nor in all the pages of *Les Grands Aliénistes Français* are there more than one or two references to England. In *Aliénistes et Philanthropes*, when dealing with Hack Tuke, Semelaigne writes:

> La question de la folie morale est une de celles qui attira plus particulièrement son attention, et il prit nettement position en faveur des idées de Prichard, celui-ci, qui décrivit avec tant de soin cet état pathologique, ne fut pourtant pas un ouvrier de la première heure. Il se refusait d'abord à admettre la doctrine de Pinel, sur la manie sans délire; ce n'est que plus tard qu'il lui reconnut une part de vérité.

Esquirol had been somewhat more charitable—quoting four cases from Prichard, and praising Prichard's work. But he considered that: "Le docteur Prichard n'a peut-être pas suffisamment distingué la folie morale, d'une autre variété de folie exempte du désordre de l'intelligence et des affections, que Pinel a nommée manie sans délire, dont je parlerai dans des chapitres suivants."

Prichard's main influence was on British psychiatry. Relatively undisturbed by extremist views, the main stream of thought in England has flowed along more equably than in other countries. Prichard with his sober industry, immense knowledge and firm religious belief typifies the Victorian psychiatrist at his best. The age could understand his views, which were kept alive until the turn of the century—the fact that Prichard was a man near 50 when Victoria came to the throne illustrates his position as a leader of psychiatric thought of the nineteenth century, if not abroad, then certainly at home.

PRICHARD'S ANTHROPOLOGICAL STUDIES

Dwarfing his psychiatric contributions were Prichard's encyclopaedic works on a wide range of subjects connected with the study of Man.

"AN ANALYSIS OF THE EGYPTIAN MYTHOLOGY, WITH A CRITICAL EXAMINATION OF THE REMAINS OF EGYPTIAN CHRONOLOGY" (1819)

In 1819 Prichard published his *Analysis of the Egyptian Mythology, with a Critical Examination of the Remains of Egyptian Chronology*. Since the discovery of the Rosetta Stone (Fig. 6) in 1799, and its lodgement in the British Museum in 1802, the world of scholarship in the early nineteenth century had sought to unravel the mystery of the hieroglyphic language of ancient Egypt. Napoleon's Egyptian expedition had been accompanied by a veritable regiment of savants, and the work of the French Scientific Commission had revealed the grandeur and extent of Egyptian civilization along the Nile Valley. The *Description de l'Égypte* was appearing in serial publications containing an immense amount of material—inscriptions from temples, funeral rolls and papyri. Thomas Young had become interested in Egyptology through writing an article on the work *Mithridates*, by J. C. Adelung, a book which had an enormous influence on Prichard, and which he translated from the German. In this book Young had noticed a reference to the Rosetta Stone, but it was not until 1814 that he settled down to the task of deciphering the hieroglyphics. The controversy over the priority of Champollion or Young does not concern us here, but the abortive attempts by de Sacy and Åkerblad, the Swede, had awakened great interest in Egyptian Research. Young's findings, published in 1819, and Champollion's great work *Précis du Système Hiéroglyphique des Anciens Égyptiens* which appeared in 1824, were not available to Prichard when he was writing his book, so that his findings were all the more remarkable.

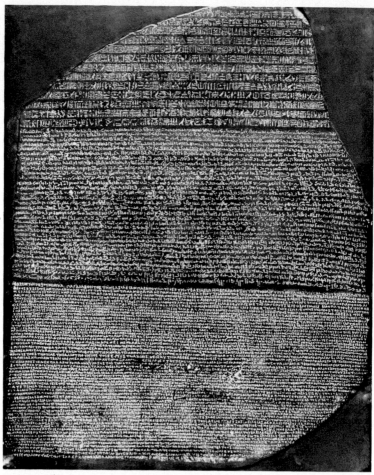

FIG. 6.   The Rosetta Stone. (*By permission of the Trustees, the British Museum.*)

Prichard's main object was to disprove Professor Murray's view that the religion and philosophy, as well as the language and all the other possessions of the Egyptian people, were peculiar to themselves and entirely unconnected with those which belonged to other nations of antiquity; and, consequently, that the Egyptians were a race peculiar to Africa. This had indeed been asserted by Champollion himself, and was strongly at variance with Prichard's own deductions from his ethnological work.

Prichard set out to compare the mythological and philosophic doctrines and civil institutions of the ancient Egyptians with those which were developed among the worshippers of Brahma in Eastern Asia. The language of ancient Egypt was so entirely unknown that no assistance could be derived from that source; Prichard therefore collected all the written evidence from pagan and Christian authors on Egyptian mythology and chronology. What follows can be no better expressed than by quoting Dr. Nash, an Egyptian scholar and a friend of Prichard,

> The treatise itself presents an ample and methodical arrangement of the authorities on the subject of Egyptian mythology and philosophy, from the writings of Pagan and Christian authors. What remains of ancient literature and philosophy, bearing upon Egyptian history, has been copiously collected and carefully applied to the illustration of this obscure and intricate branch of the history of mankind. As in all other of Dr. Prichard's writings, there is no straining of evidence to support a favourite hypothesis, but a careful statement of facts and circumstances, with a view to the elucidation of truth. The conclusion drawn from the remarkable coincidences and relations which Dr. Prichard pointed out as existing between Egyptian and Indian modes of thought, has received considerable support from a quarter the least expected. Recent investigations into the structure of the old Egyptian language, revealed to us by the successful interpretation of the hierogrammatic writing, have demonstrated an early original connection between the language of Egypt and the old Asiatic tongues. By this discovery, the Semitic barrier interposed between the Egyptian and the Asiatic races is broken down, and a community of origin established, which requires the hypothesis neither of the immigration of sacerdotal colonies, nor the doubtful navigation of the Erythraean sea. The profound views which led Dr. Prichard to assert, that "although many obstacles present themselves to the supposition that direct intercourse subsisted between the Egyptians and the nations of Eastern Asia, there appear, even on very superficial comparison, so many phenomena of striking congruity in the intellectual and moral habits, and in the peculiar character of mental culture displayed by those nations, and particularly by the Egyptians, when compared with the ancient Indians, that it is extremely difficult to refer all these analogies to merely accidental coincidence", have thus been remarkably confirmed. His comparisons of individual personages of the mythologic system of either nation may not bear

the test of measurement by the more extended knowledge of the subject which a quarter of a century has produced; but the terms of the general conclusions which are deduced from his *Analysis* may be fairly taken to be past all dispute.

The *Critical Examination of the Remains of Egyptian Chronology* is a remarkable monument of Dr. Prichard's sagacity, and of his aptitude for the elucidation of an obscure and intricate subject. The difficulty of the task which he here undertook he has not over-rated, when, after laying before the reader the lists of Manetho and Eratosthenes, the old Chronicle and the dynastic chronology of Herodotus and Diodorus, he says "nothing can be more discouraging than the first survey of the fragments we have extracted. When I first examined these fragments, with a view of computing from them the Egyptian chronology, they appeared to me to be an inextricable tissue of error and contradiction. I repeated my attempt several times at intervals, before I obtained the smallest hope of success, or a ray of light to guide me through the labyrinth. At length I thought I discovered a clue, which I have followed, and have persuaded myself that it has enabled me to unravel the mystery."

Prichard's "clue" was discovered by comparing the various lists extant of the chronology of the Pharaohs. In spite of the differences, there were nevertheless various points of agreement in all the lists which Prichard took as evidence that these lists had been compiled from a common source. He also contrasted Egyptian historians with the Hebrew, and from his consideration of all these sources arrived at a chronology of Egyptian affairs which was very nearly the same as that postulated by the Chevalier Bunsen at a later date, when a flood of light had been thrown on the subject as a result of the decipherment of the hieroglyphic language.

Prichard's book was warmly received, and was translated into German, with a preface by Von Schlegel, although the great German historian was critical of Prichard's conclusions. The Chevalier Bunsen wrote,

> simultaneously with the first steps in the progress of modern hieroglyphical discovery (in 1823), Dr. Prichard, one of the most acute and learned investigators of his time, had once more vindicated the claims of Egypt to a primeval chronology, and suggested a collation of the lists of Eratosthenes and Manetho, as the true method of elucidating the earliest period. In the work on Egyptian Chronology and Mythology he shows that the continually recurring coincidences which they offer must represent a chronological canon.

The two men became great friends, and Prichard later dedicated his *Natural History of Man* "To His Excellency THE CHEVALIER BUNSEN, Envoy Extraordinary and Minister Plenipotentiary of His Majesty the King of Prussia to the Court of Great Britain" and begins "My Dear Friend". *An Analysis* first appeared in 1819, then in 1823, and later in 1838, having been substantially enlarged.

"THE EASTERN ORIGIN OF THE CELTIC NATIONS" (1831)

Another work bearing on the same question published in 1831 was entitled *The Eastern Origin of the Celtic Nations*, "proved by a comparison of their dialects with the Sanskrit, Greek, Latin and Teutonic Languages, forming a supplement to Researches into the Physical History of Mankind". Languages display four kinds of relations— (1) As to vocabularies. If communication between nations was one of close commercial intercourse or of conquest, the words in common will be found to have reference to the new stock of ideas thus introduced. Such is the influence of the Arabic on the idioms of the Persians and Turks, and of the Latin upon some of the dialects of Europe. But if the connection was of a more ancient and intimate nature, the correspondence in the vocabularies will be found to involve words of the most simple and apparently primitive class, expressive of simple ideas, and universal objects. (2) There are languages with few words in common, but having a remarkable analogy in grammatical construction. Such are the polysynthetic idioms of the American tribes, and the monosyllabic languages of the Chinese and Indo-Chinese. (3) Some languages present both these characters of affinity, and Prichard called them "cognate". (4) There are languages in which neither of these connections can be found. Such languages are not of the same family, and generally belong to nations remote from each other in descent, and often in physical character.

Prichard proved by an elaborate comparison both of primitive words and of grammatical structure that the Celtic nations spring from a stock shared in common with those speaking the Indo-European languages.

These two works are masterly expositions of Prichard's enormous philological learning. References abound, and as may be seen from the items in Prichard's own library, range from the language of the Cree

N

and Chippeway Indians, to a vocabulary of Hawaiian words. The industry of the man was amazing, especially when seen against the background of a busy medical practice.

But his *magnum opus* is undoubtedly his *Researches into the Physical History of Mankind*, published in five large volumes.

"RESEARCHES INTO THE PHYSICAL HISTORY OF MANKIND"

As we have seen, his M.D. Thesis of 1808 was entitled "De Generis Humani Varietate", a dissertation of some 150 pages, an unusual length for an Edinburgh thesis, the average being 20–30 pages. In 1813 it was expanded into "a goodly octavo volume" with an English title *Researches into the Physical History of Man*. A second edition in 1826 was in two volumes, illustrated with plates. The first volume of a third edition was published in 1836, and this edition extended over eleven years, the fifth and last volume being published in 1847. Whilst these volumes were in preparation, Prichard produced a smaller work on the same lines designed for the general reader, with the purpose of encouraging and popularizing the study of ethnology. He called this book *The Natural History of Man* (1st Edition 1843; 2nd Edition 1845). Over a period of 37 years each edition was almost completely rewritten and "every topic comprised in it has been reconsidered, with the advantage of such additional information as I have been in the interval enabled to acquire".

When Prichard entered upon his studies, ethnology was an almost entirely uncultivated field. Camper had attempted to classify the human race according to the facial angle, having found that in the European it averaged 80 per cent, in the "Kalmuck" 75 per cent, and in the Negro 70 per cent. But his views were founded on measurements of only a small collection of skulls, and were inaccurate in other respects, particularly in relation to the difference between the infantile and adult skull. Blumenbach, to whom Prichard dedicated his work, and whom he considered the real founder of ethnology, examined a very large number of skulls, and arrived at five types of cranial configuration, which he named according to the races to which they belonged, Caucasian, Mongolian, American, Ethiopian and Malayan. In England very little had been done—in Prichard's words

The nature and causes of the physical diversities which characterize different races of men, though a curious and interesting subject of inquiry, is one which has rarely engaged the notice of writers of our own country. The few English authors who have treated of it, at least those who have entered into the investigation on physiological grounds, have, for the most part, maintained the opinion, that there exist in mankind several distinct species. A considerable and very respectable class of foreign writers, at the head of whom we reckon Buffon and Blumenbach, have given their suffrages on the contrary side of this question, and have entered more diffusely into the proof of the doctrine they advocate.

My attention was strongly excited to this inquiry many years ago, by happening to hear the truth of the Mosaic records implicated in it, and denied on the alleged impossibility of reconciling the history contained in them with the phenomena of nature, and particularly with the diversified characters of the several races of men. The arguments of those who assert that these races constitute distinct species, appeared to me at first irresistible, and I found no satisfactory proof in the vague and conjectural reasonings by which the opposite opinion has generally been defended. I was at last convinced that most of the theories current concerning the effects of climate and other modifying causes are in great part hypothetical, and irreconcilable with facts that cannot be disputed.

In the course of this essay I have maintained the opinion, that all mankind constitute but one race, or proceed from a single family, but I am far from wishing to interest any religious predilections in favour of my conclusions. On the contrary, I am ready to admit, and shall be glad to believe, if it can be made to appear, that the truth of the Scriptures is not involved in the decision of this question. I have made no reference to the writings of Moses, except with relation to events concerning which the authority of those most ancient records may be received as common historical testimony; being aware that one class of persons would refuse to admit any such appeal, and that others would rather wish to see the points in dispute established on distinct and independent grounds.

Prichard set out to enquire whether the genus Man contains more than one species. He listed the differences of colour, cranial configuration, physiognomy and stature in the different tribes of man, and compared them with similar variations in the lower animals. He concluded that these variations in man were strictly analogous phenomena to those seen in animals "depending on a principle of natural deviation, and, as such, furnishing no specific distinctions". He followed up an old idea of John Hunter's that "cultivation" is a powerful cause of variation, and suggested that civilization had been the operative cause producing the white varieties of the human species out of the original black. The arguments he put forward for this opinion were as follows:

(1) The analogy of lower species in which changes of colour are from *dark* to *lighter* hues. The lighter colours of domestic animals are the effects of cultivation.

(2) We have examples of light varieties appearing among the negro races, but not of the reverse.

(3) The dark races appear by their organization better adapted to the wild or natural state of life. Witness the easy parturition in the female, and the high development of the sense of smell, taste and hearing.

(4) All nations that have never emerged from the savage state are negroes, or very similar to negroes.

Needless to say this "bold and ingenious theory excited both surprise and interest". He disagreed with the possibility that original stocks of the same species might have arisen in different parts of the world, and after reviewing what was known of the laws governing the distribution of the mammalia concluded that—

> On the whole, it appears that it has not been the scheme of nature to cover distant parts of the earth with many animals of every kind at once; but that a single stock of each species was first produced, which was left to extend itself according as facilities of migration lay open to it, or to find a passage by various accidents into countries removed at greater or less distances from the original point of propagation. (1st edition, p. 145.)

The next stage of his enquiry was concerned with the description of various races of man. He also paid much attention to a subject which remained dear to his heart throughout his life, namely the common origin of the ancient Indians and Egyptians, and the affiliation of the European races with the Asiatic.

Some of these views were to change substantially as time went on— for instance Prichard changed his mind about the derivation of races from an original Negro stock. In the second edition of 1826 Prichard had not only collected a great amount of new material, but included a survey of the whole range of nature—beginning with the species of plants and extending to the whole of zoology. In the first volume he discussed the phenomenon of the diffusion of species, both animal and vegetable, and paid much attention to a question which had greatly concerned Linnaeus, viz. whether in every species of plants, as well as of animals, only one pair was originally produced. *Unum individuum ex hermaphroditis et unicum per reliquorum viventium fuisse primulus creatum sana ratio videtur clarissime ostendere.*

The conclusions arrived at in his previous and more limited investigation were abundantly strengthened, and Prichard concluded that

> The inference to be collected from the facts at present known seems to be as follows—the various tribes or organised beings were originally placed by the Creator in certain regions for which they are by their nature peculiarly adapted. Each species had only one beginning in a single stock: probably a single pair, Linnaeus supposed, was first called into being in some particular spot, and their progeny left to disperse themselves to as great a distance from the original centre of their existence, as the locomotive powers bestowed on each species, or its capability of bearing changes of climate and other physical circumstances, may have enabled it to wander.

The description of the numerous families of mankind was given in much greater detail He introduced some new terminology. Thus the various black-haired races of man constitute the Melanic variety. The Xanthous comprises brown, auburn, yellow, flaxen, or red-haired individuals. The Albino is distinguished by white hair and red eyes. Again, in considering the different types of skulls, he classifies them according to the form of the vertex, as meso-bregmate, steno-bregmate, and platy-bregmate; the type of the first being the Caucasian, of the second the Negro, of the third the Mongolian.

The second volume was devoted to a survey of the causes leading to the production of varieties in the human species. Is there a hereditary transmission of peculiarities of structure?

> Whatever varieties are produced in the race have their beginning in the original structure of some particular ovum or germ, and not in any qualities superinduced by external causes in the progress of its development. Yet the influence of climate and modes of life, domestication, etc. is unquestionable, and therefore according to this view it must be on the ovum that this influence is exerted.

The work concludes with a consideration of the diversity and origin of languages, and their relationships one with another. He announced his discovery of the relationship of the Celtic languages to Sanskrit and to other members of the Indo–European group. His philological investigations supported the inference drawn from other lines of argument, that the races of man have descended from a single pair.

The last edition began in 1836, the material being trebled, the whole re-cast and re-written, and the five volumes taking eleven years to appear. This is a work of enormous erudition, far exceeding in scope any previous publication. The history, physical characteristics, customs and language of each tribe is dealt with, documented from a multitude of sources. And yet Prichard never loses the general thread running throughout, that man is a single species created by God, and differing in what are only minor features. The 2,462 pages of text are for the specialist reader, and alas, it is with somewhat of relief that one can turn to the *Natural History of Man*, of only 596 pages, designed for the general reader. The book's attractiveness is enhanced by colour plates illustrating the appearance of the different races. A beautiful series of lithographs from Catlins' portraits of the American Indians is included, and the colour stands out as vivid and fresh today as it was in 1845. At the end of the book is a new section dealing with the psychology of the Negro and the ethnology of the American Indian.

Prichard's object throughout the various stages of his ethnological work was to "furnish the groundwork of a comparative inquiry into the physical and psychological characters of various races, with a view to determining how far these characters are permanent or subject to change, and whether they are in their nature specific distinctions, or merely accidental or acquired and transmutable varieties". He showed that the anatomical diversities of the human races are mere varieties and not the result of specific differences, nor was there any physiological difference except as a result of external factors. Similarly "the same inward conscious nature and the same mental faculties are common to all the races of men". All the varieties of man are derived from a single species.

> If we could divest ourselves of all previous impressions respecting our nature and social state, and look at mankind and human actions with the eyes of a natural historian, or as a zoologist observes the life and manners of beavers or of termites, we should remark nothing more striking in the habitudes of mankind, and in their manner of existence in various parts of the world, than a reference which is everywhere more or less distinctly perceptible to a state of existence after death, and to the influence believed both by barbarous and civilized nations to be exercised over their present

condition and future destiny by invisible agents, differing in attributes according to the sentiments of different nations, but universally believed to exist. The rites everywhere performed for the dead, the various ceremonies of cremation, sepulture, embalming, mummifying, funereal processions, and pomps following the deceased, during thousands of successive years, in every part of the earth,—innumerable tumuli scattered over all the northern regions of the world, which are perhaps the only memorials of races long extinct—the morais, pyramids, and houses of the dead, and the gigantic monuments of the Polynesians,—the magnificent pyramids of Egypt, and of Anahuac, the prayers and litanies set up on behalf of the dead as well as of the living in the churches of Christendom, in the mosques and pagodas of the East, as heretofore in pagan temples,— the power of sacerdotal or consecrated orders, who have caused themselves to be looked upon as the interpreters of destiny, and as mediators between the gods and men,—sacred wars desolating empires through zeal for some metaphysical dogma,—toilsome pilgrimages performed every year by thousands of white and black men, through various regions of the earth, seeking atonement for guilt at the tombs of prophets and holy persons,— all these, and a number of similar phenomena in the history of all nations, barbarous and civilized, would lead us to suppose that all mankind sympathize in deeply impressed feelings and sentiments, which are as mysterious in their nature as in their origin. These are among the most striking and remarkable of the psychical phenomena, if we may so apply the expression, which are peculiar to man; and if they are to be traced among races of men which differ physically from each other, it will follow that all mankind partake of a common moral nature, and are, therefore, if we take into account the law of diversity in psychical properties allotted to particular species, proved, by an extensive observation of analogies in nature, to constitute a single tribe.

His father had from the beginning expressed the hope that this would indeed prove to be the case, thus confirming orthodox Biblical teaching. The work grew out of the implication that the Mosaic records could not be reconciled with the facts of natural history, and ended, in the last volume of the mammoth *Researches*, with a "Note on Biblical Chronology". It is this strongly religious sentiment which also underlies his psychiatric work, and only thus can the development of his concept of the moral insanities be understood. The conclusion is worth reprinting, expressing as it so clearly does the central theme of Prichard's life and work.

CONCLUSION

It would not greatly strengthen the conclusion which I am entitled to draw from the evidence already afforded, if the limits of this work allowed me to survey the history of every particular branch of the human family. The woolly-haired races of Africa, compared with the native tribes of the New World and with the anciently civilised inhabitants of the Old Continent, furnish a sufficiently ample field for induction on this subject, since among them are comprised those human races who differ most widely from each other in structure of body and in all their physical attributes, and who have been represented as displaying the most decided contrasts in their moral and intellectual endowments. It would, indeed, be very easy to extend this research, with similar results, to all the other tribes of whose character we have yet any sufficient knowledge. Thus the nations of the great Southern Ocean might be shewn to have had among themselves, long before their discovery by Europeans, traits of a very similar kind. They had social institutions resembling those of the rest of mankind; they had universally the belief in a future life, in the protection and government of the world by Providence, in the influence of good and evil genii on human affairs, in the duty of worshipping the gods, in the efficiency of sacrifices, and obsequies, or rites performed in behalf of the dead, in the influence of priests, or human mediators. Similar observations may be made with respect to all the barbarous nations of Northern Asia. The history of the conversion of these nations to Christianity, and of the adoption among them of the ideas and practices of civilised nations, would furnish chapters, equally striking and remarkable as those to which our attention has already been directed, in the history of the human mind. The Australians as yet remain of all nations the least known, since scarcely any one has yet been able to converse with them, or to understand the expression of their thoughts. But fresh evidence is every day collected tending to raise the low estimate which had been formed, and long maintained, of their extreme mental degradation. Degraded they doubtless are: the tribes with whom the colonists have principally had intercourse are, in their external condition, perhaps, the most miserable of the human family, being destitute of the arts which could alone enable them to live with any degree of comfort in the region which they inhabit, or even to support, unless scattered in small wandering bands over a wide space, their physical existence. But there is reason to believe that we have as yet seen only the most destitute of the whole nation; and that there are tribes farther to the northward, perhaps in the inland countries of the great Austral land, who are by no means so miserable or so savage as the people near the southern shores. But even with respect to these, the opinion of the extreme stupidity of the race has been shewn to be unfounded, and the latest and most authentic statements enable us to recognise among them the same principles of a moral and intellectual nature, which, in more cultivated tribes, constitute the highest endowments of humanity.

We contemplate among all the diversified tribes, who are endowed with reason and speech, the same internal feelings, appetencies, aversions; the same inward convictions, the same sentiments of subjection to invisible powers, and, more or less fully developed, of accountableness or responsibility to unseen avengers of wrong and agents of retributive justice, from whose tribunal men cannot even by death escape. We find everywhere the same susceptibility, though not always in the same degree of forwardness or ripeness of improvement, of admitting the cultivation of these universal endowments, of opening the eyes of the mind to the more clear and luminous views which Christianity unfolds, of becoming moulded to the institutions of religion and of civilised life: in a word, the same inward and mental nature is to be recognised in all the races of men. When we compare this fact with the observations which have been heretofore fully established as to the specific instincts and separate psychical endowments of all the distinct tribes of sentient beings in the universe, we are entitled to draw confidently the conclusion that all human races are of one species and one family.

MINOR WORKS

In 1829 Prichard published his *Review of The Doctrine of a Vital Principle*—the expansion of a lecture he had given at one of the meetings of the Bristol Literary and Philosophical Society. He begins by casting doubt on a theory of evolution—then to say that there are the two great classes—the organized, i.e. the living things, and the unorganized. What produces this "organization"—what happens when death occurs? "The words anima, spiritus, the breath of life were originally allusive to the essential functions of the living body and were intended to designate the hidden cause, the principle of physical existence in which they were supposed to depend." The principle of animation was looked upon as the centre also of feeling and of inward consciousness, but unfortunately this explanation did not take into account the lowest tribes of the animal kingdom and plants. The existence of another and distant principle was at length inferred—and so as well as the anima, the source of physical life—we had the animus, the mind, or intellectual power. Lastly came mind, from *mens*, that which knows or understands. With the discovery of electricity the vital principle was imagined to be a substance of a similar kind—and it was used to explain the various physiological processes such as secretion, digestion and other functions. Prichard found this explanation also unsatisfactory. Indeed, after exploring the various theories extant, Prichard has to confess that none could embrace all the facts, only the presence of a Creator—a Divine Intelligence—can account for the wonderful manifestations of the life principle.

In addition to all this activity Prichard learnt German in order to study the many learned works on philosophy and history written in that language. As an exercise, together with his friend Tothill, he translated and published in 1815 Muller's *General History*. He wrote an article on the Mithridates of Adelung, contributed various articles to reviews and other periodicals, of which I have not been able to obtain a complete list, but the following may be mentioned: A paper on Snowden; three papers on the Mosaic Cosmogony; papers on the Universities; on the Zodiac; on Isis and Osiris; on Faln and Schlegel; articles on Delirium, Hypochondriasis, Somnambulism, Animal Magnetism, Soundness of Mind, and Temperament in the *Cyclopaedia of Practical Medicine*; and several chapters on similar subjects in the "Library of Medicine".

The study of Hebrew was alike congenial to his religious feelings and philological taste. He wrote an essay on the Song of Deborah for the gratification of his friends, and devoted much thought to Biblical criticism, as well as translating from the Hebrew Scriptures. Greek readings with a few learned friends occupied the time which other men devoted to light or frivolous pursuits, and "a poetical translation of the Birds of Aristophanes may be mentioned amongst the fruits of these horae subsecivae" (Hodgkin).

Prichard's Library

I can do no better than to conclude with a brief description of Prichard's library. Here again, as with Haslam, we are lucky in possessing a bookseller's catalogue listing some of Prichard's books. The prices might well make bibliophiles weep for times since past, and it is interesting to note the relative importance of Prichard and Jenner in the bookseller's eyes (Fig. 7).

The following are those books with inscriptions showing their provenance—they are listed with the bookseller's item number.

THE BRISTOL BIBLIOGRAPHER

BOOKS

INCLUDING A PORTION OF THE LIBRARY OF THE LEARNED

JAMES COWLES PRICHARD Esq. M. D. &c

AUTHOR OF THE PHYSICAL HISTORY OF MAN, THE EASTERN ORIGIN OF CELTIC NATIONS,
AN ANALYSIS OF EGYPTIAN MYTHOLOGY, &c. &c.

ALSO OF THAT OF

DR. EDWARD JENNER

THE DISCOVERER OF VACCINATION

AND VARIOUS OTHERS LATELY ADDED TO STOCK,

AMONG WHICH ARE

GRAMMARS, LEXICONS, BIBLES, &c.

IN LANGUAGES SELDOM STUDIED EXCEPT IN ETHNOLOGICAL PURSUITS.

THOMAS KERSLAKE
BRISTOL

"BONI IGITUR AC STUDIOSI GAUDENTO ATQUE EMUNTO."—Joh. FROBENIUS Bibliopola Basil.

9433 ACHARYA'S (Bhascona) Lilarvati, a Treatise on ARITHMETIC and GEOMETRY, translated from the Sanscrit by Jo. TAYLOR, *Bombay*, 1816, 4to. *2s 6d*

9434 ADAIR'S (Jas.) History of the AMERICAN INDIANS, 1775, 4to. *15s*

9435 ADAMS (Jos.) on MORBID POISON, (Vaccine, &c.), 1807, *coloured plates*, 4to. *boards, Dr. JENNER'S copy, 5s*

9436 ADELUNG'S (J. Ch.) MITHRIDATES, oder Allgemeine SPRACHENKUNDE, mit dem VATER UNSER als Sprachprobe in bey nahe 500 SPRACHEN und MUNDARTEN, *Berlin*, 1806-1817, 8vo. 5 vols. bound into 4, *half morocco, neat, 1l 8s*

9437 Deadly ADULTERATIONS, Death in the POT and the BOTTLE, 12mo. *2s*

9438 The Warnings of ADVENT, a Course of SERMONS, (by J. D. MAURICE, Adn. THORPE, J. KEBLE, E. MONRO, W. J. IRONS, J. R. WOODFORD, and others), 1853, 8vo. *cloth, extra, 6s 6d*

3, PARK STREET.

9439 ÆSCHYLI TRAGŒDIÆ, cum Variis Lectionibus et Notis, S. BUTLER, *Cantab.*, 1109-12, 8vo. 6 vols. *boards, 14s*

9440 Fables of ÆSOP, with Morals, &c., by Sir R. L'Estrange, 1692, folio, *newly bound, calf, gilt, neat, 9s 6d*

9441 Quarterly Journal of AGRICULTURE, 1839-41, 8vo. 3 vols. *half calf, neat, 6s*

9442 AIRY'S (G. B.) Mathematical Tracts on the LUNAR and PLANETARY THEORIES, &c., 1842, 8vo. *boards, 8s 6d*

9443 *Dutch :*—den Cleefschen Pegasus (in Praise of PRINCESS of ORANGE, &c. of V. PRINCE of ORANGE, &c.) door Margaret van AKERLAECKEN, *Niel* 1654, 8vo. *vell., with autograph of ROBERT SOUTHEY, London, Dec., 1839.*

9444 *Manuscript :*—A lithographed Epigrams, among which "Death Peach" by Dr. JENNER, a Short Dialogue, died in April," 4to. *neat, gilt edges*

9445 B. ALCHWINI Abbatis, Angli, Karoli Magni Magistri, Opera, *Lutet.-Paris.*, 1617, *port.,* folio, *calf, 18s*

FIG. 7.   The Sale Catalogue of Prichard's Library.

ITEMS FROM THE CATALOGUE OF
PRICHARD'S BOOKS

9448 Transactions (Historical and Literary,) of the AMERICAN PHILOSOPHICAL SOCIETY, Vol. 1 (HOCKEWELDER's History of the Indian Nations, Correspondence on their Languages, Words, Phrases, &c. of the Lenni Lenape,) Philad., 1819, 8vo, boards, from Dr. Prichard's library, 8s. 6d.

9464 Conversations on the ANIMAL ECONOMY, by a Physician, 1827, 8vo, 2 vols. with autograph, "J. C. PRICHARD—from the Author," 3s.

9491 D'ARVIEUX Voyage dans la PALESTINE, Paris, 1717, plates, 12mo. with autograph of Dr. "J. C. Prichard," 3s.

9530 Col. BEAUFOY's (Mark) NAUTICAL and HYDRAULIC EXPERIMENTS, with Numerous Scientific Miscellanies, vol. 1 only printed, 1834, plates of figures which cut or resist water, imperial 4to, cloth, privately printed, with gift inscription to Dr. PRICHARD, from the Author, 18s.

9614 BLUMENBACHII (J. F.) DECADES CRANIORUM, Gott., 1790-1808, Nova Pentas Craniorum, 1828, "Given to me by Professor BLUMENBACH at Göttingen,"—65 plates, 4to, 6 in 1 vol. half calf, with autograph signature of Dr. "J. C. PRICHARD," £1, 12s.

　　See Dr. PRICHARD's dedication to this author of his great work "Researches", also the Preface.

9656 REPORT of the BRITISH ASSOCIATION, 1st, 2nd, 3rd, 5th, and 6th Meetings, 1831–36, plates, 8vo, 4 vols. boards, with autograph of Dr. "J. C. PRICHARD", £1.

9687 BUSH's (Jos.) Evangelical SERMONS at L. Ashton, 1842, 12mo. with autograph gift to Dr. Prichard, 2s. 6d.

9695 CALDWELL (Chas) on the Original UNITY of the HUMAN RACE, New York, 1830, 8vo. "Dr. PRICHARD, from J. GUISCOM", 4s.

9703 Memoirs of Lant CARPENTER, LL.D., Bristol, 1842, port., 8vo, cloth, with autograph gift to Dr. PRICHARD, 3s. 6d.

9706 Dr. CARSON's (Jas) Causes of RESPIRATION, Motion of the BLOOD, ANIMAL HEAT, &c., 1833, 8vo, with autograph gift to Dr. PRICHARD, 4s. 6d.

9792 M'CORMAC's (H.) PHILOSOPHY of HUMAN NATURE, in its Physical, Intellectual, and Moral Relations, 1837, 8vo, with autograph gift to Dr. PRICHARD, 3s. 6d.

9888 EDINBURGH REVIEW, No. 40, with autograph of Dr. "J. C. Prichard", 2s.

9890 EDWARDS (W. F.) on the Influence of Physical Agents on Life, with Appendix on Electricity, Microscopic Character of Tissues, &c., 1832, 8vo, boards, with autograph gift to Dr. Prichard, 3s. 6d.

9962 GABELL's (J. H. L.) Accordance of RELIGION with NATURE, 1842, 8vo, cloth, with autograph gift to Dr. Prichard, 4s.

9966 DICTIONARY of the GALLA Language, by TUTSCHEK, Munich, 1844, 8vo, with autograph gift to "Dr. Prichard,—with Sir T. Acland's respects and kind regards", 4s. 6d.

10034 A VOCABULARY of Words in the HAWAIIAN Language, Lahainaluna, press of the High School, 1836, 8vo, with autograph gift, "Dr. J. C. Prichard, &c. &c. &c., from his obedient Servant—Jno. PICKERING", 6s.

10050 LIFE of Dr. W. HENRY, of Manchester, 1837, privately printed, royal 8vo, cloth, with autograph gift to Dr. Prichard, 3s. 6d.

10078 HOPKINS (E.) on the Connexion of GEOLOGY with MAGNETISM, 1844, plates, 8vo, cloth, neat, with autograph gift to Dr. Prichard, 3s. 6d.

10086 America:—HOWSE's (Jos.) GRAMMAR of the CREE Language, and the CHIPPEWAY Dialect, 1844, 8vo, cloth, neat, with autograph gift to Dr. Prichard, 6s. 6d.

10134 IRVING on COMPOSITION, with autograph of Dr. Prichard, 2s.

10160 KENNEDY's History of CHOLERA, 1831, 8vo, with autograph of Dr. Prichard, 3s. 6d.

10194 LASSEN's (Chr) Zeitschrift für die Kunde des MORGEN-LANDES, (vols. 1 to 4, and 2nd part of vol. 5, 1st and 2nd of vol. 6, 1st of vol. 7,) Gött & Bonn, 1837–46, 8vo. 15 parts, with Dr. Prichard's autograph, 12s.

10203 LAWRENCE's (W.) Lectures on PHYSIOLOGY and the Natural History of MAN, 1819, plates, 8vo, half calf, neat, with autograph gift from the author to Dr. Prichard, 7s. 6d.

10225 Lord LINDSAY's PROGRESSION by ANTAGONISM, 1846, chart, 8vo, cloth, autograph gift to Dr. Prichard, 4s.

10242 Report of the COMMISSIONERS in LUNACY to the Lord CHANCELLOR, 1844, with MSS. Papers by Dr. Prichard one of them, 8vo, cloth 7s.

10285 MARTIN's (B) System of MATHEMATICAL INSTITUTIONS, 1759, 8vo, 2 vols in 1, half calf, with autograph of Dr. Prichard, 4s. 6d.

10307 MERYON's (E) Physical and Intellectual Constitution of MAN, 1836, autograph gift to Dr. Prichard, 3s.

10346 MOYSANT Meilleurs Morceaux en Vers, 1800, 8vo, with autograph of Dr. "James Cowles Prichard—Staines—1804", 3s.

10416 Dr. PARRY on the Arterial PULSE, 1816, plates, 8vo, boards, with autograph of "J. C. Prichard, M.D.", 2s.

10456 PIRONDI (Sirus) de la Tumeur Blanche, Paris, 1836, 8vo, autograph gift from the author to Dr. Prichard, 1s. 6d.

10490 Dr. PRICHARD's (J. C.) Researches into the PHYSICAL HISTORY OF MANKIND, 4th edn., 1841–47, coloured plates, maps, &c., 8vo, 5 vols. cloth, £3, 12s.

10491 Dr. PRICHARD's (J. C.) Researches into the Physical History of Man, 1813, 8vo, boards, 3s. 6d.

10492 PRICHARD's (J. C.) De Generis Humani Varietate, 1808, 8vo, 1s.
This was the original sketch of his great work "Researches".

10493 Dr. PRICHARD's (J. C.) Analysis of the EGYPTIAN MYTHOLOGY with a Critical Examination of the Remains of Egyptian CHRONOLOGY, 1819, coloured plate, royal 8vo, boards, 14s.

10494 Dr. PRICHARD's (J. C.) Natural HISTORY of MAN, Inquiries into the Modifying Influences of Physical and Moral Agencies on the Different Tribes, 3rd edn., enlarged, 1848, numerous coloured plates, royal 8vo, cloth, gilt, £1, 9s.

10495 Dr. PRICHARD's (J. C.) Treatise on INSANITY and other Disorders affecting the Mind, 1835, 8vo, cloth 7s. 6d.

10496 PRICHARD (J. C.) on Sindsygdommene og andre Sygelige SJELSTILSTANDE, oversat og med Anmoerkninger af H. SELMER, Kjobenh., 1842, 8vo, with autograph gift to the author, 6s.
"To—Dr. J. C. PRICHARD—most respectfully—by H. SELMER."

10497 Dr. PRICHARD's Treatise on Diseases of the Nervous System, 1822, 8vo, boards, 3s. 6d.

10498 Manuscripts:—Eleven Thick Quarto Vols. and several smaller in the hand-writing of the late Dr. PRICHARD, a large bundle, £2, 12s.

10524 RASORI (J) Thèorie de la PHLOGOSE par PIRONDI, Paris, 1839, 8vo, 2 vols. with autograph gift to Dr. Prichard, 3s.

10552 America:—Trial of Abner ROGERS, Jun., for the Murder of Charles LINCOLN, Jun., at Boston, Boston, U.S., 1844, 8vo, cloth, with autograph gift to Dr. Prichard from Dr. Woodward and Bernard, U.S., 4s. 6d.

10556 ROMAN COINS:—Nummi Familiaries 26 plates, Nummi Imperatorium, 102 plates,—above 200 figures, 4to, half morocco, with autograph of Dr. Prichard, 16s.

10571 Bp. RUSSELL's (M.) CHARGE at GLASGOW, 1842, 8vo. with autograph gift to "James Cowles Prichard, Esq., M.D.—with the author's sincere regards", 1s.

10681 Bp. STILLINGFLEET on the TRINITY, 1697, 8vo, calf, with autograph of Dr. "J. C. Prichard", 3s.

10785 Dr. WALL (C. W.) on the Nature, Age, and Origin of SANSCRIT, Dublin, 1838, 4to, with autograph gift to Dr. Prichard, 3s.

10835 YATES (J.) on PUNIC INSCRIPTIONS, 8vo, sewed, with autog. gift to Dr. Prichard, 1.

10836 YATES (J.) on the BIBLE CHRONOLOGY, 1830, 8vo, with autograph gift from the author to Dr. Prichard, 2s.

BIBLIOGRAPHY

ADELUNG, J. C. *Mithridates, or a General History of Languages.* (Berlin) Vol. I, 1806; Vol. II continued by Prof. Vater, 1809; Vol. III, Part 1, 1812.

DAVIES, David (1826). *Letters on Medical Consultation to and from Dr. Prichard, M.D., with some observations on Medical Usage, and the Inseparability of Medical Surgery and Medicine,* by David Davies, M.D., Member of the Royal College of Physicians in London. Bristol: printed by T. J. Manchee, 30 Quay.

de SAUSSURE, R. (1946). "The influence of the concept of monomania on French medico-legal psychiatry from 1825 to 1840." *J. Hist. Med.,* **1**, 3, 365.

ESQUIROL, E. (1838). *Des Maladies Mentales.* 2 vols. Pp. xviii+678, 864. Paris: Baillière.

GEORGET, J. E. (1826). *Discussion Médico-légale sur la Folie.* Pp. 176. Paris: Chez Migneret.

HENDERSON, D. K. (1947). *Psychopathic States.* Pp. 158. New York: W. W. Norton.

HODGKIN, T. (1849–50). *The Colonial Intelligencer; or the Aborigines Friend.* Vol. II, Nos. xii–xvii, pp. 203, 217, 253, 269, 303. London: printed and published for the Society.

KERSLAKE, T. (n.d.). Bookseller's Catalogue.

MAUDSLEY, H. (1897). *Responsibility in Mental Disease.* Pp. xi+338. New York: Appleton & Co.

PRICHARD, A. (1896). *A few Medical and Surgical Reminiscences.* Bristol: J. W. Arrowsmith.

PRICHARD, A. (1898). *Some Incidents in General Practice.* Bristol: J. W. Arrowsmith.

PRICHARD, J. C. (1808). *De Generis Humani Varietate.* Edinburgh.

PRICHARD, J. C. (1813). *Researches as to the Physical History of Man.*

PRICHARD, J. C. (1819). *An Analysis of the Egyptian Mythology with a Critical Examination of the Remains of Egyptian Chronology.* London: H. Baillière.

PRICHARD, J. C. (1822). *A Treatise on Diseases of the Nervous System.* Pp. xvi+425. London: Thomas and George Underwood.

PRICHARD, J. C. (1826). *Researches into the Physical History of Man.* 2 vols.

PRICHARD, J. C. (1838). *Ibid.* 3 vols.

PRICHARD, J. C. (1829). *A Review of the Doctrine of a Vital Principle.* Pp. xii+236. London: John and Arthur Arch.

PRICHARD, J. C. (1832). *A Treatise on Hypochondriasis. From the Cyclopaedia of Practical Medicine.* Pp. 38. London: Marchant, Printer, Ingram-Court.

PRICHARD, J. C. (1832). *Abstract of a Comparative Review of Philological and Physical Researches as applied to the History of the Human Species.* Second Report 1832.

PRICHARD, J. C. (1834). *Advertisement of three lectures on Egyptian Mummies, Egyptian antiquities, and the Rosetta Stone.* Leaflet.

PRICHARD, J. C. (1834). *Soundness and Unsoundness of Mind. From the Cyclopaedia of Practical Medicine.* Pp. 16. London: Marchant, Printer, Ingram-Court.

PRICHARD, J. C. (1835). *A Treatise on Insanity and Other Disorders affecting the Mind.* Pp. xvi+483. London: Sherwood, Gilbert & Piper.

PRICHARD, J. C. (1841). *Illustrations to the Researches into the Physical History of Mankind.* London: H. Baillière.

PRICHARD, J. C. (1842). *On the Different Forms of Insanity in Relation to Jurisprudence.* Pp. xi+243. London: H. Baillière.

PRICHARD, J. C. (1843). *The Natural History of Man,* 1st edition. London: H. Baillière.

PRICHARD, J. C. (1847). *Ibid.,* 2nd edition. London: H. Baillière.

PRICHARD, J. C. (1845). *The Natural History of Man,* 2nd edition. Pp. xvii+596. London: H. Baillière.

PRICHARD, J. C. (1848). *Ibid.,* 3rd edition. London: H. Baillière.

PRICHARD, J. C. (1845). *Appendix to the First Edition of the Natural History of Man.* London: H. Baillière.

PRICHARD, J. C. (1845). *Six Ethnographical Maps.* London: H. Baillière.

PRICHARD, J. C. (1847). *On the Relation of Ethnology to Other Branches of Knowledge.* Pp. 31.
Delivered at the Anniversary Meeting of the Ethnological Society—22nd June 1847. Edinburgh: Neill & Co.

PRICHARD, J. C. (1848). *Report on the Various Methods of Research which contribute to the advancement of Ethnology, and of the Relations of that science to other branches of knowledge.* Pp. 230–253.
(From the Report of the British Association for the Advancement of Science for 1847.) London: Richard and John E. Taylor, Red Lion Court, Fleet Street.

PRICHARD, J. C. (1831). *Eastern Origin of the Celtic Nations.*

PRICHARD, J. C. (n.d.). *Researches into the Physical History of Mankind.* Vols. I–V. Vol. I, pp. xx+376; Vol. II, pp. xiv+373; Vol. III, pp. xxv+507; Vol. IV, pp. xv+631; Vol. V, pp. xv+570. London: Houlston and Stoneman.

SEMELAIGNE, R. (1888). *Philippe Pinel, et Son œuvre au point de vue de la Médicine Mentale.* Paris: Imprimeries Réunies.

SEMELAIGNE, R. (1894). *Les Grands Aliénistes Français.* Paris.

SEMELAIGNE, R. (1912). *Aliénistes et Philanthropes.* Paris: Steinheil.

SMITH, G. Munro (1917). *A History of the Bristol Royal Infirmary,* Pp. xiii+507. London: Arrowsmith; Bristol: Simpkin, Marshall, Hamilton, Lent & Co. Ltd.

SYMONDS, J. A. (1849). *Some Account of the life, writings, and character of the late James Cowles Prichard, M.D., F.R.S.* Pp. 54. Bristol.

TUKE, D. Hack. (1891). *Prichard and Symonds.* Pp. lv+116. London: J. &ʳA. Churchill.

TUKE, D. Hack. (1892). *A Dictionary of Psychological Medicine.* 2 vols. Pp. 1477. London: J. & A. Churchill.

WALK, A. (1954). "Some Aspects of the 'Moral Treatment' of the Insane up to 1854." *J. Ment. Sci.*, **100**, 807.

WEARE, G. E. (1898). James Cowles Prichard (Physician & Ethnologist of Bristol) (1781–1848). A Brief Retrospect. Reprinted from the *Bristol Times and Mirror*, 22.1.1898.

WOOD, A. (1954). *Thomas Young Natural Philosopher* 1773–1829. Pp. xx+355. Cambridge University Press.

O

CHAPTER IV

John Conolly, M.D., D.C.L.
1794–1866

JOHN CONOLLY's career, and his subsequent position in the history of psychiatry provides one of the most fascinating examples of the hair's breadth separating success from failure. A failure until the age of 45, within the space of four years he had established himself as one of the leading psychiatrists in England, and gone on to become "the chief consulting physician in this country in difficult cases of insanity and other diseases of the nervous system" (Sir James Clark).

Terms such as the English Pinel have been used to describe him, two of his books have become classics, and his name has become synonymous with the non-restraint movement. And yet

> as a practical physician, Dr. Conolly did not specially distinguish himself, either in the exact investigation of disease, or in its treatment; he had little faith in medicines, and hardly more faith in pathology, while the actual practice of his profession was not agreeable to him. I have often heard him say, that if his life were to come over again he should like nothing better than to be at the head of a large public asylum, in order to superintend its administration. His education, general and medical, had been somewhat desultory, and his reading throughout life was desultory also; he could not easily set himself patiently to master an author with whose style and sentiments he did not sympathise, or deliberately to acquire a complete knowledge of a subject that was not attractive to him. As a medical author on general diseases, his writings, though of easy and elegant composition, will be found to be somewhat vague and diffuse, wanting in exact facts and practical information—the faults felt so much in his lectures at University College. As a writer on insanity, he painted eloquently and pathetically the external features of the disease, but the philosophical depths of mental phenomena he never cared to sound, and the exact scientific investigation of mental disease he never systematically devoted himself to. Esquirol was the author whom he studied at the beginning of his career, and on him he confessedly relied almost entirely to the end of his life.

Admittedly this is written by Henry Maudsley, whose standards were high, but is it approximately correct? We must turn to the details, so that nearly one hundred years later we can perhaps re-evaluate Conolly's life and career.

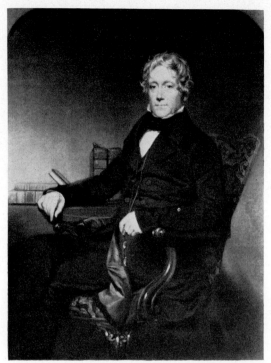

Fig. 1. John Conolly, M.D., 1794–1866.

HIS LIFE

John Conolly was born at Market Rasen, in Lincolnshire, in 1794. His father died early, and Mrs. Conolly was left with three boys to bring up, in what must have been straitened circumstances. Conolly has left an autobiographical fragment, very evocative of his early unhappiness, and only in the light of which can his subsequent career be understood.

My father was a younger son of a good Irish family, and died too early to leave any distinct impression upon my memory. He had been brought up to no profession; had no pursuits; died young; and left three boys dependent on their mother, whose maiden name was Tennyson. My eldest brother was adopted by my Grandmother Tennyson; the youngest was adopted by another relative; it was my good fortune not to be adopted by anybody, and my early days were passed with little comfort, but eventually with more advantage than the early days of my two dear brothers.

I was born in the house of my grandmother Tennyson, in the small town of Market Rasen, who lived in a small house opposite the east end of the ancient church. She was the widow of William Tennyson, of Barton-upon-Humber, who was long remembered in Lincolnshire for his high character. I fear I was an inconvenient superfluity in the family, for whom nobody cared, except my affectionate mother. We had some distant relatives in Holderness, and the result was that I was placed as a boarder, before I had completed my sixth year, with a somewhat old widow lady at Hedon; and my formal education commenced in the second week of the first year of the present century, in the small grammar-school of the decaying Borough of Hedon.

The memory, so treacherous in middle life of events of recent years, and so retentive of events and impression of those of older date, still recalls, in my own instance, my being taken from Wyton Hall on the 9th day of January, 1800—my last view of the drive past the old trees, the gardens, and all the characteristic objects of the house of an English gentleman, of all which the boyish mind has an unexpressed appreciation; and I also remember the cheerless impression ensuing from what seemed a descent from tranquil and comfortable life to the commoner arrangements inseparable from school, and to the society of a lower social kind, where nothing was tasteful, and nothing was beautiful, and nothing was cheerful. Antiquated residences, rooms of which chairs and tables constituted all the furniture, shabby neglected gardens, coarse or common companions, and general neglect of all that could promote happy feelings, were productive of a kind of desolation neither expressed nor quite understood. The same kind of objects and circumstances have, in all subsequent years, always produced the same uncomfortable feelings.

For seven years of school life at Hedon my daily life, except in holidays of three weeks at Midsummer and Christmas, was unvaried. Before nine in the morning I repaired to the school-house on the market-hill, on a spot where some trees are now planted. At nine the school-master's awful figure appeared round the corner near the church, and on his entrance I exhibited Latin exercises, written the evening before, and repeated a page or more of the Eton grammar, and construed a portion of whatever Latin author I was advanced to, or of the Greek Testament. Between eleven and twelve I construed a second lesson. At noon there were two hours unemployed, except by a frugal dinner, and more abundant play. In the afternoon more construing lessons, or, once in the week, a writing copy and some arithmetic. In all these years my schoolmaster, the vicar, never, that I remember, gave me any assistance, except by blows on the head. I read in the usual order, *Cornelius Nepos*, a book or two of *Caesar's Commentaries*, and was then promoted into poetical reading, and at the returning holidays was enabled to inform my few inquiring friends that I was in Ovid and Virgil, and latterly in Horace. Of the absurdity of such reading nothing need be said. I read with difficulty and understood nothing. I was not allowed to read an English lesson. Of the Latin authors I remained profoundly ignorant, never, I believe, except on two occasions, having even a glimmering of their meaning, one being when rather interested with the structure of a bridge over the Rhine, and another when rather excited by the catastrophe of Phaeton, on which latter occasion the exuberance of my feelings was promptly rebuked. After my school years I now and then saw my revered schoolmaster; he was tall, stout, round-faced, full-voiced, bluff in his manners. His days after leaving St. Bees' had been passed in small country places, and I never had reason to think that he ever read books. In the use of the cane and in the application of a kind of leather battledore to the palms of the hands he was expert.

At the Latin desk in the Grammar School of Hedon there were, I think, but seven scholars in the years between 1800 and 1807. Two were the grandsons of the doctor then practising at Preston; two were the grandsons of the squire whose good old house still faces the avenue at the end of the town as you go to Burstwick; one was a lively apprentice of the Hedon doctor, and came only occasionally when he had made up the medicines for the day; and one was the eldest son of a substantial burgess of Scotch extraction, I being the seventh. We formed, I believe, a little aristocracy in the eyes of the other scholars; and I found we were re-membered, and the Latin desk, by the sexton, forty years afterwards, when I was puzzling him by evoking recollections with a skill he could not account for until I mentioned a name unheard by him since the days when he was at school; he being a freeborn of the borough and educated gratis, as were, indeed, all my Hedon schoolfellows except the Latin students, who were, like myself, the sons of poor gentlefolks.

There were, indeed, in those days, few schools in all Holderness, and none so distinguished as that of Hedon: so that some half-dozen girls received instruction there in reading and writing. Their studies seemed rather troublesome to the master, who decreed that I, whom he regarded as a somewhat accomplished reader from the south, should be referred to in all verbal difficulties, thus giving occasion to many journeys on the part of the young ladies to my end of the Latin desk, and some innocent flirtations and looks from gentle eyes now dim like mine.

The daily dullness of the school was somewhat relieved on Saturdays, when part of the morning was apparently designed to prepare the minds of the scholars for Sunday. The boys were arranged in a circle, and the master moved about in the middle of it. The catechism was gone through, its questions asked sonorously, and the answers given in varied tones, more or less unmusical, and for the most part mechanical, and none of them were remarked upon or explained.

Sunday brought relief from the daily word-lessons and from the six hours' confinement in the atmosphere of the school-room. The seven o'clock morning church-bell announced the quieter seventh day; decent clothes were brought out of strange chests, the Sunday hat was brushed, and at eleven I was placed generally alone in the pew of my lately deceased great uncle, Michael Tennyson, an honour done to me, I scarcely know why, both here and at the neighbouring church of Preston, for the vicar took care of the souls of the parishioners of both Hedon and Preston. There was one service at each place every Sunday, alternately, in the morning and afternoon; and it was a great relief to me when I grew old enough to be allowed to attend the services in both places. In the other hours of Sundays I was expected to read the Bible, which I did without the remotest conception of localities and dates, an unhappiness still not unfrequent with early readers, and productive of inconveniences not easily remedied afterwards.

The state of social life in a very small town, far away from London, in the beginning of this century, afforded little opportunity for the acquirement of varied knowledge or for any kind of mental recreation. I can scarcely now believe what I too painfully remember; I could even now walk through the tranquil street (for there was but one), and name the occupant of every house at that time, on the right hand and the left; the lawyer, the tanner, the glazier, the tailor, the shoemaker, the innkeeper, the butcher, the farmer, the carrier, the blacksmith, the joiner, the sexton, besides the vicar, the two landed gentlemen, the doctor (there being but one), and the retired doctor who now and then asked me to spend Sunday with him and his family. This, and other occasional visiting, was so inconsistent with my daily wretched life, that I think it made me rather distracted than comfortable.

Reflecting often on this barren portion of my existence, the tenth portion of the years allotted to man, it has often been a question with me whether the years from six to sixteen are usually so profitless and unhappy; they are evidently not looked back upon with particular affection by many men. The fondest recollections of them which have been expressed in prose or fanciful verse, are not attractive to readers of my age, and their praises seem at the best to have been recorded in proportion to the boyish character remaining in the writers.

When in maturer years, I have heard orthodox men in English provinces declaring to country gentlemen and doctors, over excellent port (now extinct) the great importance of classical education, I have seldom dared to confess the imperfection of my own; when they have vehemently asserted its salutary subjugation of the mind, I have only assumed that the days of their youth had been more happily ordered than mine; and when, even now, a sexagenarian, I derive not unfrequent delight from the philosophical writings and letters of Cicero, I sometimes regret that I had not the admirable explanatory notes which now illustrate schoolbooks, and with the aid of which young readers may be pleased as well as instructed; and, if sometimes I find recreation in a page or two of Horace, I can but more and more be surprised that the philosophic and witty poet should have ever been made a school-book at all. I painfully remember the hours when, inexperienced in the world and its social or vicious ways, I had to translate compositions as witty and abounding in allusion to the gayest doings of ordinary life, and as elaborately elegant as those of Moore. To place Horace in the hands of an English boy seems as absurd as it would be to attempt to teach a Chinese boy our language by insisting on his reading the Fudge Family. Perhaps all this is changed: perhaps not all.

On leaving this school, he returned to live with his mother at Hull. She had by now re-married, her husband being a French émigré. A mutual affection grew up between young Conolly and his stepfather, who taught him French, and made him acquainted with French literature. This relationship seems to have had a decisive influence on Conolly, who retained his fondness for French literature throughout his life. As we shall see, Conolly even went to live in France when he married, only reluctantly returning to England when his money ran out. In a letter to his friend M. Battel, he says, "My thoughts revert more and more to my earlier days and to my education in your language, to which I am largely indebted." In another letter he writes— "When I am ill and tranquil, I have a singular pleasure in reading French. The language is associated in my mind with the early days of my life and my earliest studies. Condillac's *Essai Sur l'Origine des Connaissances Humaines* is now on my table,—the very volume put into my hands forty years ago, and of which I seem to remember every word: perhaps to it I owe the direction of my mental life."

At 18 Conolly was commissioned into a Cambridgeshire Militia regiment, which he joined at Peebles in 1812, and served with in Scotland and Ireland for four years. He seems to have thoroughly enjoyed this period of his life, and would often entertain his son-in-law

Henry Maudsley, by "lively and pleasant recollections" of his service. However, with Waterloo over, and Napoleon banished to St. Helena, dreams of military glory faded, and we find Conolly leaving the army, and marrying in 1816 the daughter of Sir John Collins, a captain in the navy. The couple, in spite of Conolly's lack of training in any profession, immediately went to France. His brother, Dr. William Conolly, was practising in Tours, and the young couple settled down in a cottage near that town. Here they passed an idyllic year, visited by friends, enjoying the wines of the country, studying French literature, and having their first baby. This latter event, and the fact that his small capital was fast becoming exhausted, determined Conolly to try his luck in medicine. In 1817 he went to Edinburgh to begin his studies, and like John Haslam before him, became one of the Presidents of the Royal Medical Society. He seems to have been popular with his fellow-students, and to have taken a prominent part in their meetings. Even at this time his future interests began to reveal themselves, he read the works of Pinel and Tuke, and was much impressed by a visit he paid to an asylum in Glasgow, whilst his "hero" was Dugald Stuart, the Professor of Moral Philosophy in the University at that time. He qualified in 1821, having taken for his thesis the subject of insanity, and given it the title "Dissertatio Inauguralis de Statu Mentis in Insania et Melancholia".

Now the problem arose as to where to practise—after a three months' trial of practice at Lewes, Conolly moved to Chichester where he remained for a year. Here he made a life-long friend, John Forbes, later to be knighted, to be one of the founders of the British Medical Association, and a prominent medical journalist. The two young men were rivals in practice, and it soon became clear that Chichester could not support them both. Conolly was

> the greater favorite in society, his courteous manner, his vivacity of character, and his general accomplishments, rendered him an agreeable companion; and he was not restrained by the gravity of the physician from joining heartily in the dances to which he was so often invited. Forbes, on the other hand, being less polished in manner, and of a somewhat reserved character, not being, indeed, apt to make many friends, though a most firm and sincere friend of the few which he had, was not so popular in society, but, as may perhaps be supposed, was more consulted as a physician. (Maudsley).

Accordingly, Conolly moved to Stratford-on-Avon, a town for

which he was always to retain an affection. Here he remained for five years, until his move to London in 1827, when he was appointed Professor of the Practice of Medicine at University College.

In Stratford he busied himself with medical journalism, a product of his friendship with Forbes. He became associated with the Society for the Diffusion of Useful Knowledge, the moving spirit of which was Lord Brougham, and later served on its Committee in London. At the same time he entered local politics, served as an alderman for several years, and was twice elected Mayor. He established a public dispensary in the town which provided a welcome service to the poor of Stratford, and being a reformer by nature and a liberal in politics, whole-heartedly supported every measure for social advance.

As well as the social reformer, Conolly always remained the romantic, passionate and impetuous in nature. It was natural for him therefore in Stratford to become an ardent Shakespearian. He invariably carried a volume of Shakespeare's plays or sonnets in his pocket as he went his rounds, and was, later in his career, instrumental in securing the preservation of Shakespeare's tomb, and the restoration of the chancel of the church. In his volume on Hamlet, published at the end of his life (1863), Conolly writes

> with every year of lengthening life, the lovers of poetry and the observers of mankind, feel the links that bind their affection to Shakespeare grow stronger . . . through all the stages of life delighted and instructed, we are disposed to yield full assent to the warmly expressed judgement of Hallam, that "the name of Shakespeare is the greatest in our literature,—it is the greatest in all literature".

Although so active in the social and intellectual life of Stratford, Conolly's professional income is said "not to have exceeded £400" per annum, and with a growing family this was not enough. His writings, although poorly paid, had made him well known, and his connection with "The Society for the Diffusion of Useful Knowledge" stood him in good stead for his next move. Chiefly through the influence of its President, Lord Brougham, he was appointed Professor of the Principles and Practice of Medicine at the newly established University College, London. At the age of 33 he moved to London, taking a house in Gloucester Place.

The next four years spent in London were once more to end in failure, and a return to practice in a country town. The patients did not arrive, his expenses were considerable and there was no hospital connected with the college. His lectures were too vague and discursive, and "were not great successes, if they were not in truth failures. His introductory and farewell addresses were published by him in a small volume; but the perusal of them will scarcely fail to strengthen the

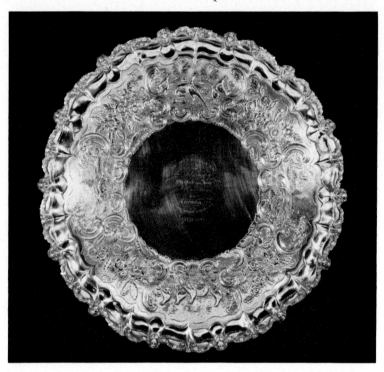

FIG. 2.   Silver Plate inscribed "To John Conolly, M.D., from the inhabitants of Stratford-upon-Avon and its neighbourhood as a testimony of their Esteem and regard. September 18th, 1828".

tradition of the somewhat vague and discursive character of the general course" (Maudsley). He was much pre-occupied with the teaching of psychiatry, and proposed to the Council of the College that the students should be given clinical teaching in insanity at one of the London lunatic asylums, but, he writes, "In that busy period of agitation and movement more important matters occupied the attention of the distinguished founders of the University, and I could not obtain attention to this suggestion."

Despite his inability to succeed in a clinical career, Conolly's social activities were as busy as ever. As a member of the Committee of The Society for the Diffusion of Useful Knowledge he took an active part in the Society's work. The following extracts from Charles Knight's *Passages of a Working Life* indicate the assistance which he rendered to the Society—

The Useful Knowledge Society had, in November, commenced the issue of a small series entitled, *The Working Man's Companion*, to be published occasionally, at the price of a shilling. The first volume, chiefly prepared by Dr. Conolly, called *Cottage Evenings*, was commended by Dr. Arnold for "its plain and sensible tone"; but he is hard upon what he calls its "cold deism". He is equally severe upon "the folly" of a little monthly publication, conducted, I believe, by a divine, who was afterwards a bishop, —*The Cottager's Monthly Visitor*. In the series of the *Working Man's Companion*, we did not neglect the occasion for combating popular errors of a social character, of inculcating the great private duties of cleanliness and of temperance as regard ourselves and our families, and of active benevolence and sympathy for our fellow creatures.

Dr. Conolly's little book on cholera was a model of what a popular treatise on the preservation of health ought to be—not leading the delicate and the hypochondriacal to fancy they can prescribe for themselves in real illness; not undervaluing medicine, but showing how rarely is medicine necessary when the laws of nature are not habitually violated. Of the fatal epidemic that had come amongst us, this wise and kind physician spoke with confidence of its speedy removal, under God's providence, in a condition of society where the principles of cordial brotherhood should more prevail than the miserable suggestions of selfish exclusiveness, where, in fact, the safety of the upper classes depended upon the well-being of the lower. The aid which Dr. Conolly rendered to the diffusion of knowledge was not special or professional. In those departments of what we now call "social science", which include the public health in its largest sense, his experience was always working in companionship with his benevolence. In 1831 we were united in the production of a series which was directly addressed to the working classes. Dr. Conolly brought to this useful labour —of which I shall have to make more particular mention—a lucid style, and an accurate conception of the true mode of reaching the uneducated. "Be thou familiar, but by no means vulgar" is as good a maxim for a popular writer, as for a young courtier going forth into the world, to deal with all sorts and conditions of men.

He frequently met Lord Brougham, for whom he always entertained a great and sincere admiration. The Committee used to meet monthly, partake of a good plain English dinner, at a moderate fixed charge, at five o'clock, there being a subscription for wine. Dinner lasted about an hour, then came two hours of solid business, the chair being generally filled by Brougham; and, in his rare absence, by the treasurer, Mr. W. Tooke, or the Vice-Chairman, Lord John Russell.

Discouraged by his lack of success both as a teacher and as a clinician, Conolly resigned his post and left London, this time for Warwick, only eight miles from Stratford, where apart from his financial difficulties, he had been so happy. The story repeats itself—after six years, struggling with difficulties,

> though much esteemed and assisted with a rare generosity, the physician-ship of the Hanwell Asylum became vacant and he, whose inclinations always leaned towards the study of insanity, made application for the office, not much encouraged thereto by his friends, who regarded such a step as the suicide of reputation and the confession of complete failure in life. On this occasion he failed, the casting vote of the chairman having determined the election in favour of Dr. Millingen, the author of *Curiosities of Medical Literature*. Another rising gleam of hope darkened; the outlook into the future black as ever; family cares increasing; and life gliding quickly on! One change more must be made, if not with hopeful expectations, yet in desperate resolve to try whether the destinies had not some place of success for one who had worked faithfully and energetically in many fields of practical activity, though hitherto with little benefit to himself. Accordingly he removed from Warwick to Birmingham in 1838, but he had not been there a year before the physicianship of the Hanwell Asylum was again vacant. He again made application for the office, and this time was happily successful. The grim destinies had not, after all, forgotten him" (Maudsley).

During his stay in Warwick he continued his literary activities, writing many articles for the *Cyclopaedia of Medical Practice*, which he jointly edited with his friend Forbes and Dr. Tweedie. They also founded the *British and Foreign Medico-Chirurgical Review*, the first number of which contained an account of Pinel releasing the lunatics from their chains. Together with Charles Hastings, he was one of the founders, in 1832, of what was to become the British Medical Association, and took an active part in its affairs. He attended the first meeting of the Association at Worcester, the second at Bristol and delivered the Anniversary Address at the third meeting in Birmingham in 1834. An extract from this address is quoted in the *History of the British Medical Association* and is a good example of Conolly's turgid style.

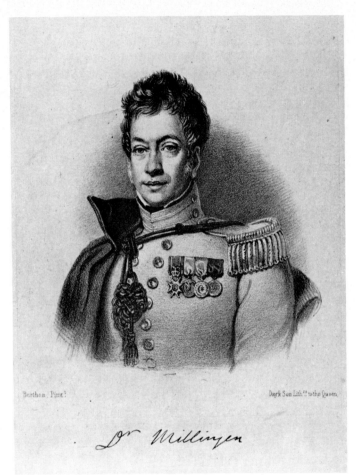

Berthon Pinx.ᵗ   Day & Son Lith.ʳˢ to the Queen.

Fig. 3. Dr. John Gideon Millingen. Superintendent of Hanwell, 1838–39.

We have no reason to apprehend that our successors will look back to the first proceedings of the Association with any feelings but those of respect, they will see that our regards, not narrowed to our own little day, were extended forward to their days, and to the hidden days beyond them. Animated by the same pure ambition as the founders, I trust they will carry on medical knowledge beyond the point at which they themselves became engaged in its pursuit, and in their turn will cheerfully transmit it, by them increased, to other generations, by whom, with the permission of Providence it may be more and more cultivated to the end of time.

Sir Charles Hastings wrote of him,

Dr. Conolly was one of the founders of the Provincial Medical and Surgical Association and took an active part in framing its laws when it was first instituted at Worcester in 1832. He was also a contributor to the first volume of the Transactions—which contained a valuable paper by him "On the Formation of County Natural History Societies".

HIS CAREER AS A PSYCHIATRIST

Whilst practising in Stratford, and again at Warwick, Conolly had held the post of visiting physician to the lunatic asylums in Warwickshire, and was so anxious to have charge of a lunatic asylum that he thought of establishing one himself. He had already written about mental disorder, and seems to have had considerable clinical experience.

Hanwell, the new County Asylum for Middlesex, had been opened on 16 May 1831, with William Ellis as its Treasurer, Medical Superintendent and Director, and his wife as Matron. Their respective salaries were £500 and £100 a year, together with certain expenses. In 1834 Ellis was knighted, and four years later resigned (Fig. 4). As we have seen, Conolly was unsuccessful, and J. G. Millingen, an ex-army surgeon, was appointed (Fig. 3). A year later he was gone, and this time Conolly was successful. On 1 June 1839 he entered on his duties as resident physician. On 21 September of the same year he announced in his first report to the Visitors the entire abolition of mechanical restraint—"No form of strait-waistcoats, no hand-straps—no leg-locks, nor any contrivances confining the trunk or limbs or any of the muscles, is now in use." And this was in an institution where instruments of mechanical restraint of one kind or other "were so abundant in the wards as to amount, when collected together, to about six hundred, half of them being handcuffs and leg-locks".

His achievements at Hanwell signalled the end of his failures and frustrations—henceforth, in spite of some difficulties, his reputation was to grow in stature, he would develop a large private practice, and become one of the most respected psychiatrists in the country. In 1843 the post of Resident Physician was discontinued and Conolly became Visiting Physician—a post he retained until 1852. Two medical officers

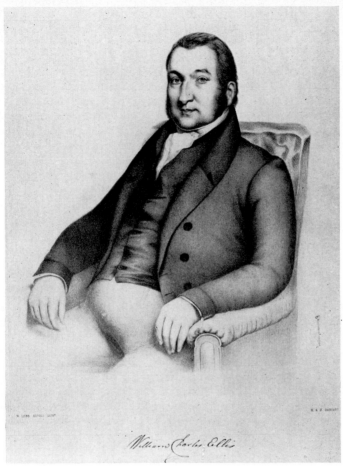

FIG. 4. William Charles Ellis. Superintendent of Hanwell 1831–1838.

were then appointed—Dr. Hitchman and Dr. Begley, one in charge of the female, and one of the male wards, instead of the Resident Physician. Dr. Hitchman, later Superintendent of the Derbyshire Asylum and an intimate friend of Conolly, has described how this system worked.

Dr Conolly visited the Asylum twice a week, spending the greater portion of the day at each visit. His interest in the patients seemed never to flag. Even cases beyond all hope of recovery were still objects of his attention. He was always pleased to see them happy, and had a kind word for each. Simple things which vainer men with less wisdom would have disregarded, or looked upon as too insignificant for their notice, arrested Dr. Conolly's attention, and supplied matter for remark and commendation—e.g., a face cleaner than usual, hair more carefully arranged, a neater cap, a new riband, clothes put on with greater neatness, and numerous little things of a like kind, enabled him to address his poor illiterate patients in gentle and loving accents, and thus woke up their feeble minds, caused sad faces to gleam with a smile, even though transient, and made his visits to the wards to be longed for and appreciated. Dr. Conolly rejoiced in acts of beneficence. To be poor and to be insane were conditions which at once endeared the sufferers to him; and when the insanity was removed, and the patient left the Asylum, he generally strove to obtain some pecuniary aid for her from the "Adelaide Fund" (a fund originated for the relief of discharged patients), and supplemented this very often indeed with liberal donations from his own purse. I believe that he gave away large sums of money in this manner.

As Resident Physician Conolly was able to begin the clinical teaching to undergraduates he had pressed for when Professor at University College, and in 1842 he began with a class consisting of two students chosen from each of the Metropolitan hospitals. William Gull was one of these students who

had the advantage of attending the clinical lectures given by Dr. Conolly at the Hanwell Asylum—we assembled at Hanwell about noon once a week. We then made a visit through the wards in company with Dr. Conolly and the medical officers of the Asylum, receiving some words of instruction upon the cases in general, our attention being especially directed to particular patients. This occupied, probably, near two hours; I believe sometimes more. We thus, from week to week, saw almost every phase of mental disorder, from acute mania to general paralysis and dementia. We also saw the application of the system of non-restraint, then on its trial, directed by that kind and calm philosophic temper so very conspicuous in Dr. Conolly. I cannot express to you the charm we felt in these visits. The asylums in the country, apart from the noise and bustle of the town; the novelty of the clinical work and teaching; the new field of facts before us, contrasting with those afforded in the routine of our other hospitals—the feeling of the peculiar advantages thus enjoyed—all combined to make us eager and thankful. (Quoted by Hunter and Greenberg, 1956.)

At this time his private practice began to grow, and from now until a few years before his death, when failing health compelled his retirement, "he was the chief consulting physician in this country in difficult cases of insanity and of other diseases of the nervous system". His opinion was particularly sought in medico–legal cases, for his evidence was always clearly and forcibly given, and he impressed the juries. He disagreed with the custom of calling experts on behalf of the defence and of the prosecution, believing that an independent medical adviser would be infinitely preferable, nor did he consider that juries were fit bodies to be entrusted with the correct assessment of soundness or unsoundness of mind.

He continued with his philanthropic work—supporting the British Medical Association, taking part in the founding of the Idiot Asylum at Earlswood, and being an active member of various societies. Thus he was one of the original members of the Ethnological Society and eventually became its President; was one of the earliest members of the National Association for the Promotion of Social Sciences; and was an active member of the Medico–Psychological Association, of which he was twice President. He visited France once again in 1845, in order to see Dr. Battel, the Inspector General of the civil hospitals.

All this activity had its effect and Conolly began to suffer increasingly from ill-health. Chronic rheumatism, neuralgia and an "irritable state of the skin", together with a progressive decline in his capacity for mental work, forced him to retire to Lawn House, his country home at Hanwell. Here he passed his time in writing, but continued to consult in difficult cases. He died there in 1866—at the age of 72, from a stroke.

It might have been naturally expected that, from his large consulting practice in cases of insanity and diseases of the nervous system generally, and the extent to which his opinion was sought in medico–legal questions, that Dr. Conolly would have died rich. It was far otherwise, however; and this may be chiefly explained by his professional position, during the greater part of his life,—a physician in small country towns, and afterwards as Resident Physician in the Hanwell Asylum, when his income was barely sufficient to maintain his family. He was also very liberal minded in his practice and otherwise, and gave little attention to financial matters. Still he had sufficient to supply all his wants during his retirement, and to leave something to his family at his death.

P

He left a son and three daughters; one of his daughters being married to a clergyman, and two to eminent psychological physicians, Henry Maudsley, and Harington Tuke.

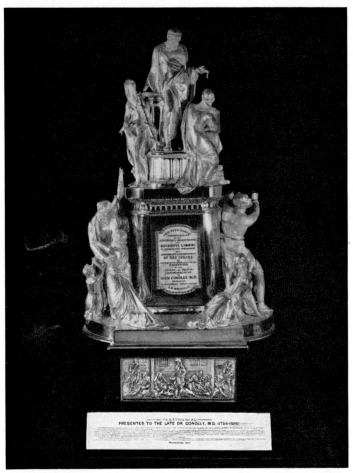

FIG. 5. "This Testimonial Commemorative of the Strenuous Persevering and Successful labours to Improve the Treatment and Ameliorate the Condition OF THE INSANE is together with a Portrait of Himself Presented by his Admiring and Grateful Contemporaries to John Conolly M.D. Physican to the Hanwell Lunatic Asylum. A.D. 1852."

"The Testimonial along with the portrait in oils by Sir John Watson Gordon, R.A. (also in the Auckland Art Gallery), was presented by his contemporaries in commemoration of his successful labours to improve the treatment and ameliorate the condition of the insane.

"The figures are intended to symbolize the doctor's labours. On the summit the god or genius of the Healing Art is represented as meditating and directing the improved treatment of the insane with Mercy on his right and Science on his left. Some of the evils to be remedied, the manner of relieving them and the results are illustrated by the groups around the pedestal and in the reliefs on the base. The groups exhibit (1) a male and female figure representing melancholy and raving madness under restraint. (2) A patient relieved from restraint in a state of partial recovery with the implements of coercion thrown on the ground. (3) The same person with his reason recovered and restored to his family to whom he is gratefully indicating the sources of his restoration in the group above. The two reliefs contrast the past and present methods of treating the insane. On the reverse the family coat of arms is shown. The plate was executed by Messrs. Hunt & Reskell, London, from designs modelled by Mr. Alfred Brown. The testimonial and portrait (along with copies of the doctor's writing on medical subjects which were placed in the library) were presented to the Auckland Art Gallery by the widow and brothers and the sisters of the late John Conolly, grandson of Dr. Conolly and a son of the Hon. Edward Tennyson Conolly, a retired Judge of the Supreme Court who died in Auckland in 1908."

The University of Oxford had conferred on him the D.C.L.; a massive silver piece comprised of an allegorical group of figures symbolizing the abolition of mechanical restraint had been presented to him when he left Hanwell; his portrait had been painted by Sir John Watson Gordon, and his bust executed in marble by the celebrated Italian sculptor Benzoni. He died, full of a fame which had suddenly burst forth in the fifth decade of his life, after over twenty years spent as an unsuccessful practitioner. The whole current of his life had been altered within the space of four years. How had this occurred—was it that the hour had found the man, or was it the culmination of a life-long striving toward a goal? Before these questions can be answered, if indeed they can, we must look further into his career and particularly to his literary work and his character, for the two are indissolubly linked.

HIS CHARACTER

Throughout his life Conolly delighted in social intercourse, and seems to have been pre-eminently a social man. He loved attending meetings, writing and lecturing, a man "who ever lived willingly in the present joy, and who had a passionate love of genial social intercourse." He made deep and lasting friendships and he and Sir John Forbes remained staunch to each other through all the phases of both their chequered lives. Sir James Clark, too, the Apothecary to Queen Victoria, was a true friend, as was Sir Charles Hastings. It is to one of his son-in-laws, Henry Maudsley, that we must turn for the best contemporary account of Conolly's character—and although drawn in the somewhat sombre and critical Maudsley manner, his memoir gives a vivid picture of the man.

> There was great energy of an impulsive kind in his character, but the anxious foresight and deliberate self-renunciation calculated to prevent the necessity of convulsive exertion, and the patient tedious labour necessary to carry an event to its best issue, were scarce so congenial to his nature. The writers whom he most admired were Pope, Bolingbroke, Addison and Cicero; he delighted in Milton's poetical works, especially "Lycidas", but his prose works were scarcely known to him; Bacon's essays he admired greatly and perused frequently, but his philosophical writings he was not familiar with. French authors and French style he esteemed highly, but German he did not read, and to German philosophy he had an antipathy, arising out of an entire unacquaintance with it. Goethe was by no means welcome to him, because this great poet's calm theory of life was repugnant to his sensibilities, and his deliberate conduct of life seemed to indicate a cold selfishness. These literary sympathies and antipathies prove, what is evident also in the character of his own easy and graceful, but diffuse style of composition, that he sometimes affected more the art displayed than the matter contained; that he was disposed to overestimate those who set forth ordinary reflections in an elegant and easy manner, and to underestimate those who broached profound thought in language sometimes neither easy nor elegant. In his youthful days he composed various slight poetical effusions; and there can be little doubt that, had he continued to cultivate his literary talents, and to labour in that direction, he might have had considerable success, either in light and easy versification, or in graceful prose.
>
> He had great sensibility of character; but his feelings were quick and volatile rather than deep and abiding. In some respects, I think, his mind seemed to be of a feminine type; capable of a momentary lively sympathy, which might even express itself in tears, such as enemies, forgetful of his character, might be apt to deem hypocritical; and prone to shrink from the disagreeable occasions of life, if it were possible, rather than encounter them with deliberate foresight and settled resolution. Consequently it

could not fail sometimes to happen that troubles, shirked at the time, were gathered up in the future, so as to demand at last some convulsive act of energy, in order to disperse them. A character most graceful and beautiful in a woman is no gift of fortune to a man having to meet the adverse circumstances and pressing occasions of a tumultuous life. He used to say, very sincerely, that he did not care for money, but that he very much liked the comforts and elegancies which money brings—an amiable sentiment, which, however, when closely analysed, might be made to resolve itself into a liking for enjoyment without a liking for paying the painful cost of it. But he truly regarded riches lightly. He was of a most liberal disposition, ever heartily rendering help, whether of money or personal service, to those who were in need of it.

Though by nature passionate and impetuous, he had great command over his manner, which was courteous in the extreme. Indeed he never failed to produce, by the suavity of his manner and the grace and ease of his address, the impression of great amiability, kindness, and unaffected simplicity; while his cheerful and vivacious disposition and his lively conversational powers rendered him an excellent social companion. His ordinary language was well chosen and elegant, and he always spoke in public with great precision and persuasive gentleness. There was a certain humility of manner, a degree of self-depreciation, in his address as in his writings, which failed not to attract men; it was none the less captivating because it might seem the form in which a considerable dash of self-consciousness declared itself. To few men was personal renunciation more uncongenial, and therefore painful; but few have been more ready to sacrifice, in a benevolent cause, those things which men commonly hold most dear.

To Conolly's gentle nature his Spartan training as a schoolboy was plainly intolerable and unprofitable, and the memory of it horrible sixty years afterwards; whatever good there was in it could not be assimilated into his nature; between his character and such discipline there was a complete repulsion. Had there happily been less repugnance some of the difficulties and trials of his subsequent life might not improbably have been avoided or lightened. But through life it may be questioned whether he ever did accept sincerely the inexorable laws of the universe; he delighted in the songs of birds, in the blossoming of trees, in genial social intercourse, in the amiabilities of human nature, in the elegancies of human life, in the graces of literary style, in the triumphs of benevolence; but he never seemed heartily to recognise or accept the stern and painful necessities of life; he so loved the gentle that even earnestness and sincerity, when rudely displayed, were distressing; he was not unamenable to the flattery which made things pleasant, and acutely pained by the harsh truth that laid bare their real relations when they were not pleasant; he shrunk from the task that was painful to him because involving pain to others, and would endure much needless imposition rather than deliberately face a difficulty and apply the effectual remedy; he would sacrifice his own serious interests rather than renounce a gratification which appealed strongly to his benevolent emotions, and could not tolerate a practice which was abhorrent to his fine sensibilities.

Sir James Clark speaks of Conolly's "moments of despondency", and that he was a great sufferer from an irritable chronic skin affection, "which often deprived him of much sleep at night, and irritated him during the day, and this sometimes caused him to appear impatient and excitable by officers and others who knew not or could not appreciate the corporeal condition and mental anxieties which produced the feeling".

HIS WRITINGS

Whilst still a student, Conolly writes, "the spectacle of a large lunatic asylum, distinguished by its excellent arrangements, awakened in me a curiosity and an interest that I had never felt before". He describes how, on entering a long gallery he met a tall, portly, good-looking man, to whom he had introduced a friend of his, a Frenchman who had served in Russia and had been on the staff of Napoleon at Waterloo. The patient's grandiose ideas and delusions intrigued both visitors. Conolly thought a good deal about this man, and consequently about psychiatry—naturally turning for information to Pinel and Tuke. He asked himself, "how does this man's mind differ from a sound mind? What effect was exercised by current views of mental disorder on the treatment and care of lunatics?" The temper of the time was reformist and men such as Prichard and Conolly turned to France for their inspiration. What had British psychiatry produced apart from restraint? "We read with almost as much amusement as wonder the respectful acknowledgment of Dr. Halloran that Dr. Cox made known to the profession the safe and effectual remedy of the circulating swing invented by Dr. Darwin". Bleeding, purges, blisters, measures to lower the strength of the patient—were they really effective? The physician had so far failed specifically to influence mental disorder and a kind of therapeutic nihilism was gaining ground. Accepted definitions and prevalent opinions were of little use—Conolly made a collection of them, "but I found them so numerous, and at the same

time so unsatisfactory that no useful object" was obtained from them.
Conolly therefore attempted to formulate his own ideas on mental
illness—his Thesis at Edinburgh was concerned with the mental state
in insanity and melancholia, and his first book, *An Inquiry concerning
the Indications of Insanity and Suggestions for the Better Protection and Care
of the Insane* published in 1830, was largely devoted to the features
distinguishing between sound and unsound mind. But as the second
part of the title shows, even at this time Conolly's mind was pre-
occupied with the ideas which, years later, were to make him famous.
The dramatic scene in the Salpêtrière appealed to a man of his temperament, whilst his admiration for the French, dating back to the
happy days with his stepfather, and his prolonged honeymoon at
Tours, predisposed him in favour of their revolutionary views.

The book begins with a review of the lamentable provisions for the
care of lunatics in England—a theme Conolly reverts to in all his books.
Insanity he considered to be often no more than an accentuation of
certain mental peculiarities widely found in the population at large.
Only when the patient becomes a danger to himself or others does
admission to an institution become necessary. Once this step was
taken, the social setting of the institution was itself responsible for a
major part of the further manifestations of disturbed behaviour. On
this account the physician must ponder most carefully before deeming
an individual of unsound mind. The state of the private madhouses,
and of the few public institutions was such that the patients' mental and
physical condition was often made a great deal worse. The dangers
inherent in "certification" made it imperative to understand the normal
mind, with all its quirks and eccentricities. The doctor must be aware
of those peculiarities of human understanding which do not amount
to insanity, such as superstitious habits, beliefs in witchcraft, delirium,
various sensory changes occurring under the influence of emotion,
and mood swings of the type which give rise to inertia and torpidity.
He stresses

> that a medical witness will never be secure from error if he forgets that
> insanity is often but a mere aggravation of little weaknesses or a prolonga-
> tion of transient varieties and moods of mind which all men now and then
> experience. An exaggeration of common passions and emotions such as
> fear, suspicion, admiration, or a perpetuation of absurdities of thought or
> action, or of irregularities of volition, or of mere sensation, which may
> occur in all minds, and be indulged in by all men, but which are cherished

and dwelt upon only by a mind diseased. A mind in which, together with the impairment of sensation, or of any mental faculty, there is (induced by that impairment or not) a loss of the power of making just comparisons.

He laid great stress on the faculty of comparison, and believed that when comparison is very much impaired then insanity is the direct and inevitable result. Activity, both mental and physical, he considered a very important factor in maintaining mental health, whilst education is nothing more than the training and exercise of the mind—to educate a man is to supply him with the power of controlling his feelings, his thoughts, his actions. It therefore follows that really educated people figure only very rarely amongst lunatics, and in Conolly's words "Everyone's recollection will convince him that of those attaining to eminence in any of the departments, even of a more imaginative character, nothing is so rare as for anyone to exhibit symptoms of insanity."

He then rather antithetically devotes several pages to the peculiarities of men of genius. Laurence Sterne for instance was very fastidious about his dress. Writing when he was ill-dressed he found that his thoughts were slovenly and ill-arranged. Haydn used to dress with particular care before sitting down to compose, for unless his hair was properly powdered and he wore his best coat he found he was unable to write. Again, if the diamond ring which Frederick II had given him was not on his finger he could not get on, nor could he write good music on any but the finest paper. The moral of all this is that just as much care must be given to the outer man as to the inner man when dealing with lunatics. The environment is likewise important. Pleasant scenery, pleasant atmospheres, lack of offensive smells, all conduce to mental calm and peacefulness. Just as the doctor must be acquainted with the range of normal behaviour, thought and activity, so must he understand the factors involved in mental health. Of these diet, physical health and education were particularly important.

> We see then that the maintaining of a perfectly sound state of mind requires not only attention to its faculties and to the feelings and emotions, but attention to the bodily health, a truth too often forgotten in the nurture of children, in the ordering of the studies of youth, and of the voluntary pursuit of studies or of business in adult age.

Conolly asks the politicians to take note of how inadequate diet acting on large masses of the population from their early to their declining years, by diminishing their mental health "enlarges the dominion of immorality and wretchedness".

Conolly was equally concerned with the importance of education in forming and strengthening the mind. Insanity had its remote origin in imperfect or misdirected education, and this was particularly noticeable in women. At that time education in the formal sense was largely a male preserve, a woman's place being in the home with her children. She was consequently more liable to mental illness than the male, for

> All who have peculiar opportunities of ascertaining the mental habits of insane persons of the educated classes, well know that, with some exceptions, their previous studies and pursuits appear to have been superficial and desultory, and often frivolous. The condition of the female mind is, even in the highest classes, too often more deplorable still. Not only is it most rare to find them familiar with the best authors of their own country, but most common to find that they have never read a really good author either in their own or in any other language; and that the few accomplishments possessed by them have been taught for display in society, and not for solace in quieter hours. All this has been said before and often, but in vain.

Worse still was the situation of the novel-reading female

> there is a frequent perversion of intellectual exercise, more fatal than its omission, which fills asylums with lady patients terrified by metaphysical translations, and bewildered by religious romances, and who have lost all custom of healthful exercise of body and mind—all love of natural objects —all interest in things most largely influencing the happiness of mankind. These evils have generally taken deep root before the patient's manifest want of reasonable constraint induces a resort to an asylum.

What made the question of feminine education so important to the psychiatrist was the belief that insanity was more frequently transmitted via the mother than via the father. Conolly's views may have had an effect more far reaching than he imagined, for they particularly impressed his friend and biographer, Sir James Clark, who as Apothecary to Queen Victoria, was in a position to influence the Queen in the way she brought up her family.

Two more controversial subjects in which Conolly was interested were physiognomy (Fig. 6) and phrenology. The facial expression in all its variety offered important clues as to the mental state, whilst phrenology, although its doctrines

> have met with little favour, and the pretensions of recent professors of

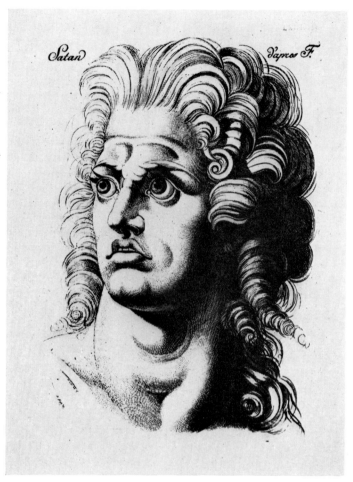

FIG. 6.   Physiognomy. The visage of Satan by Fuseli. From Lavater's
Essai sur la Physiognomie, 1783.

"Les yeux sont menacans de colère et de méchanceté; mais ils font en
même temps troublés par la crainte. Ce regard semble agité par quelque
découverte imprévue. Le haut du nez marque la violence; le bas indique
un esprit judicieux—mais devroit exprimer plus de méchanceté et de
fureur."

occult methods of acting upon the nervous system, have thrown an air of absurdity even over the truths of what is called phrenology, no person not altogether devoid of the power of observation can affect to overlook the

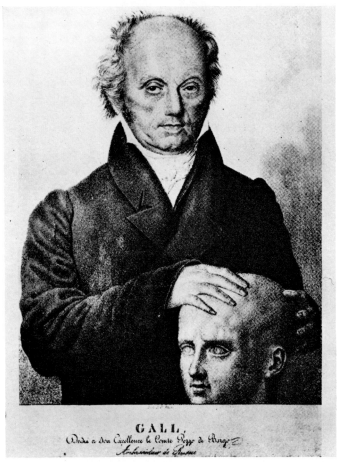

FIG. 7.   Dr. Franz Joseph Gall, 1757–1828. The Founder of Phrenology.

general importance of the shape and even the size of the brain in relation to the development of the mental faculties. It is reasonable to consider each of the large and marked divisions of the brain, and each of the convolutions, with their copious supply of grey or vesicular nerve-substance, as possessing distinct offices; and the more or less perfect development of these several masses, and the greater or less nervous energy they possess, as circumstances connected with the varieties of mental character, and with the disordered manifestations of the mind. Each mass, or each sub-division of such mass, may, like each nerve, have a distinct office. Each, however, excited, may only be capable of one kind of manifestation of the excitement. Each, when in a healthy state, may be excited simultaneously throughout; and each in disease may be excited irregularly, or too long, or lose the power of being excited altogether.

Phrenology in its present state, may be held in small estimation, yet there are not wanting grounds for the belief, that its leading principles rest on truth, and that ultimately its value may receive a general acknowledgment. It seems reasonable, indeed to expect the brain to be an aggregate of different parts, each sub-serving the manifestation of a particular mental function. Such a view has assuredly the support of analogy, being quite consistent with our knowledge of the manner in which other organs discharge complicated functions, and it also derives direct support from researches, both recent and old, into the anatomy and physiology of the brain itself.

Conolly and others founded the Warwick and Leamington Phrenological Society in 1834 and Conolly was elected its first President. Skulls and casts of skulls were collected and the members read papers to each other. In 1841 he presided at the first meeting of the Phrenological Society, and maintained an interest in the subject throughout his life. It is only comparatively recently that phrenology has taken its rightful place in the sequence of theories relating to localization of function in the brain, and Conolly's words have a very modern ring to them.

In spite of the prolixity which is the chief fault of nearly all Conolly's writings, the book's message is clear. The ignorance of the medical profession with regard to insanity must be remedied. Medical students must be admitted to the wards of mental hospitals and taught clinical psychiatry.

During the term allotted to medical study, the student never sees a case of insanity, except by some rare accident. Whilst every hospital is open, every lunatic asylum is closed to him; he can study all diseases but those affecting the understanding—of all diseases the most calamitous. The first occurrence, consequently, of a case of insanity, in his own practice, alarms him: he is unable to make those distinctions which the rights and the happiness of individuals and of families require; and has recourse to indiscriminate, and, generally, to violent or unnecessary means; or gets rid of his anxiety and his patient together, by signing a certificate, which commits the unfortunate person to a madhouse. In the plan of his medical study, therefore, attention to diseases affecting the mind forms hardly any part;

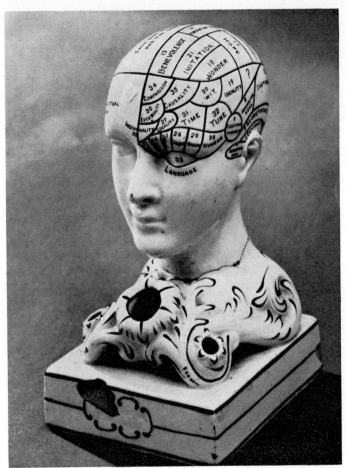

FIG. 8.   Phrenological Inkwell. (*Staffordshire Ware. From the author's collection.*)

and it has thus happened that many individuals have been ignorantly confined, and unjustly detained in houses for the reception of lunatics; and persons of all ages, suffering under temporary mental derangement, from temporary causes, shut up with the incurable: nor it is any exaggeration to say, that such treatment has in many cases destroyed all hope of recovery.

No provision of the Legislature can prevent the occurrence of these grievous mistakes, unless opportunities are at the same time given of making medical men as familiar with disorders of the mind as with other disorders; and thus of rescuing lunatics from those whose interest it is to represent such maladies as more obscure, and more difficult to manage than any other. It would be some compensation for the unavoidable evils of public lunatic asylums, if each establishment of that kind became a Clinical school, in which, under certain restrictions, medical students might prepare themselves for their future duties to the insane. It is true that insane patients are not always in a state to be visited by pupils, and that a very strict discipline would be necessary to prevent disorder or impropriety: but such discipline is quite practicable; and such arrangements might be made as would at once guard those patients from disturbance whom disturbance might injure, and present a sufficient number of instructive examples to the student. In some cases, also, the change of persons and of conversation would be actually beneficial to the patients; and would only be what they are not accustomed to, during the visits of persons who come to see them from mere curiosity. Among the many intelligent young men resorting to the London schools of medicine and surgery, some would soon be found who would zealously study mental disorders, and by acting under the physician or medical superintendent, most materially assist him. Opportunities would then be afforded of trying every variety of medical and of mental or moral treatment, and particularly of practising all those methods of influencing the mind, which, separately slight, are, in connection, very availing; and being only practicable at favourable moments, not only require great discretion, but a degree of superintendence which is at present impossible. We should then see how much could really be done in these affections, and should hear no more of mistakes which have from time to time afforded so much matter for litigation, so much personal uneasiness, and, in some cases, so much oppression and fraud.

Secondly, there must be a total abolition of restraint, restraint which in itself was inhuman and productive of reactions leading to the accentuation or continuance of the mental illness.

Let no one imagine that even now it is impossible or difficult to effect the seclusion of an eccentric man; or easy for him, when once confined, to regain his liberty. The timidity, or ignorance, or it may be, a dishonest motive, of relatives, leads to exaggerated representations; and the great profit accruing from a part of practice, almost separated from general medicine, cannot but now and then operate against proper caution in admitting such representations. When men's interests depend upon an opinion, it is too much to expect that opinion always to be cautiously formed, or even in all cases honestly given. The most respectable practitioners in this department openly justify the authorising of restraint, before the patient is seen, and on the mere report of others: and it seems that depositions to the insanity of individuals have been received in courts of law, concerning persons with whom the deponents have never had an interview; and that on these depositions proceedings have been partly founded, of which the results were the imprisonment of lunatics, and restraint over their property. When the affair is conducted with more formality, and the suspected person is visited before being imprisoned, those who visit him are often very little acquainted with mental disorders, and came rather to find *proofs* of his insanity, which, to minds prepossessed, are seldom wanting, than cautiously to examine the state of his mind. If a person of sound mind were so visited, and knew of the visit beforehand, it would not be quite easy for him so to comport himself, as to avoid furnishing *conviction* that he was *not* of sound mind. His indignation would pass for raving; his moderation, for the proverbial cunning of a lunatic. A man of an undisturbed understanding, suddenly surprised by the servants of a lunatic asylum, with handcuffs ready, and a coach waiting to carry him off, would infallibly exhibit some signs, easily construed into proofs that he was "not right in his head": a man of shy and eccentric habits, if exposed to a similar outrage, would manifest his feelings in modes still more peculiar, and furnish abundant proofs of undeniable madness: and if the attempt was made on an individual of susceptible nervous system, of irritable temperament, suffering too under some temporary cause of discomposure or affliction, no one who has ever attended to the inequalities of his own mind can doubt, that his mental government would be sufficiently shaken to warrant any restraint or coercion on the part of those who would seldom be found reluctant to restrain and coerce.

Of all these matters the public are not altogether unsuspicious, and hence arises an evil of an opposite description: for the occasional detection of mistakes, and the dread of committing a beloved relative to a lunatic asylum; the opinion that to pronounce an individual insane is equivalent to pronouncing a sentence of separation from every friend, and an abandonment of all care of him to strangers; does really prevent in some instances such interference as the interest and comfort of families require; and those to whom temporary superintendence and slight restraint would be salutary, are allowed to ruin their fortunes, or to make a whole family wretched, because restraint, when once determined on, is seldom apportioned to the individual case, but is indiscriminate and excessive and uncertain in its termination.

His attempts to implement his ideas on the training of medical students was doomed to end in a bitter personal and professional disappointment. But the total abolition of restraint was to sweep him to fame and bring about his eventual apotheosis.

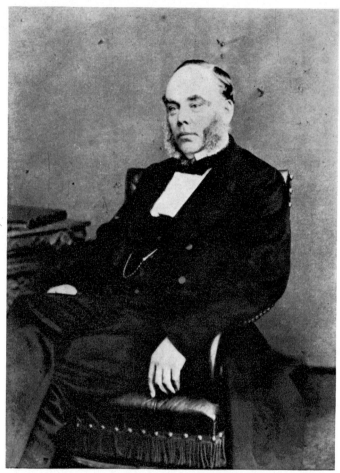

Fig. 9.   Robert Gardiner Hill, 1811–1878.

"ON THE CONSTRUCTION AND GOVERNMENT
OF LUNATIC ASYLUMS"

His next book was in some respects his most important contribution to psychiatry. Published in 1847, it was entitled *On the Construction and Government of Lunatic Asylums*, and was the first comprehensive

work of its kind by a British author. Previous publications included
the *Description of the Retreat* by Samuel Tuke in 1813; the same author's
Practical Hints on the Construction and Economy of Pauper Lunatic Asylums,
including Instructions to the architects who offered plans for Wake-
field Asylum, and a sketch of the most approved design, published in
1815; and *Remarks on the Construction and Management of Lunatic*
Asylums by Stark, the architect who had been engaged to prepare plans
for the Glasgow Asylum. There were also references to the subject in
most of the psychiatric publications from Haslam onward. The most
important factual work was, however, that by Jacobi of Siegburg—
published in 1834 and translated into English in 1841—*On the Con-*
struction and Management of Hospitals for the Insane. Although "Dr.
Jacobi's work contains a great number of useful suggestions, the reader
should be cautioned that they were written thirteen years ago, and are
all conformable to the old system of restraint and force, although
tempered by the author's evident kindness of heart and good understanding". What exerted the most powerful effect on Conolly was not
this massive German work but a 56-page essay by an obscure house-
surgeon in Lincoln.

In 1835 a young man was appointed house-surgeon of the Lincoln
Lunatic Asylum, who asserted that "in a properly constructed building,
with a sufficient number of suitable attendants, restraint is never
necessary, never justifiable, and always injurious, in all cases of lunacy
whatever". He was Robert Gardiner Hill (Fig. 9), and with the backing
of his Attending Physician, E. P. Charlesworth, within two years he
had almost completely put his ideas into practice.

A good account of the practice of restraint at this time is given in
Paul Slade Knight's *Observations on the Causes, Symptoms and Treatment*
of Derangement of the Mind, published in 1827.

ON THE METHOD OF SECURING LUNATICS

The mode of securing a mad-man, so as to prevent him from injuring
himself or others, has been the source of no slight difference of opinion;
and several years since I procured from various places, particularly recommended for their humane methods, the apparatus of restraint used in them
respectively; by which it was obvious, that the intention to avoid injury
was the leading object, but the execution of that intention singularly
deficient. Strong leather straps, carefully padded and covered with soft

Q

wash leather, were used to secure arms and legs; and as it is possible this mode may still be followed in some receptacles for lunatics, I shall point out one or two palpable defects in the construction of these straps. First—

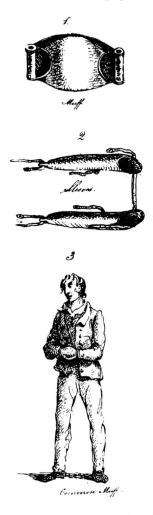

1.

Muff.

2

Sleeves.

3

Common Muff.

no padded strap can be buckled sufficiently secure round the wrist or the arm, so as to prevent a violent lunatic from working his hand out, without producing a painful pressure on the limb, and a partial stoppage at least, of the circulation; added to which, the warmth of the padding speedily produces perspiration, this soaks the leather, and makes it, in some considerable degree, stick to the skin; in this state it produces more friction, so that in fact it cannot by any means be securely used in the high state of delirium, and indeed, it has always appeared in my practice, that this padded apparatus never could be used with propriety. I never could secure the violent with it, and others of course had no occasion for it. The strap round the arms, as used in the Dublin Lunatic Asylum, is much better than these padded wrist straps, etc. but I have frequently been obliged to have this taken off, from the pressure, necessary to secure, or produced by the exertions of, very violent lunatics, being too great to permit free circulation; and the old straight waistcoat was on these accounts certainly preferable to either of these modes. But there are many powerful objections to the straight waistcoat; in hot weather particularly it is very oppressive to the patient, it cramps him exceedingly, and is at all times peculiarly offensive. After trying various methods, the most effectual as to security, the easiest as regards bodily constraint, and the least liable to erode the skin, I have represented in the lithographic sketches annexed.

Fig. *1* represents what I have termed the Muff, it consists of two strong pieces of leather sewed together at the sides, with a thinner piece of leather

Figs. 1-6. Instruments of Restraint. (From Paul Slade Knight's "*Observations on the Causes, Symptoms and Treatment of Derangement of the Mind*" (1827).)

running diagonally across, on the inside, to separate, and thus to prevent the lunatic from tearing his own hands, which he would frequently do but for this contrivance; the edges of these strong pieces of leather are secured to the patent iron wrist lock—the lock being made on purpose.[1] The hands being introduced into each pocket, the lock is shut upon the wrist, and the patient is effectually prevented from tearing or destroying things, or taking off his clothes, nor can he strike so as to effect any injury; at the same time he has nearly the full and ordinary use of his arms (see Fig. 3).

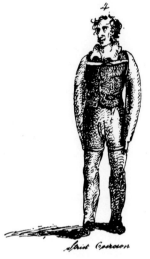

Joint Coercion

Fig. 2, represents the Sleeves, by far the best mode of securing a violent lunatic I can imagine. It simply consists of two large strong leather sleeves, closed at the bottoms, and fastened across the shoulders by a strap, and staple and lock; and again in the same manner across the back by the elbows, the sleeves being attached in front by a broad short belt across the upper part of the breast. In extreme cases where the patient makes violent exertions to break the strap across his back, I also add another strap, passing round the thigh, and through a loop sewed to the bottom of the sleeves, and then he stands with his arms, as it were loosely by his sides, in this position he can make but feeble exertions with them. It is evident, that if in addition to this, the common leg locks be added, the patient will be rendered almost powerless, without producing any injurious pressure whatever, although the exertions of the patient should be the most violent and incessant. Patients have worn these sleeves for months, without sustaining the slightest injury from them. If at any time they, or the muffs are found too warm,

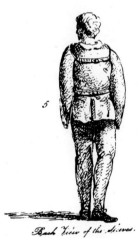

Back View of the Sleeves.

---

[1] Mr. Cornthwaite, saddler, of Lancaster, used to make the Muff, etc., that I used. I always found him a very moderate man, and a good workman.

small holes may be easily punched in them so as to admit of ventilation. See Fig. 4, front view with straps round the thighs, and Fig. 5, the back view, without straps round the thighs.

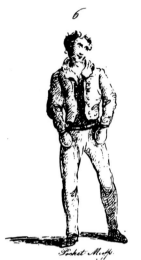

Pocket Muffs.

Fig. 6 represents a man with pocket muffs, which are made on the same principle that the other muffs are made, one is attached to each side like a pocket, and they are fastened in this position by a strap round the waist. It will frequently please a patient to give him his choice between the muff and the pocket muff.

I am firmly convinced, that leg and wrist locks are infinitely preferable to leather straps. The iron locks possess numerous advantages, but the clinking of the chain should be, by all means, prevented, for I have known it impress lunatics with the most gloomy apprehensions.[1]

In 1835, the year Gardiner Hill arrived, 80 patients were free from restraints, whilst 28 had been subject to restraint; in 1836 restraints were applied to only 12 patients, and in 1837, 2 patients only out of 130 were so treated. In 1839 he published his *Lecture on the Management of Lunatic Asylums* which he had given at the Mechanics Institution at Lincoln on 21 June 1838. In this 56-page essay he succinctly presented the arguments in favour of the total abolition of restraint, and describes how it could be effected.

But, it may be demanded, what mode of treatment do you adopt, in place of restraint? How do you guard against accidents? How do you provide for the safety of the attendants? In short, what is the substitute for coercion? The answer may be summed up in a few words, viz.——*classification— watchfulness—vigilant and unceasing attendance by day and by night—kindness, occupation, and attention to health, cleanliness, and comfort, and the total absence of every description of other occupation of the attendants.*

Gardiner Hill pointed out that several essentials must be fulfilled. The buildings must be suitable, there must be a proper classification of patients, a sufficient number of strong, tall and active attendants, well paid and of good character, and an unremitting control by the House

---

[1] "See the Particulars, etc", by a Gentleman.

Surgeon. If these conditions do not hold, "wherever restraint may become necessary, *owing to the imperfect adaptation of the Building*, or to want of sufficient *attendants*, the most simple means should be selected. On such an occasion, I do not know of any constraint which would be preferable to that of seclusion in a darkened room."

In these few pages Gardiner Hill compressed more good sense than can be found in many hundreds of pages written by some of his contemporaries—including even Conolly. Still better were his statistical tables, dealing with the numbers under restraint, admissions and discharges, causes of death, patients' occupations, and diets. Gardiner Hill's book is an outstanding piece of work formulating a definite thesis, and showing by statistics what can be accomplished if certain processes are set into motion.

This work exercised a most profound effect on Conolly; he visited Lincoln in May 1839, spoke and corresponded with Gardiner Hill and Dr. Charlesworth, so that when he entered upon his duties at Hanwell he was resolved to put their findings to the test. This story will be dealt with later—here we must now consider the ideas he put forward as to the construction and government of lunatic asylums.

The greater part of the book is a reprint from lectures Conolly published in the *Lancet* in 1846, which had been occasioned by the 1845 Act of Parliament directing that asylums were to be provided for pauper lunatics in every County and Borough in England and Wales.

The total number of insane poor in England and Wales at that time had been calculated to be about 17,000, and of these, no more than about 4,500 were provided for in asylums. The argument had been put forward in some counties that private licensed houses provided cheaper care than the county asylums, and also that the number of cures effected in private houses was greater. Conolly considered that by far the best arrangement was a large public asylum. Of recent cases sent into public asylums, if not epileptic or affected by paralysis, about 50 per cent recovered. Unfortunately the public or county asylums at that time were nearly filled with old and incurable patients, transferred from private licensed houses or workhouses when they became unmanageable, or were considered to be incurable. The cost of maintaining a patient in a private house was no cheaper than the cost of maintaining a patient in a county asylum. Conolly disapproved of the Commissioners' view that chronic cases should be cared for at much less expense than recent and curable cases, "this conclusion may, at first sight, appear reasonable to those not familiar with the insane, but I believe that by all who have lived in asylums, will be pronounced to be fallacious and not unattended with danger". Conolly speaks of the cruelty of condemning the incurable to what would appear to them to be a hopeless prison, and of the possibility of sometimes including curable patients in this condemnation. He cites a notorious event in Scotland, when 123 lunatics were quietly transported to the Island of Arran from various parishes on the mainland. The Sheriff and other authorities of the district only became aware of the importation when the dangerous appearance of certain wild persons wandering about the island brought it to their notice. The Duke of Hamilton's factor sought the advice of Dr. Hutcheson, physician to the Glasgow Asylum, who spent eleven days investigating the condition of these involuntary immigrants. As a result "twenty poor lunatics were restored to social life, and sixty-one saved from prolonged neglect and wretchedness which was the inevitable fate of all poor lunatics who, being pronounced incurable, are considered proper objects for a more rigid economy". Thirteen of the sixty-one recovered and were sent out of hospital able to support themselves; seven recovered so far as to be able to live at home; fifteen died, and twenty-six were detained in the Glasgow Asylum.

In view of the enormous amount of accommodation which would be needed to implement the Act, the main body of the book is concerned with the planning and structure of the new hospitals. Conolly was well aware of the difficulties—the lack of any uniform ideas, and the reluctance of both governors and architects to consult the medical men who had actually lived in asylums. In most of these the buildings resembled prisons, rather than hospitals for the cure of insanity.

> Even now, high and gloomy walls, narrow or inaccessible windows, heavy and immoveable tables and benches, and prison regulations applied to the officers and attendants, attest the prevalence of mistaken and limited views. It appears to me that not only should no general plan of a lunatic asylum be determined upon without being submitted to the consideration of a physician acquainted with the character, habits and wants of the insane, but that no alteration should be made in an asylum without a reference to its resident medical officers. Security does not require gloom. The buildings should be on a healthy site, admitting air and there should be a school, chapel and good hygiene. The surrounds of the asylum should be pleasant,

not too cold, not too damp and not too hot, because even if lunatics do not complain, they are still injured by severe cold.

A mistake which was committed all too often was to make no provision for the accumulation of patients.

The asylum is usually erected merely for the supposed actual number of lunatics within a county; and, in consequence of the incurable patients not being discharged, the building becomes, in the course of ten years, crowded with nearly double the number first provided for. Provision is made for these, first by means of the erection or extension of wings, to which, if the original plan has been well devised, there exists no objection; but afterwards, by piling a third story wherever it can be raised, or by excavating rooms and wards under ground. These arrangements have all the disadvantages which I have mentioned. They render proper classification, either within doors or without, almost impossible, and the preservation of order difficult. By the accumulation of so many persons, day and night, in a lofty building, many of whom can seldom leave the wards, and no one of whom is in perfect health, the asylum becomes subject to every atmospheric and terrestrial influence unfavourable to life. If no epidemic outbreak alarms the governors into an investigation and reform of buildings so arranged, or ill-placed, or otherwise unhealthy, the inmates are merely all brought to a low standard of health; to uneasiness, suffering, and a disposition to illness. There is always a risk of more active disease; and this may not only depopulate the institution to a great extent, but spread pestilence around it. Lessons of this kind are learnt with unwillingness, because they are opposed to the strong avarice which vitiates all social provision for the poor; and they are also soon forgotten. The terrible examples afforded in 1832, when the malignant cholera last visited us, are so unheeded, that when the malady comes again, it will find almost every asylum, private and public, equally unprepared with reasonable preservations against it.

The Derbyshire magistrates, finding that the number of insane paupers in their county at this time amounts to 216, have designed an asylum capable of holding 360, so that no addition to the building may be required for some time; and I regret to learn that this wise provision has constituted one of the objections made to it by the Commissioners. The Hanwell Asylum was opened in 1831, for 300 patients; it now contains about 1,000; and another asylum is already required in the county for nearly as many more.

In Conolly's opinion the optimum size of an asylum would provide accommodation for 360–400 patients. Inside the building

much ornaments or decoration, external or internal, is useless, and rather

offends irritable patients than gives any satisfaction to the more contented.
In some of the Italian asylums, busts, pictures and ornaments abound, and
the walls are painted with figures representing various allegories or
histories. These would appear more likely to arouse morbid associations
than to do any good.

Conolly has a good deal to say concerning Medical Superintendents.
In hospitals containing no more than 400 patients, all he requires is an
assistant to make up the medicines, but in a larger hospital more assistance becomes necessary, and all of these officers should be either
appointed by the physician or act under his instructions. Conolly points
out how laborious it is for one medical officer to administer to the
needs of over 300 patients, and how impossible to do so when the
number exceeds 400. Then assistants are needed. Prison discipline was
applied in too many asylums, the doctors being needlessly harassed by
rules and regulations interfering with their private life and domestic
freedom. The director of the hospital has to regulate the habits, the
character, the very life of his patients. "He must be their physician,
their director and their friend." That he should be a person naturally
benevolent is indispensable, and it is extremely desirable that he should
possess an almost inexhaustible patience. The qualities to which, of old,
much importance was attached, a commanding stature, a stern manner,
a fierce look, a loud voice, had become either unnecessary or positive
disqualifications.

There must be no misapprehension, however, as to who is the
director of an asylum.

> Seven years of close observation of the management of Hanwell have
> convinced me that no mistake can be more unfortunate than that of
> placing the direct government of an asylum for the insane in any other
> hands than that of a physician. Any other governor will find that he can
> only avoid being mischievous by avoiding all kind of interference. He
> must be idle, or he can scarcely be harmless. If he supports the physician,
> such support should not be required; if he opposes him, or controls him,
> the welfare of the patients is sacrificed, and the asylum is ruined. To put
> a gallant officer in such a position, or to transfer a governor to an asylum
> from a prison, is to place such individuals in a position in which all their
> previous experience becomes nearly useless, and for which nearly all their
> acquired habits disqualify them. To intrust such officers with the choice of
> attendants on the patients, the regulation of their duties, and even with
> the classification of the patients, can only lead, by a succession of mistakes
> of lamentable consequence, to utter confusion. It will readily be conceded

that the regulations of a camp or a garrison can have little in them applicable to an asylum; but it will not, perhaps, so easily be granted that everything, and the manner of everything, that is considered suitable to a
prison, is inappropriate and wrong as applied to an asylum for the insane.
It may be difficult for a magistrate to believe this, but nothing is more
certain.

The Matron must certainly be under the superintendent's orders.

The matron of an asylum is usually chosen by the governing body; but
it is a great evil in an asylum when this officer is made of too much importance, and led to consider herself independent of the physician, and has the
power—by sending away the attendants on his female patients, choosing
others without reference to him, and moving them from ward to ward—
to interfere in the most direct and mischievous manner with highly
important parts of his treatment. A matron to an asylum may be a valuable
auxiliary to the medical officers, and the means of doing much good; of
which I have had some personal experience. But matrons are generally
spoiled as auxiliaries to the medical officers, by a pardonable leaning to
female influence on the part of all committees, who are pleased with the
studious deference apparently paid to their opinion, and really paid to their
power; and thus the matron becomes the only companion of the governors
through the wards, and almost the only source of their information; and
it is the consequent fault of matrons of many institutions to usurp authority,
and to endeavour to exclude the medical officers from all interference with
the female side of the house, beyond that of prescribing drugs. Their
influence, also, with the governing bodies is not always exerted in the
direction of humanity or kindness, and their government of the nurses is
too often unjust and unfeeling. I am very sorry to say it, but in the generality of examinations made, or inquests held, in hospitals or workhouses, or
asylums, the matrons do not appear to advantage, and are too often found
to be the most effective agents for harsh purposes.

Conolly generally held that women on the whole did not make good
"attendants" unless they had begun their work at an early age. There
is no greater fallacy than of supposing that plain, middle-aged, ill-
dressed women are more moral or more orderly in their habits and
life than young, attractive, and well-dressed nurses.

To the building itself Conolly pays great attention, discussing the
arrangements of galleries and sleeping rooms, warming, ventilation,
hygiene, the sources of offensive smells and the different modifications
required in asylums for patients of various classes. Every detail is
discussed, from the provision of fire guards to the use of observation

panels in the doors; lighting by coal gas; and water closets, the best type being one where the stream of water is controlled by the opening or closing of the door.

He deals with wards for the elderly and feeble, the infirmaries, airing courts, evening entertainments, clothes and recreations. Restraints were commonly employed in the sick wards in order to render the patient more amenable to the various medical treatments such as poulticing or bleeding, most of which were very unpleasant and indeed painful. He quotes the case of a young woman who was found to be suffering from scabies and a breast abscess. She was strapped down in the infirmary, not because she was dangerous to herself or to others, but because she preferred to eat the poultices (which contained lead) rather than keep them applied to her skin. Despite this, Conolly released her, and with kindness and careful nursing attention was gratified to see her improve.

Conolly regarded out-door exercise, and the provision of amenities for games and for the enjoyment of the gardens as most important. The numerous lunatics of an indolent and apathetic nature who are reluctant to move out of their day rooms can often be drawn out of their sloth by an invitation to walk in the fields, gardens, or vegetable garden. At Hanwell games were organized, a band was formed amongst the attendants, and musical evenings were held once a week.

The *Illustrated London News* describes a Twelfth Night Entertainment at Hanwell in 1848.

TWELFTH NIGHT ENTERTAINMENT AT HANWELL LUNATIC ASYLUM

"Seven years have elapsed since the experiment of non-restraint has been fully tried in the Hanwell Asylum; and Dr. Conolly, in the spirit of a Christian philosopher, thanks God, with deep and unfeigned humility, that nothing has occurred during that period to throw discredit on the grand principle for which he so nobly battled."

We quote this emphatic testimony to the success of the non-restraint system of management of Lunatic Asylums from the first number of the *Journal of Psychological Medicine and Mental Pathology*, edited by Dr. Forbes Winslow: a work specially devoted to the humane treatment of the Insane and from which the most beneficial results may be anticipated.

The accompanying Engraving presents a very interesting illustration of the non-restraint system pursued at Hanwell. Among the in-door recreations for the patients during the winter days and evenings, music is the greatest favorite. There are three pianos; flutes, clarionets, and violins have been bought for patients who could play. Some of the attendants are tolerable musicians, and a small band has been formed, which contributes much to the enjoyment of the winter evening parties. It is by no means uncommon, on approaching the wards appropriated to the more trouble-some patients, on the male side of the asylum, to hear a lively performance on the fiddle, and to find patients dancing to it. The patients often have

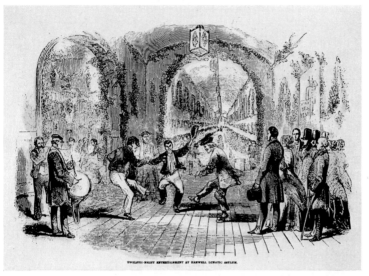

FIG. 10. Twelfth-Night entertainment at Hanwell Lunatic Asylum.

small parties for dancing, and there are some entertainments on a larger scale. One of the latter, given to the female patients, took place on New Year's Eve; and on the 6th instant (Thursday week,) the usual Twelfth Night entertainment was given to the male patients, in the institution.

They assembled, to the number of about 250, in the gallery of No. 9 ward, and in the adjoining tower, both of which were tastefully decorated with evergreens: coloured lamps were suspended from the ceiling, and the gas-burners were altered so as to appear like ornamental fan-lights; and many devices and mottoes were placed on the walls. At about half-past four o'clock these patients partook of coffee and cake in the above apartment, and all the others were similarly regaled in their respective wards, after which some danced, others sung, some played on various instruments, others amused themselves with cards, draughts, dominoes, bagatelle, &c. At eight o'clock a supper of roast beef and vegetables was served to them, with an allowance of beer and tobacco. At the conclusion of this repast they again engaged in amusements till about half-past nine, when, after singing the National Anthem, they retired to bed in tranquility and order. Good humour and mirth prevailed during the entire evening, not a single circumstance occurred to mar the happiness which all appeared to enjoy. The attendants were most zealous and assiduous in contributing to the festivity of the patients; and their exertions were, in the highest degree, praise worthy. All the officers of the Asylum, and several of the Committee of Visitors, were present.

Dr. Conolly has just published a very interesting volume on *The Construction and Government of Lunatic Asylums, and Hospitals for the Insane*, in which we find the following striking passage on these evening entertainments:—

"The first sight of three hundred persons, assembled for an entertainment, and stimulated by a lighted and decorated apartment, and the presence of strangers, and the sound of music, and allowed to dance as freely, and even as fantastically, as each may choose, is one which an unfamiliar spectator can scarcely witness without feeling some immediate trepidation. But, in an asylum where kindness is the rule, and where all the officers and the attendants, and even the visitors, are known to entertain cordial feelings towards the patients, and where the patients are unaccustomed to any kind of violent treatment, or even to sharp or unkind reproof, it is found that character of order prevails which is not lost sight of amidst the excitement of the liveliest dancing and enjoyment. What appears to be an almost unrestrained activity is moderated by the timely, kind, and judicious words: and excitement which seems likely to transgress due bounds, is suspended in a moment by friendly conversation. When the hour of separation arrives, cheerful faces and grateful expressions show the general good effect of the audience accorded, on which, usually, sound sleep is found speedily to ensue. Such are the general effects; and the especial effects on such of the patients are even more remarkable."

Our illustration shows a view of the supper and the lively dance. In the latter, the right-hand figure is poor Rayner, many years "Harlequin" at Covent Garden Theatre. The reader by the way, will find a minute account of a visit to the Hanwell Asylum in No. 55 of our Journal.

Nor was work to be neglected. "Among the means of relieving patients from the monotony of an asylum and of preserving the bodily health, and at the same time improving the condition of the mind, and promoting recovery, employment of some kind or other ranks the highest. Its regulation is proportionably important."

Sir William Ellis had introduced work therapy to Hanwell after coming from the Wakefield Asylum, where he had developed the idea. Work should be prescribed and should not be indiscriminately and, indeed sometimes, improperly used. When work has been a contributory cause towards the illness then a rest from work is indicated. In cases of mania and melancholia work is positively detrimental to the patient, says Conolly, and in chronic cases it is sometimes much objected to. In his last annual Hanwell report, of the 418 male patients then in the asylum, 219 were employed, 75 in the garden or on the farm, 40 as helpers in the wards. Of 567 women, 314 were employed, 69 in the laundry, and 49 as helpers in the wards. A large number of women were also employed on needlework.

As we have seen in his first book, Conolly believed that an adequate diet was a pre-requisite for both mental and physical health. In this he agreed with Dr. Charlesworth of Lincoln who considered that insanity was always a disease of debility. In some cases the mere diet and general comfort of the asylum is sufficient first for relief, and ultimately for cure. For the insane pauper the diet should be more liberal and nutritious than is usually found in his cottage, and for the wealthier patient simpler and plainer than that usual at his own table. Conolly allowed his patients half a pint of beer at dinner-time, and for the men who worked in the gardens as well as for the women who worked in the laundry there was half a pint of beer twice a day. Occasionally a tea-party took place following a bazaar. We have an account from the *Illustrated London News* of 1843 of such an occasion, and at the same time a vivid description of the hospital and its environs.

FANCY FAIR AT HANWELL LUNATIC ASYLUM

A bazaar, or sale of fancy work manufactured by patients of the Hanwell Asylum, was held on Wednesday, within one of the wards of the hospital. Its projectors had a twofold object in view. The first was to afford the public an opportunity of seeing the asylum, and to impress upon them the works exhibited, and the general arrangements of the place, how greatly the condition of the insane may be ameliorated, and their faculties rendered useful by kind care and judicious treatment. The second intention of the meeting was to obtain the aid of the visitors to the admirable charity for the relief of convalescent patients known as the "Queen Adelaide Fund". Unfortunately, the day turned out very wet, and the fete was shorn of many of its attractions. Notwithstanding, however, this circumstance, several hundred persons visited the asylum during the day. For a short period the sun shed its enlivening rays upon the asylum, and a number of elegantly-dressed ladies were seen promenading the grounds in various directions. The band of the 13th Light Dragoons was stationed on the lawn immediately facing the front entrance to the asylum, and during the day performed may select pieces of music. The wards of the institution, in which, owing to the wet weather, the bazaar was held, were festooned with wreaths with laurels intermingled with lilacs. With one or two exceptions, no patients were permitted to be seen in the wards. A number of male and female lunatics were, however, perambulating the most unfrequented parts of the ground under the surveillance of keepers. The bazaar during the greater portion of the day was crowded with visitors. The articles exhibited for sale were bona fide production of the patients, and appeared to give great satisfaction to the company. Mr. Sergeant Adams, the chairman of the visiting justices, and Mr. Pownall, were extremely kind and attentive to the visitors, pointing out to them every-thing that was worthy of observation. In the evening, after the stalls had been cleared, about two hundred of the female patients were regaled with tea and cake in the ornamented wards, and passed an apparently pleasant hour in singing and other recreations. It was anticipated that her Majesty the Queen Dowager, who is the patroness of the Adelaide Fund, would have paid the asylum a visit; but we learn that, being unable to do so, her Majesty, with that kind feeling which she is ever actuated, forwarded a sum of £20 to the venerable widow of the founder of the fund, Mrs. Clitherow, of Boston House, New Brentford, by whom it was expended at the sales.

Judging this to be a fit occasion to introduce our readers to the internal economy of this establishment, we inspected the whole a few days previous to the above fete, as well as on that Occasion; and we trust the result of our visit will be acceptable. For facility of access, and some interesting facts, we are indebted to the courtesy of Dr. Davy, one of the medical officers of the institution.

The asylum and its appurtenances occupy upwards of 53 acres, on the upper side of the picturesque valley of Brent, immediately to the left of the Uxbridge-road, and within a short distance of the stupendous Wharncliffe viaduct and Hanwell station of the Great Western Railway. The entrance to the asylum premises is beneath a lofty archway, of bold design, flanked by a lodge, counting-house, &c. We proceeded through the shrubberies, nearly four acres in extent; to the left lies the large western, or female airing ground, with a summer-house; and to the right the large eastern, or male airing ground, with a bowling green. In the former several patients were enjoying recreation and exercise; we learned that this salutary freedom is seldom abused, for it rarely happens that a plant or shrub is wilfully injured. This ground has lately been given up to the patients, and the levelling and laying out of the two divisions occupied many of the male patients for a considerable period; and the cheerful aspect of the front of the asylum has been very much increased by this alteration.

Our engraving, or bird's-eye view, conveys an accurate idea of the form and arrangement of nearly the entire buildings. They occupy three

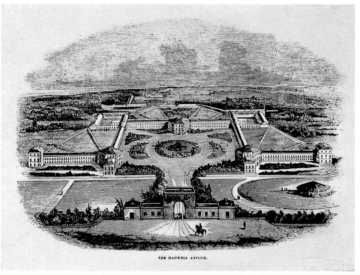

FIG. 11.   The Hanwell Asylum 1848.

sides of a large space, nearly a quadrangle; and they have lately been enlarged by the addition of wings. The structure is of brick, and simple in plan; the only attempt at ornament being in three octagonal towers; the central tower is occupied by Dr. Conolly, the resident physician, and by the matron. It may be sufficient to state that the western wing is occupied by female, and the eastern wing by male patients, classified in wards, according to the extent of their affliction. In the centre tower ward is the bazaar-room, wherein articles of fancy work, made by the better class of female patients, are exposed for sale; the produce being expended in the purchase of small articles, contributing to the comfort of the female patients, but which are not strictly within the expences payable out of the county rate. In this wing, also, is the chapel, wherein morning and evening prayers are daily read; and on Sundays Divine service is performed, the

congregation usually amounting to upwards of 300 patients. The organ
was purchased out of the procceeds of the sale of fancy work made by the
patients; and on Thursday evenings a performance of sacred music takes
place in the chapel, at which from 100 to 300 patients are present. In both
wings we were much struck with the system of prevention carried out by
means too numerous to detail; among them are the large mattresses and
padded rooms used for epileptic patients who fall out of bed; these rooms
are also used for the temporary seclusion of patients while labouring under
maniacal paroxysms. We saw several of the female patients employed in
the wash-house, drying-room, laundry, and store-room, with sane superintendents and assistants; and it was extremely difficult to distinguish the
former from the latter: amongst all reigned the utmost order and quiet.
It was a bright sunny morning, and a few male patients were in the wards:
They were amusing themselves after their own taste—some with newspapers and cheap periodical publications, others with draughts or cards,
and a party were playing at cribbage with high proficiency. Another might
be seen poring over minute calculations; and we were surprised to learn
that the figures of more than one patient were invariably correct, though
when he explained the import his statements were a strange jumble of fact
and fiction. On the walls of the department wherein we saw this calculator
hung two large kites, and these, with the bagatelle-board on the table, re-
minded us that the amusements of boyhood are encouraged by the humane
treatment evident, too, at every step throughout the establishment.

Meanwhile the system of employment is not forgotten; in the kitchen
and sculleries, all at work were patients, except the cook, two kitchen
maids, and a dairy maid; and these offices were models of cleanliness and
order, such as we rarely see equalled. The kitchen is lofty and large and
well appointed and some patients were making bread. In the courtyard
patients were also employed in the coir upholstery room, the stewards
store room, the brewhouse, and bakehouse; in two large rooms several
tailors and shoemakers were busily at work, and their methodical industry
was surprising, the only deviation being in one of the schneiders explaining
with archness and wrath the origin of the saying "nine tailors make a man",
much to the edification of one of the visiting party. In the stewards store
room are the dresses and other contrivances which have been introduced
into the asylum in lieu of mechanical restraint.

We likewise saw patients employed in the garden, the farm-yard,
carpenters and smith's shops. The coal-wharf has a basin communicating
with the Grand Junction Canal in the rear of the grounds—so that coal-
barges are unloaded on the premises. From the canal the establishment is
at present supplied with water at a heavy annual cost; but an Artesian well,
250 feet deep, has just been bored on the premises, at an expence of £8,000.

The arrangements of the airing courts will be best understood by reference to the engraving. One of these courts, on the male side has been principally planted, and is entirely kept in order by a patient, who is a gardener, and its appearance is superior to that of the rest.

Those who have had the most frequent opportunity of seeing the insane in the barren and dismal courts and yards usually allotted to them for exercise in asylums, a few years ago, can best appreciate the advantage of the present arrangement. The inducement offered by them to the listless and melancholic, to walk out of doors, is found to be in itself a valuable effect of these changes. To some of them, the large rocking-horses, so constructed that five persons can ride safely on each at one time, and one or two of which are supplied to each airing ward, offer the means of amusement, exercise, and, it may almost be said, of an alleviation of their malady; some of the patients evidently forgetting their troubles and irritations when taking this kind of exercise, and some being rocked thus to sleep. Under the large shades errected to screen them from the sun, some of the male patients are generally to be seen sitting, reading newspapers, or smoking and conversing. The female patients often take their needlework out, and thus enjoy the open air and the shade without being unoccupied.

Far is it from our wish to indulge any morbid curiosity as to the habits of the inmates of this asylum; but we could not refrain copying the following lines from the wall of one of the patients sleeping apartments:

> "Behold!
> No gloomy cell, where sullen madness pines,
> In chains and woe, where no glad sunlight shines;
> But here kind sympathy for fallen reason reigns,
> Our rule is gentleness, not force or galling chains."

These lines literally bespeak the excellent system pursued at the Hanwell Asylum. They were written by a patient of considerable intellectual attainments, but not the occupant of the sleeping-room; "he" is a pet lunatic, who attracted much attention at the fete on Wednesday; He was dressed in a mixed costume, crowned with a motley cap, bedizened with various-coloured ribands. This patient has been confined in the hospital for a period of twelve years. He is most loquacious and full of fun. He tells the story of his life with evident self-complacency. His name is William Rayner. For a number of years he was the harlequin, and his wife the columbine, at Covent-garden Theatre. He commenced his career in the character of Punch. After the death of his wife he, to use his own phraseology, "took to fretting", and was brought to Hanwell. His long residence within this establishment, and his constant association with lunatics, have not in the slightest degree affected the animal spirits. On

R

the faintest hint he is prepared to cut his capers o'er again, and to show
what he could do in early life to amuse the "quality" on the boards of
Covent-garden Theatre. "Supposing," said he, addressing himself to the
company who surrounded him, "this to be the green curtain; it rises. I
advance to the footlights and make a bow to the quality. I then go so
(cutting a most ludicrous caper), and then go so." (Attempting a most
insane pirouette), at the conclusion of which he bursts out into a most
immoderate fit of laughter making the ward ring again with its merry peal.

His chamber is, as *The Times* states, a perfect bijou; the walls are nearly
covered with coloured prints, and around, on shelves, are stuffed birds,
shells, and nicnacs, set out with extraordinary regularity, the disturbance
of which would greatly irritate the owner.

We had almost forgot to mention the burial-ground, on the south side
of the garden, wherein all patients not removed by their friends or parishes,
are buried; and here lies the individual who planned the asylum, and
eventually became one of its inmates.

The number of patients at present in the asylum is 566 females and
412 males; total 978.

Every aspect of asylum life was dealt with in Conolly's book, and
much of the contents could be reprinted today with no loss of
topicality. It is a surprisingly satisfying book, well written, free from
the turgidity of some of his other writings, and most of all, timeless in
its message. Many of the works which those who are interested in
medical history must read require a certain type of antiquarian mind, a
certain delight in the quaint, and a certain withdrawal from the
present—Conolly's book is one of those most unusual works of art which
are quite timeless. It is also, in its way, inspiring—no better illustration
of this can be given but than to reprint his concluding remarks.

I hope my concluding words will be believed, when I say, that if the
whole of the system which I have imperfectly endeavoured to sketch be
steadily persevered in, no anger—no severity—no revenge—no deception
—no disregard ever shown to the insane,—the resident superintendent will
no longer find himself living among the habitually furious, or the incurably
gloomy, or the constantly discontented. Calmness will come; hope will
revive; satisfaction will prevail. Some unmanageable tempers, some
violent or sullen patients, there must always be; but much of the violence,
much of the ill-humour, almost all the disposition to mediate mischievous
or fatal revenge, or self-destruction, will disappear. Some of the worst
habits that beset the poor lunatic will also be got the better of; cleanliness
and decency will be maintained or restored; and despair itself will sometimes be found to give place to cheerfulness or secure tranquillity. I could

PLATE I

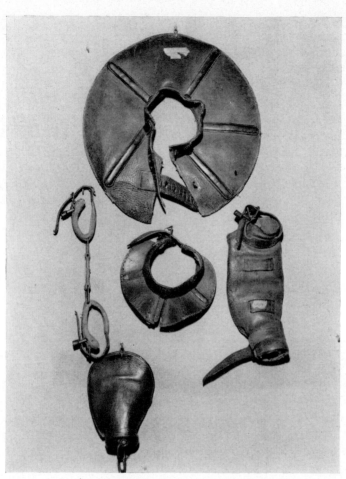

Leather instruments of restraint used at Hanwell.

walk through such an asylum as I have described, and point out illustrations
of every word in every ward.

Resolved, therefore, to make his asylum a place where everything is
regulated with one humane view, and where humanity, if anywhere on
earth, shall reign supreme, the resident medical director must be prepared
to make a sacrifice of some of the ordinary comforts and conventionalities
of life. His duties are peculiar, and apart from common occupations. His
society, even, must chiefly consist of his patients; his ambition must solely
rest on doing good to them; his happiness on promoting theirs.

None but those who live among the insane can fully know the pleasures
which arise from imparting trifling satisfactions to impaired minds; none
else can appreciate the reward of seeing reason returning to a mind long
deprived of it; none else can fully know the value of diffusing comfort,
and all the blessings of orderly life, among those who would either perish
without care, or each of whom would, if out of the asylum, be tormented
or a tormentor. Constant intercourse and constant kindness can alone
obtain their entire confidence; and this confidence is the very keystone of
all successful management.

"THE TREATMENT OF THE INSANE WITHOUT MECHANICAL RESTRAINTS"

His last major book was published nine years later (1856) and is a
review of his life work. *The Treatment of the Insane without Mechanical
Restraints* begins with a survey of the treatment of lunatics over the
centuries, always a favourite topic for Conolly. Particular tribute is
paid to Pinel and Esquirol. Conolly lists the various instruments of
restraint—the handcuffs, leg-locks, leather muffs, straps, waistcoats and
restraint chairs (Plate I), and the various treatments used—bleeding,
emesis, purgation, baths, and the more special physical treatments such
as whirling chairs, sudden immersion, the application of leeches to
the pubes and sacrum. Unfortunately these remedies are of limited
efficacy.

Young and sanguine practitioners usually feel dissatisfied with candid
statements of the possible inefficacy of medicines, resulting from experience; and probably no physician undertakes the charge of an asylum
without the pleasing belief that many of the cases considered incurable
will recover with the aid of energetic treatment. It is to be regretted that
this belief generally yields to repeated disappointments; that chronic
diseased conditions of the brain, reasonably presumed to exist, resist treatment adopted on what appear to be legitimate and reasonable grounds;

that some of the cases apparently not much removed from sanity never improve; and that others, which appeared the most unpromising, recover without our being able to explain the favourable termination. But there is still no reason to abandon the hope that fresh resources will some day be possessed by the practitioner; and that the real nature of the changes taking place in the brain may be better understood; and greater success attend medical treatment.

By far the greater number of agents which are found to be eventually remedial in insanity, are indirect in their operation, gradually influencing the mind itself. To all these the physician who wishes to maintain the non-restraint system must constantly and earnestly direct his attention.

THE NON-RESTRAINT SYSTEM

What in fact was this non-restraint system? It arose out of Conolly's interest in the experiences at Lincoln. Dr. Charlesworth, the physician to the Lincoln Asylum, had, over the course of sixteen or seventeen years before Gardiner Hill's publication in 1839, been preparing the way

for the non-restraint system by a vigilant attention to the effects of mechanical coercion, the instruments of which had been, by slow degrees, and in those long years, lessened in number at his representation, by the Lincoln Committee. A patient in that asylum had died in the year 1829, in consequence of being strapped to the bed in a strait-waistcoat during the night, and this accident had led to the establishment of an important rule, that whenever restraints were used in the night, an attendant should continue in the room; a rule which had also had the effect of much diminishing the supposed frequency of such restraint being necessary.

Various steps in the same direction had been recorded in the journals of the Lincoln asylum, and are especially alluded to in Mr. Hill's Appendix. Notice was required to be given of every instance of the application of restraints. Heavy iron hobbles and handcuffs (Plate II) were gathered and destroyed. Strait-waistcoats were torn up. Dresses of a material not easily torn were provided for patients who generally destroyed their clothes. Bedding, in similar difficulties, was protected by strong coverings or cases. At length, in August, 1834, it was reported that for many successive days not one patient had been in mechanical restraint of any kind. At that time Mr. Hadwen was the house-surgeon of the asylum. In 1835, Mr. Hadwen was succeeded by Mr. Gardiner Hill, who was soon able to say that not one patient had been in restraints, or confined to a room, in twenty-four days. In 1836, no instrument of restraint was used for three successive months;

PLATE II

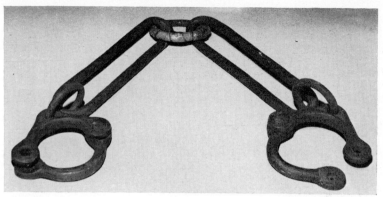

Leg locks (Hanwell).

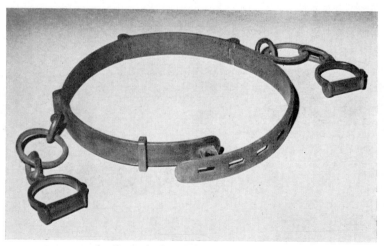

Handcuffs attached to abdominal belt (Hanwell).

and at last, in 1837, Mr. Hill expressed his confident opinion that mechanical restraints might be altogether abolished. And thus the non-restraint system became established at Lincoln.

Much interested by these details, I devoted the few weeks intervening between my appointment to Hanwell and the commencement of my residence there in visiting several public asylums; in all of which, except in that of Lincoln, various modes of mechanical coercion continued to be employed. My visit to the Lincoln Asylum (in May 1839), and conversations and correspondence with Dr. Charlesworth and Mr. Gardiner Hill, as well as frequent communications with the late Mr. Serjeant Adams, at that time a member of the Hanwell Committee, and who had been much interested by the proceedings at Lincoln, more strongly inclined me to believe that mechanical restraints might be safely and advantageously abolished in an asylum of any size; and I commenced my duties as resident physician and superintendent of the Middlesex lunatic asylum at Hanwell, on the first day of June. In various asylums, some attention had been drawn to the subject of Mr. Hill's lecture; but I had observed that his views were received unfavourably, and sometimes in a spirit of hostility, or even of ridicule; and I found them by no means favourably regarded by the medical or other officers at Hanwell. The agitation, however, of so novel a question as that of abolishing instruments of restraint which, from time immemorial, had constituted a part of the daily treatment of numerous cases of insanity, had led, at Hanwell at least, to a somewhat less extravagant employment of coercive instruments than had before been common. After the first of July, when I required a daily return to be made to me of the number of patients restrained, there were never more than 18 so treated in one day—a number which would seem reasonably small, out of 800 patients, but for the facts that after the thirty-first of July the number so confined never exceeded eight; and after the twelfth of August never exceeded one; and that after the twentieth of September no restraints were employed at all.

The principles of non-restraint had been put forward by a number of psychiatrists other than Charlesworth and Gardiner from Pinel onward. What Conolly did was to put them wholeheartedly into practice. Taking one giant stride forward, he abolished restraint throughout a large pauper lunatic hospital. Alexander Walk has pointed out that we must beware today in our interpretation of what was meant contemporarily by non-restraint—Conolly and his predecessors never left us in any doubt that a certain measure of *control* was necessary when dealing with lunatics. Seclusion, for instance, was frequently used and Conolly discussed this quite freely. "Many English superintendents speak of seclusion as something worse than mechanical restraint, seeming to forget that it is as much adapted to secure an irritable brain from causes of increased irritability as a quiet chamber, the seclusion of glare and of many visitors is adapted to the same state of brain in a fever." He speaks in favour, too, of a padded room. But he realised that a disturbed, ill-regulated environment is most productive of disturbed behaviour, and this is where Conolly's genius lay. Like the good general his strategic aim was carefully integrated with his tactics. At the outset of his experiment, the patients diet was improved, the ventilation of the wards was attended to, the number of baths increased, the staff of attendants considerably increased and better paid, and "order and regularity were everywhere enforced".

Quarrels were interrupted before words were followed by blows; and the mischievous habits of patients rendered almost harmless by constant superintendence and prompt attention. Diligent regard was paid to their clothing and bedding; and cleanliness was established and maintained to an extent which at one time it seemed nearly hopeless to expect. Those patients who were unable, or even unwilling, to be employed, were regularly taken out for daily exercise, and gloomy airing-courts were converted into gardens. Recreations and amusements were introduced for the benefit of the listless and apathetic, as well as for those the activity of whose minds required external means of relief. Considerable alterations were made in the religious services of the house; and it was required that the patients should attend the chapel neatly dressed. Prayer-books and hymn-books were furnished to them; psalmody was encouraged; and, by the appointment of a chaplain, two services were established on Sundays. Bibles, Testaments, and books of miscellaneous reading, were supplied to them under his direction and that of the physician, and the order of the chapel became much more rarely interrupted.

It was found very serviceable to institute various registers, which were required to be accurately kept; and also daily reports from each ward, by which means the state of each was made known at all times to the superintending physician, including the number of patients employed, or sick, or removed from ward to ward, or who had committed any injury or incurred any accident. No restraint and no seclusion of the patients was permitted without an immediate report being made of it. From that time the Hanwell Asylum has every year furnished statistical information of great value, in tables first constructed with the kind assistance of Dr. Farr, of the Registrar-General's office, and also of the late Mr. Serjeant Adams.

The whole-hearted support of the Committee of Management was a vital pre-requisite for the success of such a scheme. Conolly was lucky in having the right men at the right time, for both he and the Hanwell Committee were exposed to much criticism. But he has some hard things to say of Committee rule, and reverts to the theme time and time again that there must be one Director of an asylum—the Chief Physician. Even at Hanwell

> of all parts of Committee business, that which is productive of the most impatience is the medical part; and the medical suggestions are usually received with small respect. Such was too often the case, even at Hanwell, after the first enthusiasm for the new method of treatment had passed away; and propositions to increase the medical service of the house, and to make it more effective, by the aid of clinical pupils, which would have involved scarcely any expense, were rejected as not worth discussing.

He brings his book to a close on this same topic.

> To one subject I must still revert, which has long weighed upon my mind; namely, the imperfect government and organisation of all asylums for the insane in which the functions and duties of the medical officers are not regarded as of the first importance—asylums in which, if the patients are numerous, the medical officers are few in number, and without the direction of a Chief Physician. In such asylums the Committees supply, or ought to supply, the office of Superintendent or Governor. Committees vary so much in character, and are sometimes, even, so remarkably modified for a time by the predominating influence of some one individual, that what may be said with perfect truth and justice of a Committee in one year, may be inapplicable to it in the next.
>
> My personal interest in such matters has ceased. The wildest resolutions of committees can afflict me no more. But, knowing too well what rash experiments may be made by committees, and how dexterously all responsibility may be avoided, even when the comfort of a large asylum, and the discipline of the house, and the very health of the patients, are endangered by inconsiderate changes, I cannot avoid some allusion to such things, nor dismiss from my mind all anxiety about them, nor refrain from recording my opinion, founded on long observation, that the proper treatment, and the welfare, and happiness, of the insane is insecure under governing bodies constituted as those of asylums now generally are. Full security might, however, be given to the public, and every advantage to the insane surely preserved, if the control of asylums was always entrusted to intelligent superintending physicians, acting under the general inspection of a board of committee qualified for such superintendence by a liberal education, and by their habits of mind; who would entertain no

apprehension of evil from delegating such full authority to the physician as would leave him at liberty to carry out comprehensive plans, according to principles admitted and approved by them; and at the same time possessed of authority empowering him to enforce conformity to his measures among all the other officers.

MINOR WRITINGS

His first book was published only a year after he had qualified, and was prompted by his experience of an outbreak of small-pox whilst he was in practice at Chichester. Enthusiasm and strong convictions being the key to his character it is not surprising that this first book of his is *An Address to Parents on the Present State of Vaccination in this Country*: "with an Impartial Estimate of the Protection which it is Calculated to Afford Against the Small-Pox". He strongly urged parents to have their children (and themselves) vaccinated, Conolly being "perfectly sincere in his belief, that it is the only security against small-pox upon which the public ought to rely, and . . . with undiminished confidence". The discovery that this was Conolly's work we owe to Richard Hunter and Ida MacAlpine, for the book is anonymously published as by "A Candid Observer". Hunter and MacAlpine have also discovered a second book on the subject, this time published under his own name in 1824, *Observations on Vaccination and on the Practice of Inoculating for the Small-Pox* :"with an Appendix of Cases and Facts". By now he was practising in Stratford-upon-Avon, and was perhaps a little more sure of himself and in no need of anonymity. Both books have the same message—that "the discovery of vaccination is one of the most valuable acquisitions which the medical profession was ever instrumental in making for mankind, and that after more than twenty years trial of what vaccination can effect, it ought now and for ever to be cherished, as it was at first hailed, as a blessing to the whole human race".

We have already seen that whilst at Stratford, Conolly had written a popular book on cholera, and continued with his medical journalism. On his remove to London he still continued to write articles for the medical press and for the *Cyclopaedia of Practical Medicine*.

His *Four Lectures on the Study and Practice of Medicine* was published in 1832 shortly after he had resigned the Professorship of the Theory and Practice of Medicine at the London University; he dedicated them to John Forbes, his old friend of Chichester days. The book consists of four lectures delivered on 2 October 1828, 2 October 1829, 1 October 1830, and his valedictory lecture given on retiring from the University on Friday, 29 April 1831.

His first lecture followed that of Sir Charles Bell, the Professor of Surgery and Physiology, and it is written in a very turgid style. He first deals with generalities, but before long announces that "It is my intention to dwell somewhat more fully on Mental Disorders, or to speak more correctly, of disorders affecting the manifestations of mind, than has, I believe, been usual in lectures on the practice of medicine; and for many reasons". He goes on to say that he had hoped to be able to give the students opportunities to become familiar with these illnesses, and thus provide a "great impulse" to their study, "and that great general improvement will in a few years result in relation to our knowledge of these affections, to the advantage of the public, no less than to the honour of our medical school". A footnote here points out that "In this hope I was disappointed. Many circumstances conspired to render my representations to the Council of the University unavailing. The subject will I hope in time attract the attention of the medical teachers of London."

Conolly also dispenses some good advice to the students—first they should be diligent and industrious, secondly well educated—particularly in the classics—for

> Gentlemen, you cannot be familiar with the languages of Greece and Rome without at the same time becoming familiar with the characters of some of the greatest men who ever lived, and the most exalted sentiments which the human mind ever conceived: nor can you be intimately acquainted with the beauty and accuracy of expression which characterised the best Greek and Roman writers, without becoming at the same time accustomed to the most admirable order and precision of thought.

Likewise, knowledge of French and German, of how to write and speak one's own language, of Natural Philosophy, and of the Fine Arts is recommended—and where a better place to find all this than London, an "intellectual Capital, in which the student can never be driven, by the proscription of elegant and rational amusements, or the want of agreeable or virtuous society, to throw away his early life in low debauchery or vice". And lastly, religion on the seventh day, with contemplation, reading, and the conversation of wise and good associates is Conolly's prescription for peace of mind. The contents of the three remaining lectures are much the same, exhortations to the students to be gentlemen, and high flown sentiments about medicine, interspersed with some remarks on anatomy, physiology or pathology. The final lecture is his valedictory address, in which he laments the fact that after only four years he felt the need to resign his appointment, although it is not clear from what he writes as to the reasons for his decision. But if the content of these four lectures is any guide to Conolly as a teacher of clinical medicine, it is not hard to see why, in fact, he had not proved a success. As Maudsley pointed out, they are vague and discursive, as full of sentiment as they are empty of fact, and must have provided a marked contrast to the excellent lectures of the Professor of Surgery, Sir Charles Bell.

Conolly delivered the Croonian Lectures in 1848 and 1849, publishing them in an expanded form a little later, the substance of three lectures having been amplified into six. This prolixity is characteristic of Conolly's writing, and is perhaps a feature associated with any popularizer of a particular viewpoint. The lectures comprise accounts of mania and melancholy and a longer account of general paralysis, very completely described. They end with a plea for more understanding on the part of lawyers of the role of psychological factors in crime, and for a liberalization of the law in regard to responsibility and mental illness. They are undistinguished, and somewhat in line with his journalistic writings which appeared in the *Cyclopedia of Practical Medicine*, in the *Lancet*, and in other journals.

In 1863 Conolly published his last book, *A Study of Hamlet*. As we have already seen, Conolly was a fervent admirer of Shakespeare, and here he maintains that Hamlet's behaviour is that of a man who is mentally sick, and that this is a masterly delineation of madness by the great poet. The question of whether Shakespeare intended simply to portray the simulation of madness or intended to draw a true picture of a really disordered mind is one over which a great deal of controversy has raged. Hamlet himself said, "As I perchance hereafter may think meet to put an antic disposition on," and later, "I am but mad north-north-west; when the wind is southerly I know a hawk from a hand-saw." To Conolly these expressions and Hamlet's positive denial of madness constitute all the evidence giving direct support to the conclusion that Hamlet's eccentricities were merely feigned. Throughout his book quotation follows quotation to show that, in point of fact, Hamlet was mentally disordered. The constant doubts and ruminations, the melancholy that seizes him, the tendency to fantasy, the impulsive actions all betoken mental illness. Unfortunately there is little else in what is a very pedestrian account of the play, and Conolly shows no understanding of the psychopathological problems which the play so profoundly illustrates. No attempt is made even to come to a diagnosis, and Conolly rests content with showing that Hamlet was suffering from mental illness.

CONOLLY'S ACHIEVEMENT

A man's achievements, unless he be a genius, can usually best be understood in the light of his personal development and the social milieu in which he exists. Left fatherless at an early age, an "inconvenient superfluity in the family, for whom nobody cared, except my affectionate mother", sent to boarding school at the age of 6, brought up in shabby, antiquated and neglected surroundings until the age of 16, Conolly was always to remember that "the same kind of objects and circumstances have, in all subsequent years, always produced the same uncomfortable feelings". Loathing school, and finding little joy in learning, Conolly passed this "barren portion" of his existence, one-tenth of the allotted span, longing for warmth and tenderness. The world of French literature and thought opened up by his mother's re-marriage to an émigré Frenchman, and his idyllic honeymoon in France provided a sharp contrast to the drab world of a lonely schoolboy in an English village. What could be more natural than that those lonely and neglected individuals, the pauper lunatics, should be the object of his sympathy, and the subject of his life work? The time, too, was ripe. The Industrial Revolution, Chartism, and the great upsurge of humanitarianism amongst feeling men such as Brougham, Cobbett and Lord Shaftesbury provided the background upon which Conolly's emotion could so perfectly find an outlet. Conolly, unlike Prichard and Haslam, was all feeling, and the very intensity of that feeling enabled him to accomplish the total abolition of restraint, and thereby to assure himself a lasting place in the history of psychiatry. Of all his writings only two—*The Treatment of the Insane without Mechanical Restraints*, and *The Construction and Government of Lunatic Asylums and Hospitals for the Insane* are of enduring value; they place him in the forefront of what was to become a new profession—medical administration.

Although much criticized at the present time, the physician super-intendent has contributed greatly to the development of psychiatry, and seen in historical perspective, his role is still one which should not be lightly cast aside. Conolly bitterly lamented Committee control and divided councils and his admonitions must be taken none the less seriously because they were written a century ago. We can do no better than to end by quoting from his last medical work, *The Treatment of the Insane*, when he dwells on his poor "crazy children".

> No longer residing in the Hanwell Asylum, and no longer superintending it, or even visiting it, I continue to live within view of the building, and its familiar trees and grounds. The sound of the bell that announces the hour of the patients' dinner still gives me pleasure, because I know that it summons the poorest creature there to a comfortable, well-prepared, and sufficient meal; and the tone of the chapel bell, coming across the narrow valley of the Brent, still reminds me, morning and evening, of the well remembered and mingled congregation of the afflicted, and who are then assembling, humble, yet hopeful and not forgotten, and not spiritually deserted.

Gentleness and kindness were what Conolly had to give. He bequeathed to us the memory of a good and gentle man, inspired by what are perhaps the most fundamental gifts the doctor can offer to his patients.

BIBLIOGRAPHY

ANON (1866). The late John Conolly, M.D., D.C.L. Obituary Notice, *Brit. Med. J.*, March 17, p. 288.

ANON (1866). Obituary Notice, *Lancet*, March 17, p. 303.

CLARK, Sir J. (1869). *A Memoir of John Conolly, M.D., D.C.L.* Pp. xii+298. London: John Murray.

CONOLLY, J. (1821). *Dissertatio Inauguralis de Statu Mentis in Insania et Melancholia.* Edinburgh. Published in the *Edinburgh Medical and Surgical Journal* (1821), **17**, 635.

CONOLLY, J. (1822). *An address to parents on the present state of vaccination in this country: with an impartial estimate of the protection which it is calculated to afford against the small-pox.* By A Candid Observer. London: Longman, Hurst, Rees, Orme and Brown.

CONOLLY, J. (1824). *Observations on Vaccination and on the Practice of Inoculation for the Small-Pox: with an appendix of cases and facts.* Stratford-upon-Avon: R. Lapworth.

CONOLLY, J. (1828). *An Introductory Lecture* delivered in the University of London on Thursday, October 2nd 1828 by John Conolly, M.D., Professor of the Nature and Treatment of Diseases, p. 34. London: Printed for John Taylor.

CONOLLY, J. (1830). *An Inquiry concerning the Indications of Insanity.* Pp. vi + 496. London: John Taylor.

CONOLLY, J. (1832). *Four Lectures on the Study and Practice of Medicine.* Pp. viii + 177. London: Sherwood, Gilbert & Piper.

CONOLLY, J. (1842). *The Reports of the Visiting Justices of the County Lunatic Asylum, at Hanwell, to the Epiphany Sessions* 1839. London: M'Gowan & Co.

CONOLLY, J. (1842). *The Reports of the Resident Physicians of the County Lunatic Asylum, at Hanwell, to the Epiphany Sessions* 1839. London: M'Gowan & Co.

CONOLLY, J. (1845). *On the Principal Forms of Insanity.*
Lecture I.
Importance of the study of insanity; plan of clinical study at Hanwell; sound and unsound mind. *Lancet,* **ii**, p. 357.
Lecture II.
Forms of insanity; acute mania, p. 414; its treatment, p. 417.
Lecture III.
Treatment of acute mania contd; the non-restraint system, p. 467.
Lecture IV.
Cases of acute mania, with their treatment, p. 525.
Lecture V.
Treatment of acute mania contd; consideration of its causes, p. 581.
Lecture VI.
Treatment of acute mania—concluded, p. 639.

CONOLLY, J. (1847). *On the Construction and Government of Lunatic Asylums and Hospitals for the Insane.* Pp. viii + 183. London: Churchill.

CONOLLY, J. (1848). *A Letter to Benjamin Rotch, Esq., on the Plan and Government of the Additional Lunatic Asylum for Middlesex.* Pamphlet.

CONOLLY, J. (1856). *The Treatment of the Insane without Mechanical Restraints.* Pp. xii + 380. London: Smith, Elder & Co.

CONOLLY, J. (1862). Recollections in the Varieties of Insanity. Part II. Cases and Consultations. *Medical Times & Gazette,* Vol. I, pp. 27, 130, 234, 372.

CONOLLY, J. (1862). Recollections in the varieties of insanity. *Medical Times & Gazette,* Vol. II, p. 2.

CONOLLY, J. (1863). *A Study of Hamlet.* Pp. 209. London: Edward Moxon & Co.

CONOLLY, J. (n.d.). The Croonian Lectures delivered at the Royal College of Physicians, London in 1849. *On Some of the Forms of Insanity.* Pp. vi + 102. London: Savill & Edwards.

CROWTHER, Caleb (1838). *Observations on the Management of Madhouses*. Pp. 145. London: Simpkin, Marshall & Co.

CROWTHER, Caleb (1841). *Observations on the Management of Madhouses*. Part the Second. Pp. 104. London: Simpkin, Marshall & Co.

CROWTHER, Caleb (1849). *Observations on the Management of Madhouses*. Part the Third. Pp. 126. London: Simpkin, Marshall & Co.

HILL, Robert Gardiner (1839). *A Lecture on the Management of Lunatic Asylums* Pp. ix+112+36 pages of Tables. London: Simpkin, Marshall & Co.

HUNTER, R. A. and MACALPINE, I. (1959). An Anonymous Publication on Vaccination by John Conolly (1794-1866). *J. Hist. Med.*, **14**, 311-319.

HUNTER, R. A. and GREENBERG, H. P. (1956). Sir William Gull & Psychiatry. *Guy's Hospital Reports*, 105, No. 4, pp. 361-375.

KNIGHT, Paul Slade (1827). *Observations on the Causes, Symptoms and Treatment of Derangement of the Mind, founded on an extensive moral and medical practice in the treatment of lunatics. Together with the particulars of the sensations and ideas of a gentleman during his mental alienation, written by himself during his convalescence.* Pp. viii+167. London: printed for Longman, Rees, Orme, Brown, & Green.

MAUDSLEY, Henry (1866). Memoir of the late John Conolly, M.D. *J. Ment. Sci.*, **12**, 58, 151.

MILLINGEN, J. G. (1840). *Aphorisms on the Treatment and Management of the Insane.* Pp. xii. 202. London: John Churchill.

WALK, A. (1954). Some Aspects of the "Moral Treatment" of the Insane up to 1854. *J. Ment. Sci.*, **100**, p. 807.

SUBJECT INDEX

Acts of Parliament, 17 Geo. II, c. 5
  1744, 9, 47
  Gordon-Ashley Act of 1828, 158
  of 1845, 158, 245, 246
  Insane Offenders Act, 125
  Mental Deficiency Act, 1913, 186
  Mental Deficiency Act, 1927, 186
Adams, Mr. Sergeant, 254, 261, 262
Addison, Joseph, 228
Adelaide Fund, 224, 253, 254
Adelung, J. C., 189, 202
Albinus, 33
Apothecaries, 4, 5, 14
Aretaeus, 59
Arnold, Dr. Thomas, 38, 39, 44, 56-
  62, 94, 121.
Association, British Medical, 186,
  216-220, 225
  Medico-Psychological, 225
  Provincial, Medical and Surgical,
  186
  National Association for Promo-
  tion of Social Sciences, 225
Asylums, administration of, 210
  committee system in, 262, 263, 264,
  268
  county, 245
  discipline in, 246, 248
  epidemics in, 247
  optimum size of, 247, 248
  Criminal lunatic, Broadmoor, 125
  Derbyshire, 223
  Earlswood Idiot, 225
  Edinburgh lunatic, 102
  Glasgow, 216, 246
  Gloucester, 183
  Hanwell Lunatic, 220-227, 245,
  247, 248, 254-258, 261, 262, 263,
  268
  Lincoln Lunatic, 241, 260
  Swifts (St. Patrick's, Dublin), 7
  Wakefield, 253
  York Lunatic, 82, 107

Auckland, 226, 227
Australia, 142-144, 200

Bacon, Sir Francis, 228
Bath, 40, 43, 77
Battie, Dr. William, 9, 11, 48, 50, 51
  et seq., 56, 94, 144, 181
Bayle, Dr. A. L. J., 138, 139
Beck, T. R., 130
Beddoes, Thomas, 101, 115
Bell, Sir Charles, 265
Benzoni, Gav., 227
Berkeley, G., xii
Bethlem (see Hospitals)
Birmingham, 220, 221
Black, Dr. Joseph, 36
Black, Dr. William, 103
Blackmore, Sir Richard, 28, 29, 30
Blackstone, Commentaries, 125
Bleeding, 153, 154
Boerhaave, Professor H., 33, 38, 54, 59
Bolingbroke, Lord, 228
Boswell, James, 58
Boyle, Robert, 75
Brain, appearance of in insanity, 116,
  137, 138, 161, 162
Bridewell, 55
Bristol, 148, 150, 155, 158, 186, 221
Bristol College, 148, 155
Bristol Literary and Philosophical
  Society, 148, 155
British Medical Association, 186, 216,
  220, 225
Broadmoor, 125
Brodie, Sir Benjamin, 116
Brougham, Lord, 217, 220, 267
Brown, Richard, 78
Buchan, Dr. A. P., 114, 116, 140
Bunsen, The Chevalier, 192, 193
Burrows, Dr. George Man, 133, 142,
  161, 179, 181

Calmeil, Dr. L. F., 136, 138, 139

Cambridge Militia, 215
Catlin, George, 198
Celsus, 15, 122
Champollion, 189, 191
Chapters in the History of the Insane in the British Isles, ix, 95, 96, 111, 145, 157, 161, 186, 188
Charlesworth, Dr. E. P., 241, 245, 253, 260, 261
Chartism, 267
Cheselden, Dr. William, 5, 29, 33
Cheyne, Dr. George, 22, 23
Chichester, 216, 264, 265
Cholera, 219, 247
Cicero, 215, 228
Clark, Sir James, 210, 228, 230, 233
Cobbett, William, 267
Collins, Sir John, 216
Commissioners in Lunacy, 158
Condillac, 215
Conolly, John, x, 83, 94, 135, 139, 145, 161, 167, Birth and early life, 211—school, 212-215—step-father, 215—service in militia, 215-216—marriage, 216—medical studies at Edinburgh, 216—President of Royal Medical Society, Edinburgh, 216—thesis, 216—start in practice at Stratford-on-Avon, 216-217—Mayor of Stratford, 217—Professor of Practice of Medicine, London University, 217, 218—Medical Journalism, 220—Appointed Resident Physician, Hanwell, 220—Teaching of medical students, 224, 238, 236-9—ill health, 225, 230—friends and family, 226-227—honours, character, death, 227-230—Conolly on medical superintendents, 248, 249—on matrons 249—Annual Reports, 253—Croonian Lectures, 266—interest in Shakespeare, 217, 266
Conolly, Dr. William, 216
Convict ships, 142, 143, 144
Coopers Tracts, 130

Cox, Dr. J. M., 181, 230
Crichton, Sir Alexander, 44, 45, 46, 47, 161
Croonian Lectures, 266
Crowther, Dr. Bryan, 102, 104, 106, 112, 113
Croyland Abbey, xi
Cullen, William, 33, 36, 37, 38, 39, 56, 57, 59, 64, 97, 99, 122
Cupping, 66, 78, 153

Darwin, Dr. Erasmus, 79, 80, 181, 230
Defoe, Daniel, 6, 9, 47
Descartes, R., 31
Diet in mental disorders, 20, 22, 23, 31, 53, 74, 77, 232-233, 253
Duncan, Dr. Andrew, 99, 102, 103
Dunston, Thomas, 11

Education, female, 233
  classical, 215, 265
Egyptology, 189, 190
Egyptian chronology, 189, 190
Electrical machine, 79
Electricity, 78, 79
Ellis, Sir William, 222, 223, 253
Epilepsy, 20, 68, 128, 166
Erskine, Lord, 125, 181
Esquirol, Dr. J. E. D., 138, 139, 161, 168, 170, 177, 178, 184, 188, 259
Ethnology, 194
Ethnological Society, 157, 225
Exercise, in insanity, 250, 254, 255
Exorcists, Order of, xi

Facial angle, 194
Falconer, Dr. William, 40, 41, 42, 43
Falret, Dr. J. P., 161, 179
Ferriar, Dr. John, 144
Ferrus, Dr. Guillaume, 161
Fitzherbert's Pleas of the Crown, 124
Floyer, Sir John, 76
Forbes, Sir John, 216, 217, 220, 265
Fordyce, Dr. George, 97, 98
Forensic psychiatry, 116, 124-131, 164, 181-185, 225, 266
Fothergill, Dr. John, 43

Fowler, Dr. Thomas, 82, 121
Fox, Charles James, 8, 9
Franklin, Benjamin, 27, 39, 78
Frederick II, 184, 232
Friedreich, 161
Friends, Society of, 82, 148, 180
Fuller, Dr. Francis, 76
Funeral ceremonies, 199

Gainsborough, Thomas, 73
Galen, 3, 15, 59
Gall, Dr. F. J., 162, 235
General Paralysis of the Insane, 96, 100, 101, 136-139, 266
Gentleman's Magazine, 9, 47
George III, madness of, 68, 69, 70, 71, 72, 73, 74, 106, 125, 150
Georget, Dr. J. E., 139, 161, 177
Gilbert, Dr. William, xii
Gillray, Thomas, 8
Governors of Bethlem, 7, 110, 111, 112, 113, 132, 133
Gozna, Dr. John, 103
Greatrakes, Valentine, xi
Griesinger, Dr. Wilhelm, 161
Gull, Sir William, 224
Guthlac, Saint, xi

Hale, Lord, 124
Hale, Dr. Richard, 48
Hall, Dr. John, 11
Hallaran, Dr. W. S., 181, 230
Hanwell Lunatic Asylum, 220-227, 245, 247, 248, 254-258, 261-263, 268
Hare, Dr. E. H., 139
Harper, Dr. Andrew, 68, 121
Hartley, David, 59
Harveian Orators
    Richard Hale (1735), 48
    James Monro (1737), 48
    William Battie (1746), 52
    John Monro (1757), 50
    David Pitcairn (1786), 99
    Thomas Monro (1799), 73
Harvey, William, 15
Haslam, John, 6, 83, 94, 148, 181,
    s

Birth, 97—student days, 97, 98—President of Royal Medical Society, Edinburgh, 100—first writings, 100, 101—misunderstanding with manager of Royal Infirmary, Edinburgh, 101, 102—Apothecary to Bethlem 1795, 103—his duties, 104-106—evidence to Committee appointed by the House of Commons 1815, 104, 105, 106,—salary, 105—Haslam and James Tilly Matthews, 107, 108—James Norris, 107—dismissal, 113, 114—his library, 115—M.D., 114, 116—licentiate of Royal College of Physicians, 114—his friends, 141, 142—Haslam and forensic psychiatry, 124-131—Haslam and G.P.I., 96, 100, 101, 136, 137, 138, 139—President of Medical Society of London, 142—Portrait, 142—family, 142—death, 134, 143
Haslam, Dr. John Jnr., 142, 143, 144
Hastings, Sir Charles, 220, 222, 227
Hatfield, James, 125, 126
Hawkins, Sir John, 3
Haydn, 232
Henderson, Sir David, 187
Hieroglyphics, 189, 190
Hill, Dr. Robert Gardiner, 145, 240, 241, 244, 245, 260, 261
Hippocrates, 3, 15, 59
Hodgkin, Dr. Thomas, 148, 157, 158, 202
Hoffmann, Frederick, 33, 38, 56
Hogarth, William, 8
Hodd, Sir W. C., 135
Hooke, Robert, 5
Horse riding, 18, 25, 26, 76
Hospitals
    Auckland Mental Hospital, x
    Bath General Hospital, 43
    Bethlem, Moorfields 1676, 1, 3, 4, 5, 6, 11, 47, 48, 66, 80, 103, 104, 167
    St. George's Fields 1815, 104, 110

Hospitals—*contd.*
  Bicêtre, the, 73, 144, 161, 167
  Bristol Infirmary, 5, 152, 157, 162
  Chester Infirmary, 43
  Edinburgh Asylum for the Insane,
    Morningside, 102
  Edinburgh Royal Infirmary, 102
  Glasgow Medical School, 36
  Guys Hospital, 3
  London, the, 5
  Manchester Lunatic, 11, 12, 13, 14,
    48
  Maison Royale de Charenton, 167,
    178
  Maudsley, x, 135
  Middlesex, the, 5, 78
  National, the, London, 34
  Nottingham, the General Hospital,
    78, 79
  Retreat, the, York, 11, 82, 180, 241
  St. Bartholomew's, 3, 5, 62, 78, 97, 99
  St. George's, 5
  St. Luke's, 9, 10, 11, 48, 51, 52, 72,
    82, 141, 167
  St. Luke's House, Newcastle-on-
    Tyne, 1764, 11, 48
  St. Peter's, Bristol, 152
  St. Thomas's, 3, 5, 78, 150
  Salpêtrière, the, 167, 177, 178, 231
  Westminster, the, 5
House of Commons, Select Com-
    mittee, 14, 104, 109, 110, 111,
    119, 127
Howard, John, 106
Hume, David, xii
Hunter, Dr. John, 5, 140, 195
Hunter, Dr. William, 5, 36, 97
Hypochondria, 15, 16, 24, 28, 39, 202
Hysteria, 15, 16, 17, 18, 21, 25, 28, 29,
    30, 35, 39

Illustrated London News, 250-258
Impulse, irresistible, 184, 185
Insanity
  classification of, 37, 38, 44-46, 57-61
    moral, 163, 169, 170-178, 181-
    184, 186

prevention of, 61
statistics of, 10, 14, 118, 178, 179
transmission of, 233
treatment of, xi, xii, 1
  alcohol in, 27, 31, 74
  bleeding, 2, 18, 21, 54, 66, 78, 79,
    80, 106, 122, 128, 152, 162, 180
  cold bathing, 76, 67, 122
  diet, 20, 22, 23, 31, 53, 74, 77,
    233, 253
  emetis in, 2, 18, 21, 24, 54, 66,
    106
  electricity, 78, 79
  horse riding, 18, 25, 26, 76
  "insolation", 54
  music, 74, 77, 78
  purging, 2, 18, 21, 31, 54, 66,
    106, 152, 153, 166, 230
  spa, 21, 24, 36, 39, 77
  swinging, 25, 26
  work, 70, 252, 253, 255, 256

Jacobi, Dr. Maximilian, 180, 241
James I, xii
Jenner, Dr. Edward, 202, 203
Jerdan, William, 139, 142
Johnson, Dr. Samuel, 4, 5, 7, 8, 28, 77
Jones, Dr. Robert, 73, 74
Jordan, Thomas, 5

Kitchiner, Dr. William, 142
Knight, Dr. Paul Slade, 241-244
Kraepelin, Professor Emil, 187

Lamb, Charles, 126
Lancet, the, 96, 245
Lawrence, William, 106, 135, 157
Lee, Nathaniel, 8
Lewes, 216
Lincoln, 70, 244, 245, 253
Linnaeus, 197
Literary Gazette, 142
Locke, John, 59, 181
London House, Hackney, 109
London Medical Journal, 73
Lucid interval, 125, 129
Lunatic, criminal, 125

McNaghten Rules, 130, 188
Male, George Edward, 129
Mandeville, Bernard de, 23, 24, 25, 26, 27, 28
Mania sanguinis, 186
Manic, depressive insanity, 38, 46, 116, 118, 119, 128, 144
Manie sans délire, 163, 169, 171, 188
Matthews, John Tilley, 106, 107, 108, 109, 110, 111, 112, 132, 133
Matron, duties of, 249
Maudsley, Henry, 186, 187, 210, 216, 218, 220, 226, 228-230, 266
Mead, Dr. Richard, 3
Medical students and psychiatry, 51, 52, 224, 236-239
Medical superintendents, 248, 249
Melancholia Anglica, 58
Methodism and Mental illness, 64, 65, 66, 179
Millingen, Dr. J. G. V., 220, 221
Milton, John, 228
Monomania, 184, 185
Monro, Dr. Alexander, 48
Monro, Dr. Edward Thomas, 113
Monro, Dr. James, 48, 49
Monro, Dr. John, 7, 8, 48, 49, 50, 54, 55, 66
Monro, Dr. Thomas, 51, 69, 73, 104, 105, 106
Moral insanity, 163, 169, 170, 171, 172, 173, 174, 175, 176, 177, 178, 181, 182, 183, 184, 186
Moral management, 119, 122, 123, 124, 144
Moral treatment, xii
Morison, Sir Alexander, 133, 140, 141, 142, 161
Morison Lectures, Edinburgh, 141
Music therapy, 74, 78

Non-restraint, 12, 133, 134, 145, 224
Norris, James, 107, 108, 111, 112
Nursing, 2, 124, 249

Obsessional neurosis, 96
O'Donoghue, the Rev. E. C., 6, 136

Pargeter, the Rev. William, 62, 63, 64, 65, 66, 67
Paris, J. A. and Fonblanques, J. S. M., 130
Parliament
  Act of 1744, 9, 47
  Act of 1808, 125
  Act of 1828, 158
  Act of 1845, 158
  Act of 1913, 186
  Act of 1927, 186
Paulus Aeginatus, 122
Pepys, Sir Lucas, 71
Perfect, Dr. William, 62, 63, 181
Philology, 160, 193, 206
Phrenology, 233, 235, 236, 237
Physicians, education of, 3, 4
Physicans, Royal College of, Edinburgh, 34, 141
  Royal College of, London, x, 19, 47, 48, 50, 51, 55, 56, 99, 114, 155
Physiognomy, 233, 234
Pick, Arnold, 96
Pinel, Philippe, 94, 119, 120, 121, 144, 148, 161, 163, 166, 167, 169, 170, 171, 180, 181, 185, 188, 216, 230, 259
Pitcairn, Dr. David, 97, 99
Pitt, William, 9
Pole, Dr. Thomas, 150
Pope, Alexander, 7
Porpess, Anatomy of, 2
Prevention of insanity, 61
Prichard, Dr. Augustin, 152
Prichard, James Cowles, 94, 139, 145, 230, Birth and family, 148—portrait, 149—familiarity with French and other languages, 149, 150—apprenticed, studies at St. Thomas's Hospital, 150—M.D. Edinburgh, 151, 194—Trinity College Cambridge, 152—starts in practice, 152—Elected physician to Bristol Infirmary, 152—Controversy with Dr. David Davies, 155—religious doubts, 152—friends, 157—honours,

Prichard, James Cowles—*contd.*
    M.D. Oxford, F.R.S. etc, 157,
    158—leaves Bristol for London,
    158—Final illness and death, 158
    —his character, 158, 159, 160—
    religion and ethnology, 195, 199
    —religion and insanity, 179—the
    law and insanity, 130—his library,
    202—minor works, 201, 202
Provincial Medical and Surgical
    Association, 157
Pugin, 11
Purcell, Dr. John, 19, 20, 21, 40
Pygmie, Anatomy of, 2

Quakers, 106, 150, 157, 179, 188

Radcliffe, Dr. John, 3
Rake's Progress, 8
Rakewell, Thomas, 8
Religion, a cause of insanity, 58, 64,
    65, 66, 119, 178, 179
Restraint, 106-108, 110, 134, 139
    abolition of, 222, 238, 239, 241, 259
    instruments of, 241, 242, 243, 244,
    245, 259, 260-263
Revolution, French, 82
Richardson, Samuel, 7
Robinson, Dr. Nicholas, 30, 31, 77
Rose, George, 107
Rosetta Stone, 189, 190
Rowlandson, Thomas, 8
Rowley, Dr. William, 39, 40
Russell, Lord John, 220

Saussure, Raymond de, 185
Sauvages, F. B. de, 44, 58, 161
Schizophrenia, 117, 118
Schomberg, Dr. Isaac, 55
Scot, Reginald, xii
Seclusion, 256, 261, 262
Semelaigne, Dr. René, 188
Shaftesbury, VII Earl of, 133
Shakespeare, William, 66, 217, 266
Simmons, Dr. Samuel Foart, 72, 73
Sketches in Bedlam, 134, 135, 136
Slavery, abolition of, 166

Sloane, Sir Hans, 3
Smart, Christopher, 8
Societies
    American Philosophical, 158
    Bristol Literary and Philosophical,
        148, 155, 201
    Ethnological, 225
    Ethnological Society of New York,
        158
    For the Diffusion of Useful Know-
        ledge, 217, 219, 220
    For Improving the Condition of
        the Insane, 133, 134, 142
    Medical Society of London, 43, 142
    Oriental Society of America, 158
    Phrenological, 236
    Royal Medical Society, Edinburgh,
        x, 56, 97, 99, 100, 103, 216
    Royal Medico-Psychological, ix,
        186
    Royal Society of Medicine, x
    Warwick and Leamington Phreno-
        logical Society, 236
Spa treatment, 21, 24, 36, 39, 77
Spallanzani, Lazaro, 100
Specialism, the rise of, 47-62
Spleen, 23, 25, 28, 29, 30, 31, 77
Spurzheim, Dr. J. C., 142, 161, 162
Stahl, George Ernst, 31, 32, 33, 34,
    54, 56
Sterne, Laurence, 232
Stow's *Survey of London*, 2
Stratford-on-Avon, 216, 217, 218,
    220, 264
Strype, John, 2
Stuart, Dugald, 216
Suicide, 40, 179
Sutherland, Dr. A. J., 133, 141
Swift, Dean, 7
Swinging, 25, 26, 230
Sydenham, Dr. Thomas, xii, 15, 16,
    17, 18, 19
Symonds, Dr. J. A., 157, 158, 159,
    160, 186

Therapeutic nihilism, 230
Tissot, S. A. D., 47

Tuke, Dr. Daniel Hack, ix, 95, 96, 111, 145, 157, 161, 186, 188
Tuke, Dr. Harington, 226
Tuke, Samuel, 216, 241
Tuke, William, 82, 83, 230
Tunbridge Wells, 21, 77
Turner, J. M. W., 73
Tweedie, Dr. Alexander, 157, 167, 220
Tyson, Dr. Edward, x, 1, 2, 6, 48

University College, London, 210, 217, 218, 224, 264, 265
University of Aberdeen, 62, 114
University of Cambridge, 97, 152
University of Edinburgh, 5, 43, 56, 97, 99, 141, 145, 150, 151
University of Leyden, 27, 33, 43
University of London, 264, 265
University of Oxford, 48, 49, 70, 152, 227
University of Rheims, 33
University of Uppsala, 97, 103
Uterus, in mental disorder, 16, 17

Vaccination, 264
Vapours, the, 19, 20, 23, 28, 30
Victoria, Queen, 233
Voltaire, 39

Wakefield, Edward W., 106, 107, 112
Walk, Dr. Alexander, ix, 187, 261
Walpole, Horace, 7, 56
Ward, Ned (*The London Spy*), 7
Warren, Dr. Richard,
Warwick, 220
Wells, Dr. William Charles, 114, 116, 140
Wesley, John, 65, 66, 79
Whytt, Dr. Robert, 33, 34, 35, 36
Willis, Rev. Francis, 62, 69, 70, 71, 119
Willis, Dr. John, 72
Willis, Dr. Robert Darling, 72
Willis, Dr. Thomas, xii, 15, 19
Winslow, Dr. Forbes Benignus, 94, 250
Worcester, 221
Work therapy, 70, 252, 253, 255, 256

Young, Dr. Thomas, 189

Zelmanowits, Dr. Joseph, 96, 117, 136
Zilboorg, Dr. Gregory, ix, 23, 33, 61, 136, 186